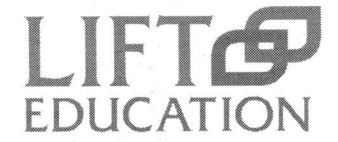

Biomedical Bootcamp
Course Companion Guide

LIFT EDUCATION

Biomedical Bootcamp Authors:

Brittany Montague B.Sc.N. - Curriculum and teachings for Pharmacology
Dana Clarkson B.Sc.N – Western diseases curriculum
Sara Bjorkquist M.A., R.Ac. – 143 Illnesses curriculum
Jeff Feltmate R.TCM.P. – 143 Illnesses Herbal Formulas & Modifications
Gillian Marsollier R.Ac., C.C.I.I. – Western dieases curriculum, editing and entirety of video recordings

I want to thank all of the contributors for your invaluable dedication to helping create the best Biomedical Exam Preparation course available. This course would not be what it is without your immense group effort. Thank you.

COPYRIGHT LIFT Education Academy, 2017

All rights reserved.

No part of this curriculum may be reproduced, stored in a retrieval system, transcribed in any form or by any means, electronic, mechanical, photocopy, recording, or any other means, or translated into any language with the prior written permission of LIFT Education Academy.

GENERAL SYSTEMS 10
GENERAL PATHOPHYSIOLOGY 11
CRANIAL NERVES 12
ORGAN SYSTEMS 14
Cardiovascular (CV) 14
Cerebrovascular 24
Dermatology 29
ENT (Ear, Eyes, Nose, Throat) 39
Endocrine and Metabolic 47
Gastrointestinal Conditions 51
Genito-Urinary Conditions 62
Gynecological Conditions 70
Hematological Conditions 78
Infectious Diseases 84
Mental and Behavioural Conditions 99
Musculo-Skeletal Conditions 103
Neurological Conditions 111
Oncology 119
Respiratory Conditions 124
Miscellaneous 130

143 TCM ILLNESSES 134
Internal Medicine 134
Abdominal Mass (Ji Ju) 135
Abdominal Pain (Fu Tong) 137
Atrophy-Flaccidity (Wei Zheng) 139
Bleeding Disorders (Xue Zheng) 141
Chest Impediment (Xiong Bi) 145
Common Cold (Gan Mao) 147
Constipation (Bian Bi) 149
Consumptive disease (Xu Lao) 151
Consumptive Thirst (Xiao Ke) 153
Convulsive Syndromes (Jing Zheng) 155
Cough (Ke Shou) 157
Depression (Yu Zheng) 159
Diarrhea (Xie Xie) 161
Drum Distension (Gu Zhang) 163
Dysentery (Li Ji) 165
Dysphagia Occlusion Syndrome (Ye Ge) 167
Dyspnea (Chuan Zheng) 169
Edema (Shui Zhong) 171

Epigastric Pain (wei tong)	173
Epilepsy (xian zheng)	175
Fainting (jue zheng)	177
Goitre (ying bing)	179
Headache (tou tong)	180
Hiccoughing and belching (e ni)	184
Hypochondrial Pain (xie tong)	185
Impediment Syndrome (bi zheng)	186
Impotence (yang wei)	188
Insomnia (bu mei)	190
Internal damage fever (FID) (nei shang fa re)	192
Ischuria (long bi)	194
Jaundice (huang dan)	196
Lumbago (yao tong)	198
Lung Distention (fei zhang)	200
Malaria (nue ji)	202
Mania (dian kuang)	203
Palpitations (xin ji)	205
Pulmonary Abscess (fei yong)	207
Pulmonary Tuberculosis (fei lao)	209
Seminal Emission (yi jing)	211
Spontaneous Sweats, Night Sweats (zi han, dao han)	212
Stranguria (lin zheng)	214
Tinnitus and Deafness (er ming er long)	217
Vertigo (xuan yun)	219
Vomiting (ou tu)	221
Watery Phlegm/sputum (tan yin)	223
Wheezing Syndrome (xiao zheng)	224
Wind Stroke (zhong feng)	226
External Medicine	**229**
Acne (fen ci)	229
Acute Mastitis (ru yong)	230
Alopecia Areata (you feng)	231
Anal Fissure (gang lie)	232
Bedsore (re chuang)	233
Boil (ding chuang)	234
Breast Cancer (ru yan)	235
Carbuncle (yong)	239
Contact Dermatitis (jie chu xing pi yan)	240
Digital Gangrene (tuo ju)	242
Drug Rash (yao wu xing pi yan)	243
Eczema (shi chuang)	244
Erysipelas (dan du)	246
Furuncle (jie)	247
Goitre (ying)	248
Hemorrhoid (zhi)	251
Herpes Zoster (she chuan chuang)	252
Phlegmon (fa)	254
Prostatic Hyperplasia (qian lie xian zeng sheng zheng)	255
Prostatitis (qian lie xian yan)	257

SCROFULA (LUO LI)	259
SEBACEOUS CYST (ZHI LIU)	260
SHANK ULCER (LIAN CHUANG)	260
TINEA (XIAN)	262
NEURODERMATITIS (NIU PI XIAN)	263
URTICARIA (YIN ZHEN)	264
VARICOSE VEINS (JIN LIU)	266
WARTS (YOU)	267
OBSTETRICS AND GYNECOLOGY (FU KE)	**268**
ABDOMINAL MASSES (ZHENG JIA)	268
AMENORRHEA (BI JING)	270
BLEEDING DURING PREGNANCY, UNSTABLE PREGNANCY (TAI LOU, TAI DONG BU AN)	273
DYSMENORRHEA (TONG JING)	275
INFERTILITY (BU YUN)	277
INSUFFICIENT BREASTMILK (QUE RU)	279
INTER-MENSTRUAL BLEEDING	280
IRREGULAR MENSTRUATION (YUE JING BU TIAO)	282
LEUKORRHAGIA (DAI XIA)	283
LOCHIORRHEA (CHAN HOU E LU BU JUE)	285
MENSTRUAL BREAST ACHING (JING XING RU FANG ZHANG TONG)	286
MENSTRUAL EDEMA (JING XING FU ZHONG)	287
MENSTRUAL HEADACHE (JING XING TOU TONG)	288
MENSTRUAL HEMATEMESIS AND EPISTAXIS (JING XING TU NIU)	289
MENSTRUAL MENTAL DISORDER (JING XING QING ZHI YI CHANG)	291
MENSTRUAL ORAL ULCER (JING XING KOU MEI)	293
METRORRHAGIA AND METROSTAXIS (BENG LOU)	294
MISCARRIAGE (ZHUI TAI, XIAO CHAN, HUA TAI)	296
MORNING SICKNESS (REN CHEN E ZU)	298
PERIMENOPAUSAL SYNDROME (JUE JING QIAN HOU ZHU ZHENG)	299
POSTPARTUM ABDOMINAL PAIN (CHAN HOU FU TONG)	300
POSTPARTUM CONVULSION (CHAN HOU JING ZHENG)	301
POSTPARTUM DIZZINESS (CHAN HOU XUE YUN)	302
POSTPARTUM FEVER (CHAN HOU FA RE)	303
POSTPARTUM RETENTION OF URINE (CHAN HOU PAI NIAO YI CHANG)	305
UTERINE PROLAPSE (YIN TING)	307
PEDRIATICS	**308**
ANOREXIA (YAN SHI)	308
ASTHMA (XIAO CHUAN)	310
INTESTINAL PARASITIC WORMS (CHANG DAO CHONG ZHENG)	312
CHICKENPOX (SHUI DOU)	314
COMMON COLD (GAN MAO)	316
CONVULSIONS (JING FENG)	318
DIARRHEA (XIE XIE)	322
ENURESIS (YI NIAO)	324
EPILEPSY (XIAN ZHENG)	326
ERYSIPELAS (CHI YOU DAN)	327
FETAL JAUNDICE (TAI HUANG)	328
FOOD RETENTION (JI ZHI)	330
MALNUTRITION (GAN ZHENG)	331
MEASLES (MA ZHEN)	332

MUMPS (ZHA SAI)	334
PNEUMONIA (FEI YAN KE SOU)	336
PURPURA (ZI DIAN)	338
RETARDATION AND FLACCIDITY (WU CHI WU RUAN)	339
RUBELLA (FENG SHA)	340
SCARLATINA (DAN SHA)	341
SWEATING (HAN ZHENG)	342
THRUSH (E KOU CHUANG)	343
WHOOPING COUGH (DUN KE)	344
INFANTILE EDEMA (XIAO ER SHUI ZHONG)	346
ORTHOPEDICS AND TRAUMATOLOGY (GU SHANG KE)	**348**
ACHILLES TENDON INJURY (GEN JIAN SUN SHANG)	348
ACUTE LUMBAR MUSCLE SPRAIN (YAO BU NIU CUO SHANG)	349
BONE FRACTURE (JU ZHE)	351
CALCANEODYNIA (GEN TONG ZHENG)	352
CARPAL TUNNEL SYNDROME (WAN GUAN ZONG HE ZHENG)	354
CERVICAL SPONDYLOSIS (JING ZHUI BING)	355
FROZEN SHOULDER (JIAN GUAN JIE ZHOU WEI YAN)	357
JOINT DISLOCATION (TUO WEI)	359
KNEE JOINT COLLATERAL LIGAMENT INJURY (XI GUAN JIE CE FU REN DAI SUN SHANG)	360
LUMBAR MUSCLE STRAIN (YAO BU LAO SUN)	361
MENISCAL INJURY (BAN YUE BAN SUN SHANG)	362
PIRIFORMIS SYNDROME (LI ZHUANG JI ZONG HE ZHANG)	365
SPRAINED ANKLE (HUAI GUAN JIE NIU CUO SHANG)	366
STRAINED NECK (LOU ZHEN)	367
TENNIS ELBOW (HONG GU WAIS HAN KE YAN)	369

PHARMACOLOGY 370

GENERAL	**370**
COMMON DRUGS	**371**
AUTONOMIC NERVOUS SYSTEM	371
CENTRAL NERVOUS SYSTEM	372
CARDIOVASCULAR SYSTEM	375
GASTROINTESTINAL SYSTEM	379
RESPIRATORY SYSTEM	382
ENDOCRINE	382
ANTI-INFECTIVE	383

BIBLIOGRAPHY **386**

Biomedical Abbreviations

Below is a list of many common abbreviations you will see in medical charts. While not necessarily examinable, these abbreviations will help you read patient files quicker, streamline your patient note taking, and allow easier inter-professional communication as they are generally understood by other medical professionals. Note: some abbreviations have multiple meanings and may differ depending on the context and country in which they are used. We have chosen the most commonly used form of each abbreviation.

Abd	Abdomen
Abn	Abnormal
ABX	Antibiotics
ADL	Activities of Daily Living
Ant	Anterior
AROM	Active Range of motion
BCP	Birth Control Pill
BID	Twice daily (*bis in die*)
B	Bilateral
BM	Bowel Movement
BMD	Bone Mass Density
BMI	Body Mass Index
BP	Blood Pressure
↑/↓ BP	High/Low Blood Pressure (note the up/down arrows, and not 'L' for 'low')
bpm	Breaths Per Minute
BPM	Beats Per Minute
BR	Breath Rate
B/O	Because of
C/O	Complains of
C/S	Cervical Spine
CBC	Complete Blood Count
CC	Chief Complaint (or Current Concerns)
CNP	Cannot Perform
CNS	Central Nervous System
CRP	C-Reactive Protein
CST	Continue Same Treatment
CT	Computed Tomography
CTS	Carpal Tunnel Syndrome
CUMX	Current Medications
CVA	Cerebrovascular Accident (*stroke*)
DDx	Differential Diagnosis
DIP	Distal Interphalangeal Joint
DM	Diabetes Mellitus (Type 1 or 2)
DOB	Date of Birth
DOE	Date of Exam
DOI	Date of Injury
d/o	Disorder
d/t	Due to
DTR	Deep Tendon Reflex
Dx	Diagnosis
Dz	Disease
ECG (/EKG)	Electrocardiogram
EEG	Electroencephalogram
EMG	Electromyography
ETOH	Alcohol (Ethanol)
FH	Family History
fMRI	Functional Magnetic Resonance Imaging
FOOSH	Fall On Out-Stretched Hand
FROM	Full Range of Motion
Frq	Frequent
F/U	Follow Up

Fx	Fracture
GERD	Gastroesophageal Reflux Disease *(acid reflux)*
GI	Gastrointestinal
HA	Headache
HEENT	Head, Eyes, Ears, Nose, Throat
HID	Headache, Insomnia, Depression
HPI	History of Present Illness
HR	Heart rate
Ht	Height
HTN	Hypertension
Hx	History (of)
IUD	Intrauterine Device
L	Left
LBP	Lower Back Pain
LE	Lower Extremity
LFT	Liver Function Tests
L/S	Lumbar spine
IBD	Inflammatory Bowel Disease
IBS	Irritable Bowel Syndrome
ICU	Intensive Care Unit
ISQ	No change (*In Status Quo*)
IV	Intravenous
Lat	Lateral
LBP	Low Back Pain
LLL	Left Lower Lobe *(of the lung)*
LLQ	Left Lower Quadrant
LMP	Last Menstrual Period
LOC	Loss of Consciousness
LUL	Left Upper Lobe *(of the lung)*
LUQ	Left Upper Quadrant
MC	Most Common
MCP	Metacarpophalangeal joint
Med	Medial
MOI	Mechanism of Injury
MI	Myocardial Infarction *(heart attack)*
MRI	Magnetic Resonance Imaging
MTP	Metatarsalphalangeal joint
MVA	Motor Vehicle Accident
MVI	Moving Vehicle Incident/Injury
Mxl	Muscle
N/A	Not Applicable
NK(D)A	No Known (Drug) Allergies
NSA	No Significant Abnormalities
NSAID	Non Steroidal Anti Inflammatory Drug
NSF	No Significant Findings
n/t	Numbness and Tingling
N&V	Nausea and Vomiting
OA	Osteoarthritis
Occ	Occasional
O/E	On Examination
O&P	Ova and Parasites
OTC	Over the Counter
Ⓟ	Pain
PBX	Probiotics
PCS	Post-Concussion Syndrome
PHN	Post-herpetic Neuralgia
PI	Personal Injury
PIP	Proximal Interphalangeal joint
PRN	When necessary (*Pro Re Nata - in reference to medication*)

© 2017 LIFT Education Academy   www.lifteducation.academy

POLICE	Protection, Optimal loading, Ice, Compression, Elevation
Post	Posterior *(or after)*
PNS	Peripheral Nervous System
Prog	Prognosis
PROM	Passive Range of Motion
Pt	Patient
PT	Physical Therapy
Px	Physical Exam
QD	Once a day (*Quaue Die*)
QH	Each hour (*Quaque Hora*)
QID	Four times a day (*Quarter In Die*)
QAM	Every morning
QN	Every night
QOD	Every other day
℞	Prescription (*Recipe*)
RA	Rheumatoid Arthritis
R	Right
Ref	Referral
ROF	Report of Findings
ROS	Review of Systems
R/O	Rule Out
RICE	Rest, Ice, Compression, Elevation
RLL	Right Lower Lobe *(of the lung)*
RLQ	Right Lower Quadrant
RML	Right Middle Lobe *(of the lung)*
RUL	Right Upper Lobe *(of the lung)*
RUQ	Right Upper Quadrant
S/S	Sprain/Strain *(or Signs & Symptoms)*
SI	Sacroiliac (Joint)
SOAP	Subjective, Objective, Assessment, Plan
SOB	Shortness of Breath
SSx	Signs & Symptoms
STD	Sexually Transmitted Disease
STI	Sexually Transmitted Infection
Sx	Symptoms
T2DM	Type 2 Diabetes Mellitus
TBI	Traumatic Brain Injury
TH	Tension Headaches
T/S	Thoracic Spine
TIA	Transient Ischemic Attack
TID	Three times a day
Tr	Tincture
Tx	Treatment
UE	Upper Extremity
US	Ultrasound
UTI	Urinary Tract Infection
VAS	Visual Analogue Scale
WNL	Within Normal limits
w/o	Without
Wt	Weight
YOA	Years of Age
YO	Years Ol

General Systems

i. **Lymphatic**: Works with other parts of immune system to help body fight off infection and disease. Made up of: lymph vessels, nodes and organs (adenoids, tonsils, SP and bone marrow). Main functions: produce, maintain, and distribute white blood cells to the body and absorb excess fluid from tissues.

ii. **Endocrine**: Regulates bodily functions through secretion of hormones. Made up of: Endocrine glands, hormones and various endocrine tissues (pancreas, ovaries, testes) that secrete hormones. Main functions: regulation of cellular activity, growth, metabolism and sexual development and function

iii. **Respiratory**: Responsible for ventilation of the body as gas exchange between the air and blood. Made up of: nose, sinuses, throat, larynx, trachea and lungs. Main functions: Move air into and out of the lungs, oxygenate and remove carbon dioxide from the blood and produce sounds for speaking.

iv. **Digestive/GI**: Provides fuel to maintain bodily functions. Made up of: Digestive tract (mouth, esophagus, stomach, small and large intestine) and accessory organs (teeth, tongue, salivary glands). Main functions: ingestions and chemical digestions of food into absorbable molecules, absorption and excretion of waste products (defecation)

v. **Urinary:** Removes toxins from the blood and produces urine. Made up of: kidneys, ureter, bladder, and urethra. Main functions: Excretion of waste products from body fluids, elimination of wastes through urine, and regulation of blood volume and concentration.

vi. **Reproductive**: Responsible for the generation of cells that enable procreation. Made up of: Breasts, ovaries, uterus, vagina, testis, and penis. Main functions: produce and maintain eggs/sperm, fertilization, and protect and nourish fetus.

vii. **Integumentary**: The body's largest system that acts as a first line of defense against pathogens. Made up of two components: cutaneous membrane (skin) and the accessory structures (hair, nails, sweat and other exocrine glands). Main functions: protection of underlying tissues, excretion of salts and organic wastes, maintenance of body temperature and detection of touch, pressure and pain stimuli

viii. **Skeletal**: Works in conjunction with the muscular system to protect and maintain body position and produce controlled movements. Made up of: bones, cartilage, ligaments and other connective tissues. Main functions: structural support and protection of soft tissues, storage of minerals, and blood cell production

ix. **Muscular**: Works together with skeletal and nervous system to produce precise body movements and circulate blood. Made up of: skeletal muscles, cardiac muscles, and smooth muscles (blood vessels, respiratory tract, intestines). Main functions: protect soft tissues, maintain posture and regulate blood flow to vital organs.

x. **Nervous**: Collects and processes information from the senses and respond accordingly connecting the person to their environment. Made up of two components: Central nervous system (brain and spinal cord) and the Peripheral nervous system (cranial and spinal nerves). Main functions: PNS - collect information from nerves and send information to the brain. CNS - interpreting information and generating an appropriate response.

xi. **Cardiovascular**: A closed system responsible for distribution of blood to body tissues and removal of metabolic waste products. Made up of: the heart, blood, arteries, veins and capillaries. Main functions: transports nutrients, oxygen and hormones to the cells of the body, removes metabolic waste from the blood, and maintains immunity and body temperature.

General Pathophysiology

Definitions

- ACUTE – sudden and short term with marked signs
- CHRONIC – long-term; more subtle
- COMMUNICABLE – infections spread from one person to another
- CONVALESCENCE – period of recovery
- ENDOCRINE - relating to glands that secrete directly into the bloodstream
- EPIDEMIC – widespread outbreak in a localized region
- EPIDEMIOLOGY – the science of tracking patterns of disease
- EPITHELIUM - outer layer of skin
- ETIOLOGY – cause/origin of disease
- EXACERBATION – a worsening from triggers; influences
- EXOCRINE - relating to glands that secrete to ducts at the epithelium layer
- HOMEOSTASIS - state of equilibrium of the internal body environment
- IATROGENIC – doctor/treatment caused
- IDIOPATHIC – unknown cause
- INCIDENCE - # of new cases/year
- INCUBATION – in the process of development ex) infection without signs or symptoms
- INSIDIOUS – proceeding in a gradual, subtle way, but with harmful effects.
- LATENT – silent; no outward signs or symptoms
- LESION – local tissue change
- LOCAL – specific site ex) swelling from a wasp sting
- MANIFESTATION – signs that show themselves
- MORBIDITY – how often a disease occurs in a specific group/area (rates/%s)
- MORTALITY – death rates
- NOTIFIABLE – a disease that one must report
- ONSET – when the disease starts (gradual or sudden)
- PANDEMIC – everywhere outbreak ex) AIDS, plague
- PATHOGEN - bacterium, virus or other microorganisms capable of causing disease
- PATHOGENESIS – evolution/development of a disease
- PREDISPOSING FACTOR – tendency or high risk ex) smoking; age
- PRODROMAL – the period between initial symptoms and full development. Ex) dizzy before a migraine
- PROGNOSIS – the probability of a recovery
- SEQUELAE – potential outcome of a primary disease ex) HBP can lead to KI issues
- SICKNESS = DISEASE (objective, quantifiable signs) + ILLNESS (subjective experience of the patient)
- SUBCLINICAL – disease not severe enough to present signs/symptoms
- SYNDROME – a collection of signs and symptoms ex) multiple sclerosis
- SYSTEMIC – affecting the entire body ex) wasp sting causes full body allergic reaction
- THERAPY – treatments taken to help alleviate signs/symptoms

Cranial Nerves

	Cranial Nerve Functions & Tests			
CN#	Name	Sensory/Motor	Function	Associated Exam(s)*
I	**Olfactory**	Sensory	Smell	Smell Test
II	**Optic**	Sensory	Vision	Visual Acuity / Visual Fields Confrontation Test
III	**Oculomotor**	Motor	Pupillary constriction, opening the eyelids, most extra-ocular movements	Pupillary Reflex Test Cardinal Fields of Gaze Accommodation Test
IV	**Trochlear**	Motor	Downward/inward movement of eye	Cardinal Fields of Gaze Accommodation Test
V	**Trigeminal**	Sensory + Motor	3 sensory branches: Ophthalmic, Maxillary, Mandibular Temporal & masseter mxls	TGN Touch Test Jaw Clenching Test
VI	**Abducens**	Motor	Lateral deviation of eye	Cardinal Fields of Gaze Accommodation Test
VII	**Facial**	Sensory + Motor	Taste to anterior 2/3 of tongue Mxls of facial expression	Taste Test (anterior portion) Facial Expression Test
VIII	**Acoustic/Vestibulocochlear**	Sensory	Hearing Balance	Gross Hearing Tests Balance Test
IX	**Glossopharyngeal**	Sensory + Motor	Sensation of part of ear canal & taste to posterior 1/3 of tongue Motor control of pharynx	Taste Test (posterior) Gag Reflex/Speech
X	**Vagus**	Sensory + Motor	Sensory to pharynx and larynx Motor to palate, pharynx, larynx	Gag Reflex/Speech Vernet Rideau (lifts soft palate when you say "Ahhh")
XI	**Spinal Accessory**	Motor	SCM & trapezius muscle movement	SCM/Trapezius Muscle Resistance Test
XII	**Hypoglossal**	Motor	Tongue movement	Tongue Motor Test
*	*While you are not required to know these tests, they are helpful in understanding what the cranial nerves do. Search examples on YouTube to further your understanding of this subject.*			

General Use	Mnemonic	Meaning
Cranial Nerves - Names *While you can just memorize the numbers of the cranial nerves, the names actually tell you what they do (if you know latin, that is). Remember the names of the cranial nerves with either of these unforgettable sentences!*	**Oh Oh Oh, To Touch And Feel Very Green Vegetables, AH!** **On Old Olympus' Towering Top, A French And German Vault And Hop!**	**Olfactory** **Optic** **Occulomotor** **Trochlear** **Trigeminal** **Abducens** **Facial** **Vestibulocochlear** **Glossopharyngeal** **Vagus** **Accessory** **Hypoglossal**
Cranial Nerves - Type *If you're struggling to remember whether a cranial nerve is sensory, motor, or both, use this crude sentence to stimulate your memory.*	**S**ister **S**ays **M**arry **M**oney, **B**ut **M**y **B**rother **S**ays **B**ig **B**oobs **M**atter **M**ore	Sensory, Motor, or Both (**S**, **M**, or **B**)

Organ Systems

Cardiovascular (CV)

Please follow along with the course audio

ii. <u>General Pathophysiology:</u>

- **Claudication** – cramping in the leg induced by exercise (usually due to arterial obstruction)
- **Hypoxia** – deficiency of O2 reaching the tissues
- **Infarct** – The area of HT tissue permanently damaged by an inadequate supply of O2
- **Ischemia** – Decreased blood flow to an organ, usually due to constriction or obstruction of an artery.
- **LOC** – Loss Of Consciousness.
- **mm Hg** – Millimeters of mercury. The units that blood pressure is measured in.
- **Murmur** – Cause by congenital defects or damaged HT valves that do not close and allow blood to flow back into the chamber from which it came.
- **Necrosis** – Death of tissue within a certain area.
- **Orthopnea** – SOB while lying flat
- **Paroxysmal** - Sudden recurrence or intensification of symptoms, such as a spasm or seizure
- **PND (Paroxysmal nocturnal dyspnea)** – severe SOB/cough attacks at night that wakes one up
- **Stenosis** – The narrowing or constriction of an opening, such as a blood vessel or heart valve.
- **Syncope** – A temporary, insufficient blood supply to the brain which causes LOC (usually cause by a serious arrthymia)

ii. **Common Western Tests**
- Blood pressure cuff (sphygmomanometry) – Cuff on arm pumped up to check the systole over diastole.
- Chest x-ray – Still pictures of HT and LU to check for enlargement
- Computerized tomography scan (ct or cat) – Several x-rays to provide cross-sectional view
- Coronary angiogram – Studies blood flow through HT and vessels using dye and special x-rays.
- Doppler ultrasound – Non-invasive diagnostic procedure that changes sound waves into an image that can be viewed on a monitor (esp. Good for measuring blood flow and pressure)
- Echocardiogram – Creates moving picture of HT using high-pitched sound waves. Finds areas of poor blood flow, abnormal HT valves and m.
- ECG – Electrocardiogram. Electrodes on chest and arms record HT activity
- Electrophysiological test – Catheters tipped with electrodes inserted into groin, arm or neck through blood vessels to HT. Maps electrical impulses to identify abnormalities.
- Event monitor – Portable ECG device to be worn over weeks/months (push button to start it when experiencing sxs)
- Holtor monitor – Portable ECG device worn for 24 hours
- Magnetic resonance imaging (MRI) – Provides still or moving pictures of blood flow through HT
- Stress test – Electrodes placed on chest to monitor HT function during exercise or when medication given.
- Ultrasonography - a technique using echoes of ultrasound pulses to delineate objects or areas of different density in the body.

iii. **General Red Flags**: (not all need to be present – these are just general to indicate CV issues. Red flags indicate a potentially serious condition that must be reviewed by a medical doctor. While one red flag symptom does not necessarily indicate an emergency situation, attention must be paid to red flag signs and serious conditions systematically ruled out).
- *Local heart symptoms*: Chest pain, irregular heartbeat, tachycardia, palpitations
- *Circulatory symptoms*: Cyanosis, cold hands/feet, leg cramps, varicose veins, phlebitis (blood clots in veins), leg edema
- *Respiratory symptoms*: dyspnea, orthopnea,
- *Others:* Light-headedness, syncope, weakness, fatigue, possible anemia

Common Diseases + Specific Red Flags

NCCAOM: All conditions listed in chart, with varying levels of importance listed below:
Frequent ***
Moderately common **
Least frequent *
Pan-Can: Common diseases are placed on a grey background

Condition **Symptoms and signs** **Related TCM Illness**	**Causes & Diagnostic tests**	**Red flags (and what to do about them)** *Please fill this section out as you listen to your videos!*
Aneurysm (Aortic) ** *A bulge in a section of the aorta (main artery in body) that could burst due to weakness (fatal)* **SSx:** Asymptomatic – may be abdominal, chest or back discomfort, pulsating sensation in abdomen, cold foot or a black/blue toe (means that a clot has formed), fever or weight loss if due to inflammatory reasons OR chest pain, SOB, dysphagia (difficulty swallowing) if thoracic **TCM Illness: Abdominal Pain (fu tong); Abdominal Mass (ji ju) OR Chest Pain (xiong bi)**	**Causes:** HBP, atherosclerosis, aging, smoking **Diagnosis:** Often found by chance during a routine exam or during a screening test for aneurysms; x-ray, ultrasound, echocardiogram, MRI, CT scan **Tx:** Surgical repair if aneurysms over 5.5cm, causing sxs and rapidly growing; if smaller – statins, beta-blockers, quit smoking, exercise	**Red flags:** **Refer to GP (General Practitioner)/PCP (Primary Care Physician) immediately or ER if severe.**
***Arrhythmias**		
Atrial fibrillation (Afib) *Disorganised electrical signals in the HT atria lead to fast and irregular heartbeats* **SSx:** Rapid, irregular heart rate and rhythm -Palpitations (forceful heartbeats) -Feeling of HT racing -Fainting/light headedness -Fatigue, SOB or weakness -Exercise intolerance -May have chest pain *Similar to 'atrial flutter': abnormally rapid heartbeat with a regular pattern* **TCM Illness: Palpitations (xin ji)**	**Causes:** May be a problem of the heart itself and/or linked to cardiovascular disease -HBP, HT attack, Coronary artery disease, abnormal HT valves (mitral stenosis), HT defects, hyperthyroid, stimulants, LU disease, viral infections, previous HT diseases, Sick sinus syndrome (improper function of HT pacemaker), stress, sleep apnea **Types** -Occasional: symptoms come and go. Last from a few minutes to hours and stops on its own. -Persistent: HT rhythm will not go back on its own. Need electric shock or meds to restore. -Long-standing persistent: continuous; lasts > 12 months -Permanent: - normal HT rhythm cannot be restored – need meds. **Possible diagnostic tests** ECG, transthoracic echocardiogram,	**Red Flags:** Persistent, long-standing, or permanent arrhythmias indicate a serious heart problem that requires medical intervention. Persistent arrhythmias increase the risk of cardiovascular disease and stroke Be sure to assess pulse speed and rhythm before and after treatment

	CBC, exercise stress testing **Tx:** Electrical cardioversion (a shock to chest to stop HT electrical activity for a moment – hopefully resets); anti-arrhythmic drugs, catheter ablation to cauterize 'hot spots' causing afib, warfarin/Coumadin to prevent blood clots	to rule out arrhythmias. If you find anything unusual, record your findings and refer on for medical treatment. **Refer to GP/PCP soon.**
Premature ventricular contractions (PVC) *Extra beats of the lower heart chambers (ventricles) that are common in otherwise healthy people, but can be a sign of underlying heart disease if persistent.* **SSx:** Rapid, irregular heart rate and rhythm -Palpitations (forceful heartbeats) -Feeling of 'flip-flopping' 'fluttering' or 'jumping' heartbeats -Sometimes described as an 'odd feeling in the chest' or simply increased awareness of the heartbeat **TCM Illness: Palpitations (xin ji),**	**Causes:** Abnormal (premature, or early) ventricular contractions leading to extra out-of-sync contractions and a 'stuttering' heartbeat. Persistent PVCs eventually result in less effective pumping of blood **Possible diagnostic tests** ECG, Holter monitor (24hr continuous ECG), exercise stress ECG (treadmill or bike test to challenge the heart) **Tx:** Stop alcohol, caffeine, nasal decongestants with adrenaline, drug abuse and smoking. Ca+ channel blockers, anti-arrhythmic drugs, radiofrequency catheter ablation (to destroy HT tissue areas causing issues)	**Red Flags:** Persistent PVCs increase the risk of chronic heart rhythm problems and strain the heart muscle over time. Look out for very fast, forceful, or chaotic arrhythmias - a sign of more severe heart disease. **Refer to GP/PCP very soon.**
Tachycardia *-Very rapid, racing heart rate (>100BPM)* **SSx:** -Palpitations (forceful heartbeats) -Fainting/light-headedness/SOB **TCM Illness: Palpitations (xin ji)**	**Causes:** Something that disrupts normal electrical impulses. Exs) HT disease/tissue damage, congenital, anemia, exercise, shock/fright, HBP/LBP, smoking, fever, excess alcohol/caffeine, meds, drug abuse, electrolyte imbalance, hyperthyroid **Diagnosis:** ECG, Holter or Event monitor, Electrophysiological test, cardiac imaging, MRI, CT scan, chest x-ray, coronary angiogram, stess test **Tx:** Vagal maneuvres (calm vagus nerve – coughing, bearing down, ice pack on face), cardioversion, catheter ablation, anti-arrhythmic meds or Ca+/beta-blockers, pacemaker, surgery (to destroy extra electrical pathway	**Red Flags:** **Refer to GP/PCP very soon or ER if severe.**
Bradycardia *Slow heart rate (<60BPM)* **SSx:** -Fainting/light-headedness -Fatigue, SOB or weakness -Exercise intolerance	**Causes:** Disruption of normal electrical impulses controlling HT rate and pumping action. Exs) HT damage, HBP, congenital, infection (myocarditis), hypothyroidism, electrolyte imbalance, sleep apnea,	**Red Flags:**

TCM Illness: Vacuity Taxation (xu lao)	inflammatory disease (SLE,ex), hemochromatosis (build up of iron in organs), meds **Diagnosis:** ECG, Holter or Event monitor, exercise test, lab test **Tx:** Adjust meds, pacemaker, treat underlying disorder	**Refer to GP/PCP if you cannot obtain results or if severe.**
Blood Pressure		
Hypertension *Sustained elevation of resting systolic BP (>140mmHg), diastolic (>90mmHg) or both.* • Essential or Primary: No known cause (most common) • Secondary: Hypertension as SECONDARY to an identified cause (usually KI disease) SSx: Often asymptomatic until complications. Dizziness, flushed face, h/a, fatigue, epistaxis, nervousness, papilloedema Secondary: cardiovascular, neurologic, renal sxs TCM Illness: According to sxs. Ex) Headache (tou tong)	**Causes:** Heredity, dietary, lack of exercise, stress, alcohol, BCP, secondary to KI disease, Cushing's syndrome, hyperthyroid, meds, drugs, licorice **Diagnosis:** Multiple BP measurements, urinalysis, renal ultrasonography, blood tests, ECG, evaluate for sleep disorder **Tx:** Weight loss, exercise, smoking cessation, decrease salt/alcohol, meds/statins, tx secondary cause	**Red Flags:** **Refer to GP/PCP soon.**
Hypotension *BP lower than 90/60mmHg* SSx: Often association with good health, but can be problematic: -syncope, light-headedness, palpitations, dizziness, confusion, blurred vision, can be seizures TCM Illness: Vacuity Taxation (xu lao) or symptoms: Dizziness (xuan yun), Palpitations (xin ji)	**Causes:** Hypovolemia (excessive diuretic use), bed rest, haemorrhage, severe vomiting, diarrhea or sweating, diabetes). Also decreased baroreceptor responsiveness, some psychiatric meds **Diagnosis:** Sphygmomanometer reading **Tx:** Remove alcohol, re-evaluate diuretics, tx underlying disease, salt, meds with ephedra, NSAIDS that retain renal sodium, caffeine	**Red Flags:** **Refer to GP/PCP if you cannot obtain results.**
Coronary artery disease (CAD)		
Atherosclerosis*** *Plaque build-up in the wall of an artery. Often causes PAD (Peripheral Artery Disease)* SSx: Asymptomatic until growth or	**Causes:** high cholesterol, inflammation of vessels, smoking, familial, sedentary lifestyle, HBP, obesity, diabetes **Diagnosis:** angiography, ultrasonography, MRI imaging	No **Red Flags**: Asymptomatic until growth or rupture of plaque reduces blood flow. Then will see sxs of decreased flow to areas.

rupture of plaque reduces blood flow. THEN, may see: chest pain, pain in leg, arm, SOB, fatigue, confusion if blocking to brain, m. weakness to blocked area **TCM illness: According to symptoms. Chest Impediment (xiong bi); Impediment syndrome (bi zheng)**	**Tx**: treat risk factors, lifestyle, diet meds, increase physical activity, antiplatelet and antiatherogenic drugs	**Refer to GP/PCP very soon.**
Buerger's Disease *Poor circulation to the periphery (beginning at the hands and feet), leading to gangrene and ischemia (tissue death)* **"When you have small burgers stuck in your vessels you cannot get circulation to your limbs."** **SSx**: Claudication, non-healing foot ulcers, rest pain, pain worse with stress or exposure to cold, Raynaud's, absent pulses at affected extremity, gangrene **TCM illness: Impediment syndrome (bi zheng)**	**Causes**: Blood clots (thrombi) occlude peripheral vessels, reducing blood supply and leading to infection and tissue necrosis, -Smoking is primary risk factor **Diagnosis**: non-invasive vascular testing, angiography, exclusion of other causes **Tx**: Quit smoking, amputation	**Red Flags:** **Refer to GP/PCP very soon.**
Angina Pectoris *Lack of blood perfusion and therefore O2 to the myocardium (heart m.) due to atherosclerosis of the coronary arteries* **SSx**: Exertional tight chest pain, can radiate to throat, jaw, shoulders, arms, back, cold or extreme heat and stress can trigger attack, pain disappears completely within minutes of rest and nitroglycerin **TCM illness: According to symptoms. Chest Impediment (xiong bi)**	**Causes**: Secondary to atherosclerosis, occlusion of coronary artery due to a clot **Diagnosis**: ECG, myocardial imaging **Tx: Drugs: Sublingual nitroglycerin,** antiplatelets, beta-blockers, Ca+ channel blockers, ACE inhibitors, statins, coronary angioplasty or coronary artery bypass graft surgery	**Red Flags:** **Refer to GP/PCP very soon or ER if severe.**
Congestive Heart Failure (CHF)** *Failure of the heart muscle pump to circulate blood effectively. Often secondary to a heart illness. Either left or right ventricles fail.* **'When the HT fails, congestion is everywhere!'** **SSx**: Swelling (edema) of the legs/ankles -Rapid, irregular heartbeat	**Causes** Narrowed blood vessels (coronary artery disease), hypertension, or other chronic heart conditions weaken the heart muscle or stiffen the blood vessels, worsening the strain on the heart **Possible diagnostic tests** CBC, ECG, echocardiogram, exercise stress test, CT/MRI, coronary angiogram	**Red Flags:**

-SOB (with exertion and when lying down) -Fatigue, weakness -Reduced exercise tolerance -Increased urinary frequency at night -Sudden weight gain from fluid retention (ascites) -Lack of appetite, nausea -Possible cough with foamy pink (blood-tinged) mucous **TCM illness: Heart Palpitations (xin ji), Vacuity Taxation (xu lao), and Coughing and Panting (ke shou)**	**Tx**: diet and lifestyle changes, treatment of cause, drugs	Severe complications of untreated heart failure include: kidney or liver damage or failure, heart valve problems, heart rhythm problems (arrhythmias) **Refer to GP/PCP very soon.**
Corpulmonale *Right ventricular enlargement secondary to LU disease. Causes pulmonary artery hypertension and eventually right ventricular failure.* 'Cor = HT Pulmon = LU HT/LU disease!' **SSx:** Exertional dyspnea, syncope and angina, fatigue, ascites, spleno-/hepatomegaly, weight gain, edema, distended jugular veins, fatigue, increased peripheral venous pressure, parasternal heave/lift **TCM Illness: Vacuity Taxation (xu lao), Coughing and Panting (ke chuan), Lung Distention (fei zhang)**	**Causes:** Usually a result of COPD or pulmonary embolism, injury due to mechanical ventilation, alveolar hypoxia **Diagnosis:** Chest x-ray, ECG, cardiac MRI, right heart catheterization **Tx:** Diuretics, O2, treatment of CAUSE	**Red Flags:** **Refer to GP/PCP very soon.**
Heart Failure** **See above (CHF) – same thing!**		
Infective Endocarditis *Infection of the endocardium, usually with bacteria (streptococci or staphylococci) or fungi.* 'Infections signs + HT signs' **SSx::** *(non-specific and vary greatly)* Fever, heart murmur, petichiae, fatigue, night sweats, weight loss, anemia, endocardial vegetations (abnormal growth) **TCM Illness: Internal Damage Fever (nei shang fa re)**	**Causes:** Abnormality of endocardium, microorganisms in bloodstream (bacteremia – from infections, dental procedures, drug use, injuries, wounds, etc.) **Diagnosis:** Blood cultures, echocardiography **Tx:** IV antibiotics, valve repair or replacement	**Red Flags:** **Refer to ER.**
Ischemic Heart Disease (CAD – Coronary Artery Disease) *Impairment of blood flow through the*	**Causes:** Atheroscleosis, variant angina	**Red Flags:**

coronary arteries commonly due to atheromas (arterial wall degeneration due to fatty deposits or scar tissue leading to restricted circulation and possible thrombosis) **SSx:** Angina sxs, SOB, myocardial infarction, silent ischemia, sudden cardiac death **TCM illness: Chest Impediment (xiong bi)**	**Diagnosis:** ECG, stress tests, coronary angiography **Tx:** Drugs: antiplatelets, statins, beta-blockers -coronary artery bypass surgery -if thrombosis – fibrinolytic drugs	**Refer to GP/PCP very soon or ER if sxs are severe. May call 9-1-1 if sxs very severe.**
MI (Myocardial Infarction – Heart Attack)** *Ischemic myocardial necrosis due to abrupt decrease of myocardial blood flow in the coronary artery. NOT relieved by nitroglycerin.* **SSx:** Chest discomfort with or without dyspnea, nausea, syncope and diaphoresis. **TCM illness: Chest Impediment (xiong bi)**	**Causes:** One or more blocked coronary arteries; OR spasm of coronary artery which shuts down blood flow (often caused by stress, smoking or drugs) **Diagnosis:** ECG, coronary angiography, lab: cardiac markers **Tx:** O2, aspirin, nitrides, opioids, drugs: antiplatelets, antianginals, anticoagulants, possible fibrinolytics	**Red Flags:** **Call 9-1-1.**
Viral Myocarditis *Inflammation of the myocardium (heart muscle) due to a virus* **'Flu virus + HT sxs'** **SSx:** variable – flu-like sxs and/or sudden severe chest pain, difficult breathing, fatigue, palpitations, lethargy, syncope (sudden onset heart failure) **TCM illness: Chest Impediment (xiong bi)**	**Causes:** virus (over 20 – ex) flu, HIV, measles, rubella, parovirus, adenovirus, TSS, Lyme's (last 2 bacterial) **Diagnosis:** Cardiac MRI, chest x-rays, echocardiograms, endomyocardial biopsy **Tx:** IV cardiac meds, temporary pacemaker insertion, ventricular assist device (VAD), immunoglobins, corticosteroids, cardiac transplant	**Red Flags:** **Refer to ER.**
Peripheral vascular disorders		
Chronic Cardiomyopathy *Chronic HT disease causing the HT to become enlarged, thick, or rigid. HT weakens over time and can lead to failure or arrhythmias.* **SSx:** Asymptomatic OR, SOB, dyspnea (esp. upon exertion), fatigue, edema, light-headedness, syncope, chest pain, HT murmurs, palps.	**Causes:** Familial, aging, HBP, thyroid issues, diabetes, poor diet, excessive alcohol, toxins, CHD, MI, viral hepatitis, HIV, drug use, viral infection inflaming the HT **Diagnosis:** CBC, Chest x-ray, ECG, Holter and event monitors, echocardiography, stress test, cardiac catheterization, coronary angiography, myocardial biopsy,	**Red Flags:**

TCM illness: Chest Impediment (xiong bi), Palpitations (xin ji),	genetic testing **Tx:** Stop smoking/drinking, diet/lifestyle change, meds to reduce BP, blood thinners, surgery, surgically implanted devices, HT transplant	**Refer to GP/PCP soon.**
DVT (Deep Vein Thrombosis)** *Clotting of blood in a deep vein of an extremity (usually calf or thigh) or the pelvis. Primary cause of pulmonary embolism.* **SSx:** Asymptomatic OR, Swelling in affected limb, warmth, pain/tenderness, redness, pallor or other skin colour changes **TCM illness: Blood Impediment (xue bi)**	**Causes:** Aging, prolonged sitting/inactivity, traumatic injury (includes surgery), secondary to chronic disease, toxins/drugs, iatrogenic. **Diagnosis:** History, ultrasonography, **Tx:** Anticoagulants	**Red Flags:** **DO NOT NEEDLE until cleared by GP/PCP. Refer immediately.**
Orthostatic Hypotension *Excessive fall in BP when an upright position is assumed (by >20mmHb systolic, 10 mmHg diastolic, or both.* **SSx:** Faintness, syncope, light-headedness, dizziness, confusion, blurry vision (all resolved w lying down). **TCM illness: Dizziness (xuan yun), Palpitations (xin ji), Vacuity Taxation (xu lao)**	**Causes:** Hypovolemia, drugs, prolonged bed rest, adrenal insufficiency, aging **Diagnosis:** Physical exam measuring HT rate after 5 min. supine and at 1 and 3 min. after standing, tilt table **Tx:** Patients on prolonged bed rest must sit up and exercise more often, increasing sodium and water intake, loose fitting pants, avoid alcohol and large meals, meds to cause sodium retention (fludrocortisone) or arterial and venous constriction (midodrine), NSAIDS	**Red Flags:** **Refer to GP/PCP if you are unable to obtain results.**
Peripheral Atherosclerotic Disease (PAD) *Occlusion of blood supply to extremities resulting from underlying atherosclerosis.* *"There is a pad blocking the blood flow to my feet"* **SSx:** Intermittent claudication, pain, achiness, cramping all better with rest and worse going uphill, popliteal, post-tibial or dorsal pedis pulse may be absent, painful, cold and numb limbs, poor capillary refill, poor hair growth, dry & scaly skin on extremities, prone to leg, toe or heel ulcers **TCM illness:** None that match (Lower Limb Aching and Pain - xia	**Causes:** Aging, HBP, diabetes, smoking, familial, obesity, CAD **Diagnosis:** Arteriography, Doppler ultrasound **Tx:** Walking→resting→walking to decrease further occlusion, stop smoking, elevate head of bed, angioplasty, may need amputation	**Red Flags:** **Refer to GP/PCP soon.**

zhi teng tong)		
Raynaud's Disease** *Idiopathic spasm of arterioles in hands causing them to become pale/cyanotic* N.B. Raynaud's PHENOMENON is the same condition, but secondary to an identified cause ex) SLE, RA **SSx:** Pale, cyanotic hands (from finger tips to palm – can become smooth, shiny and tight in chronic), parasthesia, if severe: ulcers on finger tips, possible pain (but uncommon) **TCM illness: Blood impediment (xue bi)**	**Causes:** Smoking, stress, prolonged exposure to cold, SLE, trauma, Buerger's disease, RA, RSS, exposure to some chemicals, some meds (inlc. Beta-blockers and BCP) **Diagnosis:** Intake, if phenomenon, assess for identified cause **Tx:** Avoid any vasoconstrictors (cold, nicotine, stress), niacin, nerve block	**Red Flags**: Refer to GP/PCP if you are unable to obtain results.
Rheumatic Fever *Non-suppurative (inflamed but no pus) acute inflammatory complication of group A streptococcal infection. Possible sequela = carditis* **'A sore throat can lead to a broken heart.'** **SSx:** Migratory polyarthritis, chorea, erythema marginatum, subcutaneous nodules, skin rash, sore throat, abdominal pain, epistaxis **TCM illness: Internal Damage Fever (nei shang fa re), Fever (fa re), Impediment Condition (bi zheng), can lead to Vacuity Taxation (xu lao)**	**Causes:** Malnutrition, overcrowding increases susceptibility to strep **Diagnosis:** 1 or 2 (or more) of the major manifestations present (migratory polyarthritis, chorea, erythema marginatum, subcutaneous nodules) **Tx:** Aspirin, corticosteroids, penicillin, antibiotics (make sure that strep throat and scarlet fever are txed quickly!)	**Red Flags**: **Refer to GP/PCP immediately or ER if sxs are severe.**
Rheumatic Heart Disease *Long-term consequence of rheumatic fever during childhood due to one or more valves (usually mitral) in HT damaged (scar tissue).* **SSx:** Chest pain, excessive fatigue, palpitations, SOB, edema and PREVIOUS RHEUMATIC FEVER **TCM illness: Impediment Condition (bi zheng), Palpitations (xin ji), Vacuity taxation (xu lao)**	**Causes:** Rheumatic fever affecting MITRAL valve **Diagnosis:** History of rheumatic fever, HT murmur as result, ECG, x-ray, echocardiogram, cardiac catheterization **Tx:** Sxs dependent – meds for arthritis or arrhythmias	**Red Flags**: **Be sure that they are being monitored by their GP/PCP.**
Thrombophlebitis *Inflammatory condition causing a blood clot in the superficial veins.* **SSx:** Warmth, tenderness and pain in affected area, redness and	**Causes:** Aging, immobilization, **pregnancy**, major surgery, plane trips over 4 hours, cancer, previous DVT, CVA, MI, CHF, ulcerative colitis, spinal injury, SLE, Behcet's, blood clotting disorder	**Red Flags**:

swelling **TCM illness: Blood impediment (xue bi)**	**Diagnosis:** Ultrasound, blood test **Tx:** Blood-thinners, clot-dissolvers, compression stockings, varicose vein stripping, filter (inserted in vein until healed)	**Refer to GP/PCP on same day.**

Please go to your online course to answer your Know Your Stuff questions!

Cerebrovascular

Definition: Cerebrovascular disease refers to a group of conditions that affect the supply of blood to the brain, causing limited or no blood flow to the affected areas.

i. <u>General Pathophysiology:</u>
- Aneurysm – weak parts in arteries can develop protrusions with a very thin wall, which can tear and cause brain bleeding
- Ataxia – loss of full control of body movements
- Cerebral Embolism – blood flow is blocked by a clot or air bubble that traveled from somewhere in the body
- Cerebral Haemorrhage – escaping of blood from a ruptured blood vessel wall
- Cerebral Thrombosis – a blood clot/plaque that forms in the brain's blood supply
- Cerebral Insufficiency/Ischemia – inadequate blood supply to the brain/heart
- Embolic – blood clot or other debris swept through bloodstream to lodge in a narrower artery (often a piece of a thrombus)
- Infarction – cessation of blood flow
- Thrombotic – blot clot (thrombus) forms in an artery

ii. <u>Common Western Tests:</u>
- Carotid Ultrasound – sound waves create detailed images of the carotid arteries in neck. Can see plaques blocking blood flow.
- CAT/CT (Computerized Axial Tomography) Scan – employs multiple x-rays to emit a cross-sectional imaging technique (sometimes a dye is injected first)
- Cerebral Angiography – x-ray and injected dye to detect blood flow in brain
- Chemotherapy – the use of powerful drugs to kill tumour cells
- ECG – Electrocardiogram. Electrodes on chest and arms record HT activity
- Electroencephalogram (EEG) – electrodes affixed to scalp to record electrical activity of brain
- Electromyography (EMG) – translates electrical signals that cause muscles to contract – can asses health of muscles and nerve cells (motor neurons)
- Evoked Potentials (EP) – measures speed of nerve impulse conduction
- MRI Scan – imaging technique using radiology to visualize the internal function and structure of the body.
- Radiotherapy (Radiation) – high-energy rays to kill tumour cells to stop them from growing and multiplying
- Spinal Tap (Lumbar Puncture) – small needle inserted at base of spine and small amount of CSP collected for testing
- Transcranial ultrasound – detects blood flow in arteries within brain

ii. <u>General Red Flags:</u>
- Dysphagia (difficulty swallowing)
- Aphasia (difficulty putting thoughts into words)
- Dysarthria (difficulty articulating speech or slurred speech)
- Apraxia (difficulty planning or performing tasks)
- Vomiting
- Seizures
- Fever
- Confusion
- Irregular breathing
- Apnea (pauses in breathing)
- Bowel/bladder incontinence

Common Diseases + Specific Red Flags

Condition / Symptoms and signs / Related TCM Illness	Causes & Diagnostic tests	Red flags (and what to do about them)
ALS (Lou Gehrig's) *A progressive nervous system disease that destroys nerve cells and causes disability* **'A Lively Symphony of colour in the brain, yet unable to walk'** **SSx:** Difficulty walking, tripping/falling easily, weakness in legs, feet, ankles, hand weakness (often starts in periphery), slurred speech, trouble swallowing, m. cramps/twitching in arms, shoulders and tongue, difficulty holding up head and posture, unaffected thinking ability **TCM Illness:** Atrophy-Flaccidity (wei zheng)	**Causes:** -5-10% inherited -Remainder idiopathic **Diagnosis:** EMG, MRI, muscle biopsy, spinal tap, blood and urine tests **Tx:** Medications (Rilutek) to reduce chemical glutamate levels in brain) + meds for ALS symptoms, physio, breathing care, occupational therapy, speech therapy, nutrition, psychological support	**Red Flags:** **Refer to GP (who will probably refer to a Neurologist)**
Bell's Palsy *Damage to facial nerve (usually inflammation) on one side of face causes paralysis and drooping. Sudden onset over hours or days.* **'The Bell swung cold air at my face and paralyzed it!'** **SSx:** Unilateral facial paralysis, may affect sense of taste, tears and saliva, difficulty eating and closing affected eye, weakness or inability to raise eyebrow on affected side **TCM Illness:** None that match	**Causes:** Lowered immunity and exposure to wind and cold, possible herpes virus **Diagnosis:** History + facial nerve neurological exam **Tx:** Usually eventual recovery over 1-2 months. Prednisone within 3 days of onset. Occasional use of anti-viral medications.	**Red Flags:** **Refer to GP if in the initial stages (within 2-4 weeks).**
Brain Tumour *A mass of tissue formed by an accumulation of abnormal cells in the brain. Can be benign (slow growth) or malignant (Cancer - often not noticed until pressing on a structure – if metastasizes, often stays in the CNS).* **SSx:** H/a, n/v, balance issues, increase intracranial pressure, seizures, 'mental' sxs, difficulty walking, blurry or double vision, sleepiness, speech or expression issues **TCM Illness:** None that match (would be Shi Yong – Stone	**Causes:** Idiopathic. Possible genetics, environmental toxins, radiation to head, HIV, and smoking. **Diagnosis:** CAT scan, MRI, analysis of blood, electrolytes and liver function, biopsy **Tx:** Surgery to remove tumour, chemotherapy, radiation, dietician, physio, counselling.	**Red Flags:** **Refer to GP ASAP for assessment.**

Carbuncle)		
CI (Cerebral Insufficiency – STROKE. Also called a CVA – Cerebrovascular Accident) *** *Blood supply to part of brain is interrupted or severely reduced, depriving brain tissue of O2 and nutrients. Brain cells die within minutes.* **TIA:** *'Baby stroke' – sudden/brief ischemic condition. Often no cumulative effect but can herald an upcoming stroke.* **SSx:** Dysarthria, paralysis/numbness/weakness of one side of face and body, sudden vision difficulty, h/a, ataxia **TCM Illness:** Wind Stroke (zhong feng)	**Causes:** Either ISCHEMIC (blocked artery – can be thrombotic or embolic) or HAEMORRHAGIC (leaking/bursting blood vessel), smoking, obesity, sedentary lifestyle, heavy drinking/drugs, HBP, high cholesterol, diabetes, sleep apnea, cardiovascular disease, over 55, African-American, male **Diagnosis:** Blood pressure, blood tests, CAT scan, MRI, carotid ulatrasound, echocardiogram, cerebral angiogram **Tx:** Depending on type of stroke: aspirin, TPA (clot-busting drug), medications to brain, mechanical clot removal, angioplasty (balloon used to expand a narrow artery or a stent inserted), warfarin, surgery vessel repair/clipping/embolization,	**Red Flags:** **Think FAST:** **F**ace – does one side of face droop with smiling? **A**rms – can one arm not function properly with lifting? **S**peech – is speech slurred? **T**ime – call 911 immediately **Call 9-1-1.**
Haemorrhage *Intracerebral bleeding often due to a ruptured vessel.* **SSx:** Sudden/severe h/a, n/v, seizures, LOC **TCM Illness:** Headache (tou tong)	**Causes:** HBP, atherosclerosis, thrombus, occ. aneurysm **Diagnosis:** CAT scan, MRI **Tx:** Surgery	**Red Flags:** **Call 9-1-1.**
MS (Multiple Sclerosis) *Demyelination disease in which the insulation covers of the nerve cells in the brain and spinal cord are damaged/inflamed, therefore nerve impulses are distorted/interrupted. Often in patches.* **'Multiple Patchy Numbness'** **SSx:** Parasthesia in face, trunk, extremities, weakness/clumsiness in hands/legs, visual disturbances (possible blindness), fatigue, dizziness, mood swings, loss of bladder control, affected gait/balance, dry mouth, dysphagia, apathy, m. weakness, impotence, affected speech, tremors, shooting pains **TCM Illness:** Atrophy-Flaccidity (wei zheng)	**Causes:** Idiopathic. Possible lifestyle, environmental, genetic and biological. Usually affects woman (3x more chance) and those of ages btwn 15-40. **Diagnosis:** MRI, spinal tap (lumbar puncture), EP. Must have lesions in two separate areas of CNS + lesions formed at different points in time for dx (therefore can take a bit to dx) **Tx:** Difficult to treat, often managing symptoms -diet changes, prednisone, adrenocorticotrophic hormone (regulates cortisol), physio,	**Red Flags:** **Refer to GP/PCP ASAP for assessment.**
Parkinson's Disease *Slow, progressive, degenerative CNS dysfunction that affects mov't.*	**Causes:** Loss of pigmented neurons of the substantia nigra, locus ceruleus and other brain stem cell groups. Dopamine def.	**Red Flags:** 4 main sxs: i. Slow, poor mov'ts ii. Muscle rigidity iii. Resting tremor

'His parking job is always slow and jerky. His face always looks blank and back bent while concentrating on his parking.' **SSx:** Resting 'pill rolling' tremor (worse at rest, better with movement, none while sleeping), gradually rigid muscles, bradykinesia, akenesia (difficulty starting mov't), fixed eyes, mouth open, stooped posture, arms don't swing, jerky mov'ts, often dementia, constipation, orthostatic hypotension **TCM Illness:** Atrophy-Flaccidity (wei zheng)	Idiopathic, but possibly CVA disease resulting in blocked of blood vessels in brain, side effects of some antipsychotics, CO poisoning, drug abuse, or even from a rare form of encephalitis. **Diagnosis:** With medical history, review of signs and symptoms + neurological tests. CAT scan or MRI may be used to rule out other diseases. **Tx:** Medication – levodopa common, physio, speech therapy, surgery – deep brain stimulation implant to reduce symptoms (using electrical impulses)	iv. Postural instability **Refer to GP/PCP ASAP for assessment.**
Peripheral Neuropathy*** *Damage to peripheral nerves causing weakness, numbness and pain (usually in the hands/feet). Can be mono-, multiple mono- an polyneuropathies (one nerve;, many single nerves; many nerves)* **SSx:** Very dependent on types of nerves affected: gradual onset numbness/parasthesia, sharp/jabbing/throbbing/freezing/burning pain, extreme sensitivity to touch, lack of coordination, m. weakness/paralysis (if motor nerves affected). If autonomic nerves: heat intolerance, altered sweating, incontinence, changes in BP **TCM Illness: Atrophy-flaccidity (wei zheng)**	**Causes:** *Mono*: RSS, trauma, pressure on nerve *Multiple Mono*: Effects of metabolic diseases (ex) diabetes or hypothyroidism *Poly*- nutritional deficiencies, malignancy, metabolic causes, toxicity, autoimmune, bone marrow disorders, infection **Diagnosis:** CBC, chem screen, thyroid function tests, EMG, History, neurological exam, CAT scan, MRI, nerve or skin biopsy **Tx:**, Meds – pain relievers, anti-seizure meds (may relieve nerve pain), topicals, antidepressants, TENS, immune suppressions, physio, surgeries	**Red Flags:** **Refer to GP/PCP ASAP for assessment if unable to obtain results.**
Subarachnoid Haemorrhage *Bleeding in subarachnoid space due to trauma or aneurysm.* **"A bloody spider is crawling under my skull!"** **SSx:** Sudden and severe h/a, vomiting, altered consciousness, dizziness, fainting, stiff neck, photophobia **TCM Illness: None that match – can use other symptoms like Fainting (jue zheng)**	**Causes:** Trauma, aneurysm, results of bleeding disorder **Diagnosis:** CT scan, cerebral angiography, transcranial ultrasound **Tx:** Anticoagulants, surgery (craniotomy) to relieve pressure and stop bleed (clip aneurysm), bed rest, avoid bending over	**Red Flags** **Call 9-1-1.**
Trigeminal Neuralgia *Chronic pain condition affecting the trigeminal nerve (nerve that carries sensation from your face to your brain)*	**Causes:** Compression of trigeminal nerve often by a blood vessel. Or can be from aging, MS, tumour, brain lesion, prior surgery in area or facial trauma, tension	**Red Flags:**

SSx: Paroxysms of spontaneous pain in face lasting from several seconds to minutes, constant aching, often unilateral, can become more freq. and intense over time **TCM Illness:** Headache (tou tong)	**Diagnosis:** Based on pain description – type, location and triggers, neurological exam, MRI **Tx:** Meds – anticonvulsants, antispasmodics, botox, surgery, rhizotomy (surgeon destroys nerve fibres – residual facial numbness)	**Refer to GP/PCP ASAP for assessment if unable to obtain results.**
Viral Encephalitis (Aseptic Meningitis) *Inflammation of the brain due to a virus.* *"The virus is in my meninges! OUCH!"* **SSx:** flu-like sxs (fever severe h/a), achy m./jts/), stiff neck, photophobia, fatigue, weakness, diplopia, perception of foul smells, confusion, seizures, issues with senses/mov't, LOC Children: may also have bulges in fontanels, n/v, body stiffness, inconsolable crying, not feeding **TCM Illness:** None that match. Can use sxs (ex) Headache (tou tong)	**Causes:** Primary: virus/infection directly infects brain Secondary: faulty immune system reacting to an infection elsewhere in body Herpes simplex (HSV), enteroviruses, mosquito-borne illnesses, tick-borne illnesses, rabies, childhood infections such as measles/rubella **Diagnosis:** MRI, CAT scan, spinal tap, blood/urine tests, EEG, brain biopsy **Tx:** Fluids, anti-inflamms, antivirals	**Red Flags:** **Refer to ER or call 9-1-1 if severe.**

Dermatology

Definition: Dermatological disease refers to a group of conditions that affect the skin, scalp, hair or nails causing decreased functionality, pain, and/or cosmetic defects.

i. **General Pathophysiology:**

<u>Types of Lesions:</u> Lesions can be grouped in: clusters; linear (a line); or annular (in a ring). The can be distributed locally (one area) or generalized (whole body)

- Adipose - Fat tissue
- Atrophy - Paper thin + wrinkly skin
- Bulla - Vesicle with free fluid (big zit)
- Crust - 'Scab' - dried serum, pus or blood
- Erosion - Loss of part or all of epidermis or epithelium
- Excoriation - Linear or hollowed out, crusted area caused by rubbing, scratching or picking
- Lichenification - Thickened skin with accentuated skin markings
- Macule - Flat + discoloured
- Malignant - Cancer causing tumor/mass
- Neoplasm - A new and abnormal growth of tissue; typically on the skin
- Nevi - Mole
- Nodule - Palpable + solid
- Papule - Solid + elevated
- Pustule - Superficial + elevated + pus (zits)
- Pruritis - Itching
- Scales - Heaped up particles or cornified epithelium
- Scars - Fibrous tissue replaces normal skin - results in destruction of epidermis + part of dermis
- Telangiectasia - Dilated + cluster of superficial blood vessels
- Tumour - Nodules over 20mm diameter
- Ulcer - Erosion that extends into dermis
- Vesicle - 'Blister' - well circumscribed and elevated + contains serous fluid
- Wheal - 'Hive' - Transient + elevated from local edema - no free fluid

2 Major layers:
1. <u>Epidermis:</u>
   I. Superficial/outer layer = dead cells
   II. Inner cellular layer = keratin + melanin
   III. No blood vessels

1. <u>Dermis:</u>
   I. Deep
   II. Highly vascularized
   III. Contains: Connective tissue; sebaceous (oil) glands; hair follicles

Underneath the dermis = subcutaneous tissue: Fat; sweat glands; hair follicles

ii. **Common Western Tests**

Never touch a patient's skin condition and always use clean clinical practices

- Biopsy - tissue sample obtained to determine diagnosis
- Cytology - To test changes in cell structure
- Patch Testing - If allergies suspected
- Skin Scrapings – Scraping of full epidermis and hair follicles
- Skin cultures - Of discharges, skin swab, or nail clippings (to test for bacteria, viruses or fungi)
- Wood's Lamp - UV light over suspicious area (fungus will fluoresce)

iii. General Red Flags

- Skin ulcers
- Jaundice
- General pruritus
- Hair loss
- Discoloration of skin
- New, fast growing, or oddly shaped nevi or lumps/bumps

Common Diseases + Specific Red Flags

Condition **Symptoms and signs** Related TCM Illness	**Causes & Diagnostic tests**	**Red flags (and what to do about them)**
Acne Vulgaris** *Whiteheads, blackheads, or pimples* **SSx:** Whiteheads, blackheads, pimples, cystic lesions, usually on top of body, can cause scarring **TCM Illness:** Acne (fen ci)	**Causes:** Oily skin from hormonal imbalance (clogs pores); genetics; bacteria from touching face or cosmetics Inflammatory condition from dead skin cells and oil (sebum) clogging the pilosebaceous glands around the follicles. **Diagnosis:** Visual observation **Tx:** Keep skin clean, don't pick at acne, blemish washes, oil free lotions, antibiotics, vitamin A derivatives (like Acutane)	**Red Flags:**
Actinic Keratosis *Pre-cancer patch of crusty scaly patch of skin caused from long term sun exposure* **SSx:** rough scaly patches of raised skin that can be brown, black, or red. Often found on the scalp, hands, arms and face **TCM Illness:** None that match	**Causes:** long term exposure to sun/radiation **Diagnosis:** physical examination and skin biopsy **Tx:** surgical removal of growth, topical agents to reduce incidence	**Red Flags:** **Refer to GP/PCP ASAP for assessment**
Alopecia** *Hair Loss* **SSx:** patches of uneven hair loss, thin brittle hair **TCM Illness:** Alopecia Areata (you feng)	**Causes:** Genetic influence, use of heated hair products, tight braiding/extensive wearing of hats, some medications, parasitic, stress **Diagnosis:** Visual observation for patterns of hair loss **Tx:** avoid harsh hair treatments and practices, possible pharmacological interventions	**Red Flags:** **Refer to GP/PCP ASAP for assessment**
Atopic Dermatitis (Allergic Rash) *Chronic itching and superficial inflammation of the skin usually in skin folds (elbows, knees, etc.)* 'Allergy-Topical Dermatitis.' **SSx:** Redness, itching, may be weepy/crusty lesions (all eczema) worse with stress or environmental changes or application of irritants or allergies (Eczema + itching + allergies)	**Causes:** Idiopathic; emotions; allergies; irritants; environmental changes; immune deficiency; genetic **Diagnosis:** *Observation + history intake;* may perform biopsy (rare); skin swab; blood test for elevated igE and eosinophils **Tx:** Remove offending agent and soaps with SLS (sodium lauryl sulphate); antihistamines; topical corticosteroids; lotions to lock in	**Red Flags:** Severe and spreading, not alleviated by normal treatment (usually topical corticosteroid) - refer to dermatologist

TCM Illness: Eczema (shi chuang)	moisture	
Basal Cell Carcinoma (BCC)* *Skin cancer from overexposure to sun (LEAST risky of skin cancers) - rarely metastasizes* "This is your BASic skin cancer. No worries! Just get early treatment!" **SSx:** Dome-shaped skin growth with blood vessels in it (pink, brown or black), waxy and hard skin growth, bleed easily, develop gradually TCM Illness: None that match (considered a 'wind-poison/toxin)	**Causes:** Overexposure to sun; fair complexion and sun exposure **Diagnosis:** Skin biopsy **Tx:** Tumour excision, curretage and desiccation (scrape and burn), cryosurgery, radiation on area, Moh's surgery (removes tumour in layers and stops once cancer is gone), medicated creams	**Red Flags:** ABCs of melanoma: ● Asymmetrical ● Borders (uneven/blurred) ● Colour (multiple/variegated) ● Diameter (>6mm) ● Evolving Refer to GPPCP who will probably refer to a skin cancer specialist if unsure
Burns* *Injury to the tissues of the body caused by heat, chemicals, electrical current or radiation* **SSx:** red scorched skin, blisters, severe pain, impaired function TCM Illness: None that match	**Causes:** heat, chemicals, electrical current or radiation **Diagnosis:** physical examination and review of history **Tx:** dependent on the origin of the burn, extent and depth. Small burns often treated with cold water/compress, flushing of the chemical that caused the burn, removal of electrical current	**Red Flags:** **Call 9-1-1 immediately if severe.**
Candidiasis Albicans *Yeast infection affecting the skin and membranes, includes: athlete's foot, oral thrush, vaginal yeast infection, nail fungus, jock itch, diaper rash* **SSx:** Well demarcated, red, itchy patch(es), exudate, small red pustules along edge of lesion, often in folds (warm and moist areas), white, flaky substance over affected areas, skin cracks 'Why is your red CANDy cracked and has a white substance on top of it?' TCM Illness: Thrush (e jou chuang - only if in mouth); Tinea (xian), Eczema (shi chuang)	**Causes:** -Overuse of antibiotics, systemic corticosteroids (ex. inhalers), and/or immunosuppressive therapies -Pregnancy -Obesity -Diabetes -HIV -Overexposure to warm, wet environments **Diagnosis:** Observation and/or skin/nail scraping **Tx:** Antifungal topicals, antifungal oral	**Red Flags:**
Carbuncles *Cluster of infected boils surrounding hair follicles - multiple and interconnecting furuncles* **SSx:** Clusters of red painful boils, pimple/blisters containing pus, often found at the nape of the neck TCM Illness: Carbuncle (yong)	**Causes:** Often associated with severe acne or seborrheic dermatitis, poor hygiene, obesity, irritations or abrasions to the skin surface **Diagnosis:** Observation of affected site, possible pus sample from boil/blister	**Red Flags:**

	Tx: incision and drainage of infected area, antibiotics, meticulous skin care, frequent cleansing, application of moist compress	Refer to ER or call 9-1-1 if severe.
Cellulitis** *Common bacterial skin infection that can go much deeper* **SSx:** Red, swollen, hot and tender skin area or rash that develops quickly, usually on the lower legs, appears 'tight and glossy', may be a central area with pus, fever; can spread to lymph nodes and bloodstream → life threatening *"My skin is very embarrassed. It has a lot of cellulite that is doesn't like to show because it could be life-threatening to its self-esteem"* **TCM Illness: Phlegmon (fa)**	**Causes:** Staph or strep bacteria enter the skin through a cut or lesion or skin condition; immunosuppressed; diabetes; IV drug use **Diagnosis:** Observation, palpation of glands **Tx:** Antibiotics; raise legs	**Red Flags:** Refer to ER or call 9-1-1 if severe.
Contact Dermatitis (Skin Hypersensitivity) *Skin inflammation due to various substances in contact with skin* **SSx:** Transient redness, severe swelling, itching (all eczema) blister formation, can be acute or chronic; exposure to irritant **TCM Illness: Contact dermatitis (jie chu xing pi yan); Eczema (shi chuang)**	**Causes:** Chemical irritants; soaps (SLS esp.); detergents; organic acids; drugs; plants (ex. poison ivy), metals, synthetic fabrics, dyes, cosmetic, industrial agents **Diagnosis:** Observation and history; skin patch testing **Tx:** Remove offending agents; hydrocortisone; cold water to remove agent; lotions to lock in moisture (once agent removed)	**Red Flags:**
Dermatitis *Inflammation and irritation of the skin due to external agents* **SSx: itchy red rash, raised/ swollen areas of skin, blisters** **TCM Illness:** Closest is Contact Dermatitis (jie chu xing qi yan) – but isn't an exact match, possibly - Drug rash (yao wi xing pi yan)	**Causes:** Contact with skin irritants, venous stasis, dry skin, exposure to ultraviolet light (photosensitivity reactions) **Diagnosis:** Physician will diagnose after reviewing signs and symptoms, possible skin biopsy to rule out different conditions **Tx:** Removal/avoiding known skin irritants, cleanse area thoroughly, topical corticosteroid ointments	**Red Flags:** Refer to GP/PCP ASAP for assessment
Dermatophytosis (Ringworm/Tinea) *Superficial fungal infection in dermis. Many different types of tinea and can be on many places on the body* **SSx:** Pink to red papulosquamous (papules + scales) annular lesion with scaling, raised borders	**Causes:** Dermatophytes (a group of fungi) invade and grow in dead keratin; exposure to infected humans, soil or animals.; immunocompromised **Diagnosis:** Observation; skin scraping (can look like other skin conditions, so a scraping can help	**Red Flags:**

Dermato = skin Phyt = plant Osis = condition *"There is a blooming, round skin plant on me!"* TCM Illness: Tinea (xian)	differentiate); Wood's light **Tx:** Topical and systemic antifungals; avoid prolonged exposure to moist/warm (ex) keeping running shoes or work out clothes on too long	
Eczema** *Inflamed/irritated skin* **SSx:** Itchy, very dry, slightly thickened or scaly, 'burnt' looking, can be red or even pale-red, sometimes has vesicles that may ooze *"EcZEEEEEEEEEEEEEEEEEEEmely itchy!"* TCM Illness: Eczema (shi chuang)	**Causes:** Overactive immune response; genetics (even of allergies/asthma); poor diet; stress; some is contact; SLS (sodium lauryl sulfate in soaps) **Diagnosis:** Observation and history **Tx:** DO NOT SCRATCH!, corticosteroid creams, cold compresses, antihistamines, antibiotics if infected	**Red Flags:** DO NOT SCRATCH!
Erysipelas (St. Anthony's Fire) *Superficial cellulitis (affects upper layers of skin)* **SSx:** Swollen, shiny, red, very tender and well demarcated lesions usually on face, arms or legs, often break into vesicles, fever, chills, malaise Ery (thema) = reddening of skin Pelas = skin (think pelt) 'Red Pelt' TCM Illness: Erysipelas (dan du)	**Causes:** Streptococci and can develop with risk factors of: lymphatic obstruction/edema, nephrotic syndrome, immunocompromised, skin trauma, insect bites, IV drug use **Diagnosis:** Observation and history **Tx:** Elevate affected area, antibiotics (penicillin), antifungals, surgery (rare), amputation (rare)	**Red Flags:** **Refer to GP/PCP ASAP**
Folliculitis *Bacterial infection of the hair follicles* **SSx:** Raised bump and/or pustule surrounding a hair(s) *Follicle + itis (inflammation)* TCM Illness: Furuncle (jie)	**Causes:** Staph aureus; yeast; fungus; wearing tight clothes too long; old make-up; dirty hot tubs/pools; thick creams/lotions; immunodeficiency **Diagnosis:** Observation & history **Tx:** Usually goes away within 2 weeks on it's own; warm compresses; medicated ointments; antibiotic if a fever persists	**Red Flags:** Any signs of systemic infection **Refer to GP/PCP**
Furuncles (Boils) *Deep infection with staphylococci around hair follicle* **SSx:** tender red areas surrounding the hair follicle, draining pus on rupture TCM Illness: Furuncle (jie)	**Causes:** most commonly caused by bacteria staphylococcus aureus (present in normal skin flora) **Diagnosis:** Observation & history **Tx:** incision and drainage of infected area, antibiotics, meticulous skin care, frequent cleansing, application of moist compress.	**Red Flags:** **Refer to ER or call 9-1-1 if severe.**

Fungal Infections* Infection of body tissue area with fungal causative agent SSx: itchy, reddened areas on the skin, scalp or nails TCM Illness: None that match	Causes: contact with infective agent within the environment Diagnosis: physical examination followed by microscopic examination and culture Tx: antifungal treatments, topical creams and ointments	Red Flags: **Refer to GP/PCP ASAP for assessment**
Impetigo *A highly contagious, superficial skin infection - most common in children* SSx: Itchy, honey-coloured scab with red edges, sores pop easily and form a crust, itchy, swollen lymph nodes *'These scabs are impetigoing (impeding) my ability to get a date!'* **TCM Illness: Boils (ding chuang) and carbuncles (yong), may even been furuncle (jie)**	Causes: Bacterial - either staph aureus, or streptococcus pyogenes, skin-to-skin contact, bites or injury (allow bacteria in), immune deficiency or diabetes Diagnosis: Observation, skin culture Tx: Don't share towels, etc!, simple hygiene if mild, vinegar solution, not touching area, topical antibiotics, warm compresses to soak off scabs	Red Flags: Don't share towels, etc., simple hygiene
Lice* *Parasitic insect that lives on humans/animals* SSx: itching at the hairline, small bites behind the ears and at hairline TCM Illness: None that match	Causes: Contact with human/animal already infected - lice need a source of human blood to survive Diagnosis: Observation and review of history, visual inspection for lice and/or eggs (small oval particles, look similar to dandruff) Tx: Use of medicated shampoo to eliminate lice, manual removal using fine toothed comb	Red Flags: If treatments ineffective refer to GP
Lipomas *Benign tumor of adipose (fat) tissue encapsulated found just below the skin* SSx: Rubbery, compressible mass of adipose tissue, variable in size TCM Illness: None that match	Causes: Unknown, minor soft tissue injury may lead to development Diagnosis: Biopsy to differentiate from malignant mass Tx: Usually no treatment unless it interferes with daily life	Red Flags: **Refer to GP/PCP ASAP for assessment**

Malignant Melanoma* *Skin cancer (neoplasm of melanocytes). This cancer can be fatal, but has good results when excision of tumour is early* **SSx:** Maculo-papular rash/lesion, irregular borders that are raised, may be coloured spots around borders, changing size, shape, texture and colour (ABCD - Asymmetry; Border irregularity; Colour changes; Diameter over 6mm), often on men's torsos or women's legs **TCM Illness:** None that match (considered a 'wind-poison/toxin'; May be boil (ding chuang); carbuncle (yong)	**Causes:** Family history, overexposure to sun, previous melanoma **Diagnosis:** Observation, CBC, chem panel, biopsy, ultrasonography (best imaging for lymph node involvement), PET scan for metastases **Tx:** Surgical excision of tumour, chemo/radiation, elected lymph node dissection, lymph biopsies	**Red Flags:** Maculo-papular rash/lesion, ABCD - **A**symmetry; **B**order irregularity; **C**olour changes; **D**iameter over 6mm
Nevi *Grouping of normal skin cells (moles and/or birthmarks)* **SSx:** Hyperpigmented areas that vary in shape and color, **TCM Illness: None that match**	**Causes:** hereditary predisposition possible **Diagnosis:** Visual observation **Tx:** No treatment necessary	**Red Flags** **Refer to GP/PCP ASAP for assessment**
Psoriasis** *Chronic skin condition caused by abnormal growth of skin cells* **SSx:** Thick, silvery, scaly and inflamed patches of skin commonly found on knees, elbows, scalp and chest **TCM Illness:** None that match (actually called Pine Skin Tinea – song pi xian)	**Causes:** cause is unknown **Diagnosis:** Difficult to diagnose due to its similarities to eczema and dermatitis **Tx:** avoidance of triggers (excessive alcohol, smoking stress, sun exposure)	**Red Flags:** **Refer to GP/PCP for assessment if not responding**
Rosacea *Chronic inflammation of face (usually) with prominent capillaries (telangiectasia) and papules* **SSx:** Redness of face (esp. central region - esp. nose), easy flushing, tiny red pimples, fine, red lines, bulbous nose, red/swollen eye issues, small and dilated blood vessels *"You got a rosy-face-ya!"* **TCM Illness: None that match**	**Causes:** Hot/spicy foods, middle age, fair complexion, emotions, sun-damaged skin. alcohol **Diagnosis:** Observation **Tx:** Low dose tetracycline; identify food allergies; oral and topical antibiotics; sulpha-based skin washes; emotional release	**Red Flags:**

Scabies* *A skin infestation caused by a tiny mite. Can take 6 weeks to appear after exposure and 2 months to disappear* **SSx:** ITCHING (esp. at night), scratch marks on skin, pimple-like rash, usually on non-hairy body parts, often line on skin ¼" -1" long **TCM Illness: None that match**	**Causes:** Mites; mite burrows in skin, makes a tunnel and lays eggs; prolonged skin-to-skin contact or exposure to infected objects such as bed linens **Diagnosis:** Skin scraping **Tx:** Various ointments that are applied at night (when mites most active), antihistamines to reduce itch	**Red Flags:** **Refer to GP/PCP ASAP. Highly contagious!**
Seborrheic Dermatitis *Inflammatory scaling disease usually of the scalp and face (sometimes called dandruff or 'cradle cap' in infants)* **SSx:** Itchy, greasy, scaling of scalp, dandruff, red/yellow scaling papules (hairline, behind and in ears, eyebrows, nose ridge and nasolabial folds - can be on body as well), can lift scales off and squeeze greasy residue *'I look like a dragon with these scales - where is my dragon saber!!?? ROAR!'* **TCM Illness: None that match**	**Causes:** Stress, genetics, yeast, cold and dry weather, medications, diet alcohol **Diagnosis:** Observation **Tx:** Dandruff/tar shampoo (infants need a special shampoo from pediatrician), sun exposure, antifungals, corticosteroids, sulphur topicals	**Red Flags:** **Refer to GP/PCP for assessment if not responding to treatment**
Shingles** *Painful rash caused the varicella-zoster virus (dormant chickenpox virus)* **SSx:** 1) Flu-like symptoms → 2) Prodromal pain and hypersensitivity along site of the future eruption → 3) lesions/blisters 2-3 days later that erupt a few days later → Crusts forms and takes 2-4 weeks to heal; vesicles on an erythematous base with normal skin in between -Post-herpetic pain possible - pain in same area after lesions healed *"It was like I hung a shingle off a dermatome announcing- HEY EVERYBODY! CHECK OUT MY SKIN RASH. YOWCH!"* **TCM Illness: No exact match; related to chicken pox (shui dou)**	**Causes:** Vesicular eruption and neuralgic pain in the dermatome of the root ganglia affected by the varicella-zoster virus Immunosuppressed; high stress (decreasing immune system); over 50 years old **Diagnosis:** Observation, serological, skin culture **Tx:** Wet compresses, analgesics, medications to treat viruses, shingles vaccine for those looking to avoid it	**Red Flags:** Can lead to Persistent chronic nerve pain (called 'post-herpetic neuralgia') if left untreated. Important to refer to medical doctor very soon.
Squamous Cell Carcinoma* *Malignant tumour of squamous cells from the epidermis*	**Causes:** Long time exposure to sun/other forms of radiation **Diagnosis:** Biopsy of skin cells	**Red Flags:**

SSx: Firm nodules with indistinct borders, scaly opaque areas of skin, advanced cases - lesions and open sores to affected areas **TCM Illness: None that match**	**Tx:** Surgical removal, radiation therapy (chemotherapy) *High cure rate with early detection and treatment*	**Refer to GP/PCP ASAP for assessment**
Thrush *Infection of the mouth caused by the fungus candida albicans* **SSx:** White, cheesy plaque resembling cheese curds within the oral cavity **TCM Illness: None that match (actually called Goose Mouth Sore – e kou chuang)**	**Causes:** Candidiasis infection **Diagnosis:** Microscopic examination and sample collection **Tx:** Oral antifungal treatments, frequent mouth care	**Red Flags:** **Refer to GP/PCP for assessment**

ENT (Ear, Eyes, Nose, Throat)

i. General Pathophysiology:

- Infection: viral or bacterial agent, characterized by severe pain, discharge, changes in hearing
- Trauma: outer ear (lesions), or inner ear (burst eardrums, blunt force injuries)
- Polyps: small fleshy 'blobs' inside nose
- Abnormal exudate: pale-gray may indicate allergies
- Deviated septum: can affect breathing and trapping of pathogens
- Swelling inside nose: viral or bacterial infection

ii. Common Western Tests

Ear:
- Weber test: testing hearing using tuning fork to detect one-sided, middle, or inner ear hearing loss
- Rinne test: Sensorineural loss (hearing loss from sensory organ, Ex) cochlea OR hearing loss from cranial nerve VIII, vestibulocochlear nerve) – again using a tuning fork
- Cultures of discharges
- Otoscopy: Visual examination of ear canal using an otoscope (medical device specifically for ears with built in light)

Eye:
- Wall eye chart
- Tonometry: measures intraocular eye pressure (IOP)
- PERRLA (Pupils Equal Round Reactive to Light and Accommodating)
- Fundoscopy (ophthalmoscopy) exam: evaluates back of eye (retina, blood vessels, optic disc)
- Slit lamp

Nose:
- Cultures of nasal discharge
- X-rays on sinuses
- Ultrasound

Throat:
- Culture/swab
- Laryngoscopy - usually the fibre-optic kind. Small camera goes through nose and down throat to inspect vocal cords/larynx

iii. General Red Flags

Ear:
- Trauma
- Sudden and severe ear pain (usually not an emergency, but will require an evaluation)
- Possibly vertigo

Eye:
- Foreign body in eye
- Sudden, acute visual loss or disturbance
- Sudden and severe eye pain
- Flashing lights and/or seeing dark lines in vision
- Inflamed eye

Nose:
- Severe epistaxis that won't abate
- Trauma

Throat:
- Epiglottitis (epiglottis swells and covers windpipe – emergency!)

iii. General Red Flags

- Persistent unilateral hearing loss/tinnitus
- Blood stained mucous
- Dysphonia (difficulty speaking) for more than 1 month
- Facial palsy
- Sudden hearing loss
- Septal deviation
- CSF (cerebrospinal fluid) leak (persistent clear dripping from nose)
- Dysphagia
- Persistent and growing lumps

Common Diseases + Specific Red Flags

Condition Symptoms and signs Related TCM Illness	Causes & Diagnostic tests	Red flags (and what to do about them)
Blepharitis Inflammation of the eyelids due to tiny oil glands at base of eyelashes becoming clogged Symptoms: Itching, swelling, redness, burning, gritty feeling in eye, irritation, loss of eyelashes, photophobia, tearing, eyelids appear greasy, crusty eyelashes in morning "It looks like someone BLEPHED on my eyelids!" TCM Illness: None that match	Causes: Staph introduction into eye; can be part of symptom set of sebborheic dermatitis; rosacea, allergies, old makeup (bacteria), eyelash mites or lice -Very rare: skin cancer Diagnosis: Eyelid swab to check for bacteria/fungi; eyelid visual exam Tx: Antibiotic ointments; warm compresses to soak the area; steroid eye drops	**Red Flags:** None. Often a chronic condition that is difficult to treat, but not dangerous.
Cataracts Painless clouding of the internal lens of the eye blocking light from passing through (blurring vision) Symptoms: Progressive and painless loss of vision (blurry vision), photophobia, diplopia, reduced colour vision, IMPROVEMENT in vision with up-close objects, 'milky-opaque' film over pupil (lens portion), later stages - blindness + 'milky-opaque' film over pupil (lens portion) "I can't see because there is a giant, white CAT in front of my eye!" TCM Illness: None that match	Causes: Aging; long-term exposure to UV light; diabetes; prolonged corticosteroid use; smoking, trauma Diagnosis: Retinal exam + slit lamp or ophthalmoscope Tx: Surgery to replace lens	**Red Flags:** Surgery is required to replace the lens.
Chalazion Painless, slow-growing, hard mass in eyelid due to a blocked oil gland Symptoms: Small, hard bump on eyelid "I feel like I have a chunk of chorizo sausage on my eye." TCM Illness: Sebaceous cyst (zhi liu)	Causes: *Unclean hands (most common, rosacea; seborrheic dermatitis; TB; viral infections; hx of having chalazions increases risk for future ones, old make-up -Very rare: skin cancer Diagnosis: Visual observation Tx: Warm compresses to soak the area; steroid injection; surgical removal	**Red Flags:** They usually clear up in a month on their own.

Conjunctivitis *Inflammation of the conjunctiva* Ssx: Burning and itchy eyes, mucous secretions from eyes, redness of conjunctiva, lymphadenopathy (swollen lymph nodes), photophobia, blurry vision Conjunctiva- + -itis (inflammation of something) TCM Illness: None that match	**Causes:** Virus; bacteria (including some STDs); allergies; irritants (consider shampoos, pool chlorine, any outside factors) **Diagnosis:** Usually just observational diagnosis, but can be a swab test sent to a lab to find the cause as well **Tx:** Antibiotic drops; herbal washes; ask patient not to share their personal items as it can spread easily to others if bacterial (not with the allergic kind)	**Red Flags:** Differentiate between topical irritant and serious cause (infection, STI). Clean surface of the eye with sterile water if caused by irritant. Medical attention required immediately for antibiotics if caused by an infection.
Dacryocystitis Pain, swelling, redness, a mass or lump associated with the lacrimal gland (tear duct). Secondary reaction to obstruction of the nasolacrimal duct (most common in infants) Symptoms: Pain, swelling, redness (erythema), fever, tearing, conjunctivitis, inflammation of the lid margins, edema, may be a mass or lump associated with the lacrimal gland 'I fell and hit right below my eye with my daiquiri straw! Close call! All swollen now. I guess I had one too many…' OR Dacryo = tear -cyst = sac -itis = inflammation TCM Illness: Sebaceous cyst (zhi liu)	Causes: Trauma; deviated septum, rhinitis; polyps Diagnosis: May need neuroimaging and surgical exploration if unresolvable; blood cultures; culture of lacrimal fluid Tx: Depends on if acute (severe) or chronic: Antibiotics (both oral and topical); hot compresses	**Red Flags:**
Epistaxis Nosebleed Symptoms: Bleeding from the nose TCM Illness: Bleeding disorder (xue zheng)	Causes: Blunt force injuries causing blood cells in the nasal cavity to burst, inflammatory disease, tumours, dry nose, nose picking, deviated septum Diagnosis: Physical examination Tx: Head tilt forward and pinch bridge of the nose, apply ice to the area.	**Red Flags:** Refer to GP/PCP for assessment if bleeding will not abate
Glaucoma Progressive loss of peripheral vision, vague visual disturbances, frequent changes in eyeglass prescriptions due to increased IOP. 2 types: Open-angle – fluid doesn't flow out of the eye drain structure properly; or	Increase in intraocular pressure causing mild visual loss or even blindness due to optic nerve atrophy Causes: Idiopathic. May be a secondary issue to diabetes.	**Red Flags:**

Closed-angle – angle btwn iris and cornea too narrow so cannot drain Symptoms: Progressive loss of peripheral vision, mild h/a or eye pain, vague visual disturbances (may see halos around light), frequent changes in eyeglass prescriptions, poor adaptation to low light "The pressure has 'glommed' on to my optic nerve. I can't see very well!!" TCM Illness: None that match	Diagnosis: Tonometry Tx: Eye drops to decrease pressure in anterior chamber; surgery if canal of Schlemm is blocked (drains the anterior chamber of eye)	Immediate medical attention required (likely surgery) to prevent permanent loss of vision
Hordeolum Red, swollen, bump with pus in centre Symptoms: Painful, red, swollen, bump that has pus at centre, gritty feeling in eye, photophobia 'My eyelid is hoarding all of the pus!' TCM Illness: Sebaceous cyst (zhi liu)	AKA 'Styes' – infection of an oil gland(s) in eye along eyelid margin. Causes: Staph is most common Diagnosis: Observational diagnosis Tx: Warm compresses; can be lanced if chronic	**Red Flags:** Avoid squeezing or bursting styes or you can cause infection – which would be a referral to GP ASAP
Laryngitis Loss of, or, unnatural change in voice, hoarseness Symptoms: Loss of, or, unnatural change in voice, hoarseness, tickling sensation in throat, raw or sore throat, dry throat and/or cough TCM Illness: None that match	Inflammation of the voice box (larynx) and vocal cords Causes: Overuse; allergic reactions; infection; polyps, cold or flu Diagnosis: Laryngoscopy if chronic or recurrent (usually just diagnosed from symptoms though) Tx: RESTING voice, steam inhalation, antibiotic if from bacteria, corticosteroids if voice needs immediate recovery	**Red Flags:** None, unless throat is rapidly swelling from an allergic rxn.
Macular Degeneration Gradual, painless loss of visual acuity, blurry vision, dark areas or distortion in central vision Symptoms: Progressive loss of visual acuity (affects one eye at a time), blurry vision, dark areas or distortion in central vision (peripheral vision not usually affected), hazy vision Macula: responsible for acuity of vision (fine details)	Atrophy of the maculae (area around fovea at back of eye that is area of highest visual acuity) Causes: Yellowish spots (drusen – which may be deteriorating tissue deposits behind retina) accumulate in and around the macula OR abnormal blood vessels under the retina; age; UV exposure; may be genetic; obesity; HBP; smoking Diagnosis: Have vision checked with Amsler grid	**Red Flags:**

Degeneration: we all know what this means! TCM Illness: None that match	Tx: Laser on macular site to stop abnormal blood vessel growth; vitamin supplement; medication to stop abnormal blood vessel growth (anti-VEGF drug)	
Meniére's Disease Recurring vertigo, tinnitus and hearing loss (aural fullness) Symptoms: Sudden, severe vertigo from hours to days (usually one-sided), progressive hearing loss, n/v, intermittent or constant tinnitus, sense of fullness/congestion in ear, can cause permanent hearing loss "Argh! There are MEN in my ear - yelling and making me dizzy!!" TCM Illness: Vertigo (xuan yun), tinnitus and deafness (er ming, er long)	Inner ear disorder that causes recurring vertigo, tinnitus and hearing loss (aural fullness) Causes: Idiopathic Possibly: increased fluid in inner ear (endolymph); allergies; viral infection; abnormal immune response; genetic; head trauma; migraines Diagnosis: Intake to confirm the 3 main sxs + hearing test (often issues with hearing low frequencies); balance tests; blood test to rule out other conditions (like brain tumour or MS) Tx: No cure, but reduced sxs with: motions sickness meds (ex) Valium; anti-nausea meds (ex) Gravol; diuretic; steroids; rehab for balance; surgery is last resort (one is to cut the vestibular nerve; the other is to remove the labyrinth of the ear - causes permanent hearing and balance loss in that ear)	**Red Flags:**
Otitis Externa Inflammation or infection of the external auditory canal Symptoms: Pain, redness and swelling to the area, itchy, pressure within the ear, discharge TCM Illness: None that match	Causes: Exposure to infectious agent, compromised skin integrity in the ear, irritation or allergic reaction Diagnosis: Otoscopy, review of patient symptoms and history, culture of discharge, swabs of ears Tx: Antibiotics for infection, analgesic for pain, topical agents for redness/swelling	**Red Flags:** **Refer to GP/PCP for assessment**
Otitis Media Inflammation or infection of the middle ear space Symptoms: 'Plugged' ears, decreased hearing, hearing loss, ear pain, pressure within the inner ear, headache, fever, irritability, loss of appetite (very common in children and infants)	Causes: Allergies, other illnesses such as flu and cold, sinus infection, respiratory illnesses Diagnosis: Otoscopy, review of patient symptoms and history, culture of discharge, swabs of ears Tx: Antibiotics for infection, analgesic for pain, topical agents for redness/swelling	**Red Flags:** **Refer to GP/PCP for assessment** Signs of worsening infection high fever, flushed skin, decreased consciousness - **Refer to ER**

Pharyngitis Inflammation of the pharyngeal walls, may include tonsils, palate and the uvula Symptoms: Complaints of scratchy/sore throat, red swollen throat on inspection with patchy yellow or white exudates TCM Illness: None that match	Causes: Bacterial, fungal or viral infections, prolonged antibiotic use or inhaled corticosteroids, immunosuppressed individuals Diagnosis: Cultures of throat swabs/exudate to determine root cause Tx: Antibiotic/antiviral/antifungal depending on the cause	**Red Flags:** **Refer to ER if red flags present**
Retinal Detachment Separation of the retina from underlying epithelium from a break, hole or tear Symptoms: 'Curtain folding over visual field', floaters, blurry vision, flashes of light, loss of vision TCM Illness: None that match	Causes: Trauma; HBP, medications; eye surgery; chronic eye inflammation/diseases Diagnosis: Eye examination; ultrasound Tx: If just a tear: laser surgery or freezing to fix the tear If detached - surgery	**Red Flags:** **Emergency situation - immediate surgery required!**
Rhinitis Irritation and/or inflammation of the nasal cavity Symptoms: Stuffy and/or runny nose, sneezing, coughing, excess mucus in the nose and/or throat 'I feel like a have a rhino horn in my nose.' TCM Illness: None that match	Causes: Environmental irritants, allergic reactions, infections (cold/flu) Diagnosis: Skin/blood test to rule out allergic reactions, possible nasal endoscopy (severe cases) Tx: Antihistamines, nasal sprays,	**Red Flags:** None
Serous Otitis Media Decreased hearing after a cold/allergy attack, aural fullness Symptoms: Decreased hearing, aural fullness, if a young child and chronic - difficulty learning speech "Otis seriously couldn't hear the media blasting" TCM Illness: None that match	Collection of middle ear serous fluid. Can be acute or chronic. Most common cause of hearing loss in children. Often happens during/after a cold or allergies. Cause: Cold/allergy attack Diagnosis: Blocked eustachian tube from a recent cold/allergy attack Lab: Hearing test; impedance tympanometry (check mov't of eardrum when pressure is applied)	**Red Flags:** **Antibiotics and surgery may be required**
Sinusitis Runny, stuffy nose, facial pain, may	Inflammation or swelling of the tissue lining the sinuses - often due to blocked	**Red Flags:**

be purulent discharge Symptoms: Cold-like symptoms (for acute sinusitis) + runny, stuffy nose, facial pain, loss of smell, cough, congestion, may be fever and fatigue as well, pus in nasal cavity (purulent discharge) TCM Illness: Nasal congestion (bi yuan) - not on Pan-Can list	fluid allowing bacterial growth Causes: Common cold; allergic rhinitis; polyps; deviated septum; immune deficiency Diagnosis: Observation and intake; may press on sinus areas or tap teeth near nose to see if they are sore Tx: Decongestants, nasal saline sprays, antibiotics, warm compresses, antihistamine if from allergies, immunoglobulin if due to immune deficiencies, may need surgery if polyps or deviated septum	
Tonsillitis Inflammation of the tonsils Symptoms: Throat pain and tenderness, swelling of the tonsils, difficulty swallowing, headache, loss of appetite, white/yellow exudate on tonsils, fever, chills, bad breath TCM Illness: None that match	Causes: Bacterial/viral infections, most commonly the streptococcus bacteria Diagnosis: Culture of throat swab to determine cause, then the appropriate antibacterial/antiviral Tx: Antibiotic/antiviral	**Red Flags:** Refer to ER if cannot swallow

Endocrine and Metabolic

i. **General Pathophysiology:**
- Diabetes - type I in which the body cannot produce insulin, type II in which the body develops a insulin resistance
- Diabetic Ketoacidosis – body starts burning fat due to lack of glucose to burn. Fat releases keytones, which makes the blood acidic. Sxs include: vomiting, fruity smelling breath, confusion, difficulty breathing
- Hyper____ - refers to overproduction of hormones/substances caused by endocrine/metabolic influences
- Hypo____ - refers to underproduction of hormones/substances caused by endocrine/metabolic influences

ii. **Common Western Tests:**
- Endoscopy - a non-surgical procedure using an endoscope (flexible camera with light) to view the digestive tract
- TSH test - measure amount of thyroid stimulating hormone in blood, indicative of many endocrine disorders
- Blood Glucose test ex) A1C test (tests over 3 months time) - measure blood sugars

iii. **General Red Flags:**
- Unexplained weight gain or loss
- Feeling of fatigue/lethargy, intolerance to regular activities
- Vomiting

Common Diseases + Specific Red Flags

Condition / Symptoms and signs / Related TCM Illness	Causes & Diagnostic tests	Red flags (and what to do about them)
Addison's Disease* *Adrenocortical insufficiency from atrophy of adrenal gland that causes insufficient production of steroid hormones* **Ssx:** Extremely slow onset of progressive weakness, fatigue, weight loss, skin hyperpigmentation, maybe body hair loss *'Please add some adrenal additions to add to my energy.'* **TCM Illness:** Consumptive disease (xu lao)	**Causes:** Most commonly an autoimmune response, tumour, adrenal gland infection, TB, bleeding into adrenal gland, pituitary disease, taking corticosteroids and then abruptly stopping **Diagnosis:** Confirmation of physical symptoms, test of cortisol levels **Tx:** Hormone replacement to replace the lack of steroid hormones	**Red Flags:**

Cushing's Syndrome* *Range of abnormalities caused by excess corticosteroids* **Ssx:** Weight gain (particularly in the face), pronounced back hump, hyperglycemia, thinning/fragile skin, prolonged wound healing, easy bruising *'Actually, being swollen and overweight like this feels quite cushy! Thank you steroids!'* **TCM Illness: Edema (shui zhong)**	**Causes:** Prolonged use of corticosteroids, tumour on adrenal gland **Diagnosis:** Physical examination, cortisol level test **Tx:** Surgical removal of tumour in addition to radiation, drug therapy to inhibit adrenal function	**Red Flags:** **Be aware of clinical manifestations so as to refer to GP if you suspect this condition**
Diabetes Mellitus (I&II)* *Disease of the pancreas that inhibits the body's ability to produce insulin* Type I: the pancreas cannot produce insulin Type II: the body develops insulin resistance **Ssx:** Increased thirst and hunger, sweating, weight loss or gain, blurred vision, impaired wound healing, nausea, fatigue, increased urination *'Ok, so... FIRST you won't produce the insulin... and THEN you won't even accept it? Come on!'* **TCM Illness: Consumptive thirst (xiao ke)**	**Causes:** Type I: cause is unknown, the immune system attacks the pancreas. Usually develops in children Type II: poor nutrition, sedentary lifestyle, high sugar and carbohydrate intake **Diagnosis:** Review of symptoms, blood sugar test, A1C test, urine test **Tx:** Continual blood sugar monitoring and anti-diabetic drugs (metformin), extreme cases daily insulin injections	**Red Flags:** Shakiness, sweating, loss of consciousness, fatigue, pale skin are signs of hypoglycemia (low blood sugar) and is a medical emergency. Check the blood sugar and get the person to eat/drink sugar, **if unconscious call 911**
Hyperlipidemia*** *High cholesterol - abnormally high concentration of fats (lipids) within the blood* **Ssx:** Increased blood pressure, symptoms in areas of blockage **TCM Illness: MAY be chest impediment (xiong bi) if affecting HT**	**Causes:** High intake of fatty foods, lack of exercise, genetics, inflamed body and vessels- **Diagnosis:** Blood test **Tx:** Largely lifestyle changes, improved diet, exercise, cholesterol lowering drugs	**Red Flags:** Watch for HT symptoms or signs of circulatory issues. **Refer to GP if present.**
Hyperglycemia *Abnormally high blood sugar levels in diabetics* **Ssx:** Increased thirst, trouble concentration, blurred vision, frequent urination	**Causes:** Too low of an insulin/antihyperglycemic dose, lack of exercise, poor diet, having an illness such as flu or cold **Diagnosis:** Blood glucose test (finger prick rapid testing)	**Red Flags:** Chronic hyperglycemia has negative

TCM Illness: Symptom based – h/a (tou tong), palpitations (xin ji)	Tx: Administration of insulin/oral antihyperglycemics, lifestyle changes such as increase exercise, improved diet low in sugar	long-term effects on overall health - be aware of long term elevated blood sugars.
Thyroid Disorders*		
Hyperthyroidism (Grave's Disease) *Overactive thyroid gland producing excessive amounts of thyroid hormone* Ssx: Decreased appetite, weight loss, fatigue, thick brittle nails, heart palpitations, nervousness, irritability, heat intolerance, warm, moist skin, exophthalmos *'I am so hyper that it is going to put me in an early Grave!'* TCM Illness: Goitre (ying bing)	Causes: Most commonly Graves Disease (hormonal disorder that produces excess thyroid hormone) Diagnosis: Thyroxine and TSH (thyroid stimulating hormone) blood test Tx: Antithyroid medication, radioactive iodine	Red Flags: **Refer to GP if cardiac symptoms.**
Hashimoto's thyroiditis Autoimmune disease in which the body attacks and eventually destroys the thyroid gland - replaced by fibrous tissue Ssx: Early on no symptoms, as disease progresses weight gain, fatigue, sleepiness, depression, decreased libido, difficulty sleeping, muscle aches and pain TCM Illness: Goitre (ying bing)	Causes: Unknown cause - autoimmune response Diagnosis: Thyroid stimulating hormone (TSH) test and antibody test, review of patient history Tx: Thyroid hormone replacement (usually levothyroxine sodium)	Red Flags: People with autoimmune disease are more susceptible to other illnesses and other autoimmune disease - such as Addison's disease. Watch for more symptoms.
Hypothyroidism *Disease of the thyroid in which the thyroid does not produce enough hormones, resulting in a hypometabolic state* Ssx: Fatigued and lethargic, impaired memory, slow speech, decreased initiative, low tolerance to activity, anemia, constipation, weight gain TCM Illness: Consumptive disease (xu lao)	Causes: Autoimmune component, treatment for hyperthyroidism, thyroid surgery, certain medications Diagnosis: Blood tests for thyroid function (TSH), physical examination and review of history/symptoms Tx: Hormone replacement (usually Synthroid)	Red Flags: Watch for palpitations and cardiac symptoms. **Refer to GP if present.**
NKHHC (Non-Ketonic Hyperglycemic Hyperosmolar coma) *LIFE THREATENING condition in which a patient produces enough insulin to prevent ketoacidosis however still suffers from severe hyperglycemia and*	Causes: Impaired thirst sensations, functional inability to replace fluids, inadequate fluids intake, fever/additional illness with history of type II diabetes, poorly managed diabetes, low KI function, aging,	Red Flags:

extracellular fluid depletion **Ssx:** High blood sugar reading, decreased level of consciousness, confusion, hallucinations, excessive thirst, dry mucous membranes, warm dry skin, fever **TCM Illness: Symptom dependent**	diuretics **Diagnosis:** Blood and urine tests, review of symptoms **Tx:** IV fluids to treat dehydration and fluid deficit, insulin infusion to reduce blood sugar, continual monitoring for electrolyte levels and patient status until past acute phase	**This is a medical emergency and prompt diagnosis is KEY for survival - call 911 immediately if suspected**
Obesity*** *Abnormal or excessive adipose accumulation* **Ssx:** High Body Mass Index (BMI), large amount of adipose tissue **TCM Illness: None that match**	**Causes:** Poor diet, lack of exercise, some genetic risk factors, hypothyroid **Diagnosis:** Measure of BMI, physical examination by physician **Tx:** Lifestyle changes - decrease caloric intake, increase exercise	**Red Flags:** **Refer to GP for further assessment if patient suffering from side effects**
Pheochromocytoma *Tumour of adrenal medulla that results in excessive production of epinephrine* **Ssx:** Severe and episodic hypertension, pounding headache, high heart rate, profuse sweating, heart palpitations *'Pheo needed a new chrome adrenal in order to calm him down'* **TCM Illness: Palpitations (xin ji), headache (tou tong)**	**Causes:** Exact cause unknown, benign tumour that develops **Diagnosis:** Urine test for elevated epinephrine levels, most accurate during episodes of hypertension **Tx:** Surgical removal of tumour, medications to lower blood pressure	**Red Flags:**

Gastrointestinal Conditions

General Pathophysiology:
- Stomach ulcers - often caused by stress, acidic food, and h-pylori bacteria
- Gallstones - hard deposits of material in the gall bladder
- Constipation - difficulty/inability to empty bowels
- Diarrhea - frequent, liquid bowel movements
- Indigestion - pain and discomfort due to decreased ability to digest
- Bowel obstruction - part of small or large intestine becomes blocked and digested material cannot pass
- Pyrosis - heartburn
- Dysphagia - difficulty swallowing

Common Western Tests
- Colonoscopy - examination of colon using a probe inserted through the anus
- Gastroscopy - examination of stomach and intestines using a probe inserted through the mouth
- Occult blood - test of blood in the stool
- Barium swallow - used to detect abnormalities in the upper GI. Swallow liquid barium and then x-rays taken to follow the barium

General Red Flags
- Hemafecia
- Melena (dark, tarry, sticky stool)
- Vomiting blood
- Severe abdominal pain

Common Diseases + Specific Red Flags

Abdominal Pain *Pain in the abdominal area* **Ssx:** Onset of pain to the abdomen **TCM Illness: Abdominal Pain (fu tong)**	**Causes:** Indigestion, illness, medications, bowel obstruction, ulcers, acute appendicitis, acute pancreatitis, upper GI haemorrhage, chronic esophagitis, renal calculi, cancer of colon/rectum, Irritation of abdominal peritoneum lining **Diagnosis:** Variety of tests, abdominal x-ray, lab tests, review of medications and history to determine cause **Tx:** Will depend on cause	**Red Flags:** **Refer to GP for further assessment or ER if severe**
Appendicitis* *Inflammation of the appendix* **Ssx:** Dull pain near naval (to the right and inferior), loss of appetite, nausea/vomiting, fever **TCM Illness: Abdominal Pain (fu tong)**	**Causes:** Blockage of appendix, often from stool or other organic material **Diagnosis:** Abdominal exam (rebound pressure), urine test to rule out UTI, if necessary CT scan **Tx:** Surgical removal of appendix	**Red Flags:** **Refer to ER immediately**

Condition	Causes / Diagnosis / Tx	Red Flags
Ascites *Accumulation of fluid within the abdominal cavity* **Ssx:** Increased abdominal girth, abdominal discomfort/pressure, shortness of breath *"I would get more ascited, but my belly feels too heavy"* **TCM Illness: Abdominal Pain (fu tong), Edema (shui zhong)**	**Causes:** Advanced liver disease, portal hypertension, salt/water retention, advanced kidney and/or heart failure **Diagnosis:** Physical examination, ultrasound of the abdomen, CT scan **Tx:** Treatment of the underlying cause i.e. HT failure, cirrhosis, medication to reduce water retention (diuretics), paracentesis (removal of fluid)	**Red Flags:** **Refer to GP for further assessment**
Cholestasis *Blockage or reduction of bile drainage/flow from the liver to the stomach* **Ssx:** Severe itching of the skin without skin rash (usually hands and feet – may be due to bile salts deposited in skin), yellowing of eyes/skin, pale stool, dark concentrated urine *'Chole = bile* *Stasis = blockage/stoppage'* **TCM Illness: Jaundice (huang dan)**	**Causes:** Gallstones, hepatitis, abdominal tumours **Diagnosis:** Blood tests to determine liver function/level of bile products in the blood **Tx:** Meds to decrease bile in bloodstream (usually cholestyramine), soaking of itchy areas, endoscopy or surgery to unblock bile ducts	**Red Flags:** **Refer to GP ASAP for further assessment**
Cholecystitis** *Inflammation of the gallbladder* **Ssx:** Sudden extreme upper right or central abdomen pain, pain between shoulder blades or back, pain in right shoulder *'Chole = bile (think GB)* *itis = inflammation'* **TCM Illness: Abdominal Pain (fu tong), Epigastric Pain (wei tong)**	**Causes:** Gallstones, high fat diet, low fibre intake, tumour, bile duct blockage **Diagnosis:** Abdominal CT and/or ultrasound **Tx:** Removal of gallstones, antibiotics to prevent infection	**Red Flags:** **Refer to ER**
Cholelithiasis** *Gallstones - hardened deposits of digestive fluids (bile)* **Ssx:** Sudden extreme upper right or central abdomen pain, pain between shoulder blades or back, pain in right shoulder *'Chole = bile (think GB)* *lithiasis = stone formation'*	**Causes:** Unknown, caused by a backup of bile - gall bladder isn't draining properly, high fat diet, diabetes **Diagnosis:** Abdominal ultrasound or CT **Tx:** Surgical removal of gallbladder	**Red Flags:**

'Poor John Lithgow always seems so perturbed because of his gallstone pain' **TCM Illness:** Abdominal Pain (fu tong), Epigastric Pain (wei tong)			**Refer to ER**
Hepatocirrhosis* *Accumulation of scar tissue within the liver cells* **Ssx:** Constipation, diarrhea, abdominal pain, weight loss, muscle weakness, bleeding gums, unexplained bruising, jaundice **TCM Illness:** Abdominal Pain (fu tong)	**Causes:** Long term alcoholism, chronic liver infections, obesity **Diagnosis:** Liver biopsy, upper abdomen CT scan, review of symptoms **Tx:** Lifestyle changes, reduction of alcohol intake, avoidance of infection	**Red Flags:** **Refer to GP very soon for further assessment**	
Colon Cancer *Cancer of the colon* **Symptoms:** Change in bowel habits (can be either diarrhea OR constipation - something out of the ordinary routine), rectal bleeding, abdominal pain and/or cramps, fatigue, weight loss **TCM Illness:** Abdominal Pain (fu tong)	**Causes:** Uncontrolled cell growth (as is the case with ALL cancers), family history, poor diet, smoking **Diagnosis:** Abdominal ultrasound/MRI/CT, colonoscopy, biopsy of colon **Tx:** Chemotherapy, radiation, surgical removal of cancerous material	**Red Flags:** **Refer to GP very soon for further assessment**	
Colorectal Cancer *Cancer of the colon and/or rectum* **Symptoms:** Change in bowel habits (can be either diarrhea OR constipation - something out of the ordinary routine), rectal bleeding, abdominal pain and/or cramps, fatigue, rectal pain **TCM Illness:** Abdominal Pain (fu tong)	**Causes:** Uncontrolled cell growth (as is the case with ALL cancers), family history, poor diet, smoking **Diagnosis:** Abdominal ultrasound/MRI/CT, colonoscopy, biopsy of colon **Tx:** Chemotherapy, radiation, surgical removal of cancerous material	**Red Flags:** **Refer to GP very soon for further assessment**	
Constipation *Difficulty/inability to pass stool* **Ssx:** Prolonged period of no bowel movements, lower abdominal pain, abdominal pressure, feeling bloated and/or full **TCM Illness:** Constipation, (bian	**Causes:** Low fibre diet, medications (pain medications especially), iron, pregnancy, neurological diseases **Diagnosis:** Review of symptoms, abdominal x-ray **Tx:** Stool softeners, laxatives, enemas (instillation of fluid into the rectum to stimulate bowel	**Red Flags:**	

bi), Abdominal Pain (fu tong)	movement), increase fluids and fibre in diet	**Refer for GP and/or ER**
Crohn's (Regional Enteritis)*** *Chronic inflammatory disease of the intestine that can affect any part of the GI tract from mouth to anus* **"Gum to Bum"** **Ssx:** Abdominal pain, weight loss, fever, fatigue, abdominal cramping, diarrhea (may have blood or mucous in stool), dehydration, impaired nutritional absorption **TCM Illness: Abdominal Pain (fu tong), Diarrhea (xie xie)**	**Causes:** Idiopathic **Diagnosis:** History of symptoms, blood work, colonoscopy **Tx:** Corticosteroid therapy, antibiotics, nutritional therapy, worst case scenario surgery	**Red Flags:** **Refer to GP for further assessment**
Diarrhea *Watery stool* **Ssx:** Frequent loose bowel movements, liquid, watery stool **TCM Illness: Diarrhea (xie xie)**	**Causes:** Illness, antibiotic use, reaction to medication, gastric disorder, food poisoning **Diagnosis:** Visual examination and review of symptoms **Tx:** Imodium, modification of medications	**Red Flags:** **Refer to GP when necessary**
Diverticulosis/it is** *Outpouching of the mucosa through the muscle of the intestinal wall* **Ssx:** Majority have no symptoms, lower abdominal cramps (left lower quadrant), alternating constipation and diarrhea *'The intestine has diverted out to catch it's own food particles'* **TCM Illness: Abdominal Pain (fu tong)**	**Causes:** No known cause, possibly fibre deficiency **Diagnosis:** CT scan with oral contrast dye, colonoscopy **Tx:** Uncomplicated cases are treated with high fibre diet, laxatives	**Red Flags:** **Refer to ER for further assessment if acute**
Fatty Liver *Reversible condition of excess fat cells in the liver, 5% adipose or more* **Ssx:** Fatigue and generalized abdominal pain, poor appetite, weakness, confusion, jaundice *'Your LR needs to lose weight – it is possible!'*	**Causes:** Obesity, malnutrition and starvation, rapid weight loss, chronic alcohol use, diabetes, insulin resistance **Diagnosis:** Physical examination for enlarged liver, blood test for liver function, abdominal ultrasound, liver biopsy **Tx:** Lifestyle modifications and reduction of risk factors (alcohol,	**Red Flags:** **Refer to GP for further**

	drugs)	assessment
TCM Illness: Abdominal Pain (fu tong)		
Fibrosis of Liver *Excessive accumulation of scar tissue within the liver as a result of long term inflammation* Ssx: Fatigue, easy bruising/bleeding, yellowing of skin, itchy skin, loss of appetite, ascites *'The LR fibre has been woven too tightly and doesn't allow for bile to flow'* **TCM Illness: Jaundice (huang dan), Edema (shui zhong)**	**Causes:** Obesity, chronic alcohol and/or drug use, chronic hepatitis B or C infection **Diagnosis:** Review of medical history and symptoms, blood tests for liver function, abdominal CT **Tx:** Lifestyle modifications, improved diet and exercise, treatment of underlying causes	**Red Flags:** **Refer to GP for further assessment**
Food Sensitivities/Allergies (Celiac, Lactose Intolerance)*** *Allergic reaction or intolerance to certain foods* Ssx: Itchy skin/throat, fever, development of rash abdominal pain, diarrhea severe case - anaphylaxis flushing of skin, swelling of throat and mouth and tongue, rapid rash development, difficulty talking and breathing **MEDICAL EMERGENCY** **TCM Illness: Abdominal Pain (fu tong)**	**Causes:** Immune response is triggered in response to antigen **Diagnosis:** Review of history and exposure to certain foods, allergy test **Tx:** Avoiding said foods, antihistamines, epinephrine pen for anaphylaxis	**Red Flags:** **Signs of anaphylaxis - call 911 immediately**
Gastritis *Inflammation of gastric mucosa* Ssx: Nausea/vomiting, abdominal discomfort and pain, hiccups, heartburn, indigestion **TCM Illness: Abdominal Pain (fu tong), Epigastric Pain (wei tong)**	**Causes:** Excessive aspirin use, alcohol, spicy food, h-pylori bacteria, smoking, hiatal hernia, chronic acid reflux, endoscopic procedures **Diagnosis:** History of drug and alcohol use. endoscopy, blood tests **Tx:** Antibiotics if caused by bacterial agent, proton pump inhibitors to decrease acid, TUMS	**Red Flags:** **Refer to GP for further assessment**
Gastro-enteritis *Stomach flu* Ssx: Diarrhea, vomiting, fever, headache, loss of appetite, chills, aches and pain, epigastric pain	**Causes:** Virus most often the cause **Diagnosis:** Review of physical symptoms **Tx:** Fluids, rest, tylenol for	**Red Flags**

'The gastro is trying to enter the outside' **TCM Illness: Abdominal Pain (fu tong), Epigastric Pain (wei tong), Diarrhea (xie xie), Vomiting (ou tu)**	fever/headache	**Refer to GP for further assessment**
Gastric Ulcer *Ulcers to the upper part of the GI tract, most common in women and older adults* **Ssx:** Dull stomach pain, weight loss, loss of appetite, bloating, hiccups, stomach pain improves with food **TCM Illness: Epigastric pain (wei tong)**	**Causes:** H-pylori bacteria, chronic drug use (aspirin), smoking, alcohol, stress **Diagnosis:** Endoscopy, biopsy of material if necessary **Tx:** Reducing aspirin intake, treating bacterial infections, reducing stress	**Red Flags:** **Refer to GP for further assessment**
GERD (Gastro-Esophageal Reflux)*** *Chronic reflux of stomach contents into the lower esophagus* **Ssx:** Heartburn, irritation of esophagus, mild difficulty swallowing, regurgitation of food **TCM Illness: Epigastric pain (wei tong)**	**Causes:** Impaired lower esophageal sphincter, decreased esophageal clearance, high acid intake **Diagnosis:** Endoscopy, barium swallow **Tx:** Diet modifications, medications (antacids - decrease acidity of stomach)	**Red Flags:** **Refer to GP for further assessment**
GI Bleeding *Bleeding in the upper or lower GI tracts* **Ssx:** Hematemesis, melena, occult stool, fresh blood in stool **TCM Illness: Closest is Bleeding Disorders (xue zheng)**	**Causes:** NSAIDS (non steroidal anti-inflammatory drug), gastric cancers, ulcers, lesions in GI tract, polyps, cirrhosis **Diagnosis:** Endoscopy to determine origin, barium swallow **Tx:** Antacids, proton pump inhibitors, repair during endoscopy, surgical repair	**Red Flags:** **Refer to GP ASAP for further assessment**
Haemorrhoids** *Swollen, inflamed veins in the rectum or anus. Can be internal or external* **Ssx:** Pain to the rectum/anus, itching and discomfort during bowel movement, fresh red blood **TCM Illness: Haemorrhoid (zhi)**	**Causes:** Common in elderly people and during pregnancy, straining while defecating, holding breath during physical labour **Diagnosis:** Physical examination of anus/rectum **Tx:** Topical creams to reduce size, fibre	**Red Flags:** **Refer to GP for further**

		assessment if bleeding is profuse.
Hepatitis* *Inflammation of the liver, various forms - Hep A,B,C,D,E* **Ssx:** Yellowing of skin, nausea/vomiting, loss of appetite joint pain, fever, weakness/fatigue **TCM Illness:** Jaundice (huang dan)	**Causes:** Viral infection is most common cause, chronic alcohol and drug use, autoimmune disease Hep A = contaminated water/food Hep B = infective blood, semen, body fluids Hep C = infective blood Hep D = from Hep B (more serious) Hep E = contaminated food/water **Diagnosis:** Review of symptoms and history, confirmed by blood tests **Tx:** Vaccination against Hep A & B, lifestyle modifications, medications to manage symptoms and prevent advancement of disease	**Red Flags:** **Refer to GP for further assessment**
Hepatic Carcinoma (Primary – Liver Cancer) *Cancer of the liver* **Ssx:** Ascites, upper abdominal pain, weakness and fatigue, yellowing of skin, nausea, white chalky stool, swellings *'A yellow person with lots of white chalk is reason to be scared!'* **TCM Illness: Abdominal Pain (ji ju), Jaundice (huang dan), Edema (shui zhong), Drum Distension (gu zhang)**	**Causes:** Prolonged alcohol/drug use, chronic hepatitis infections, hemochromatosis (unusually high levels of iron in liver) **Diagnosis:** Review of physical symptoms and history, abdominal CT/ultrasound, liver biopsy **Tx:** Surgery to remove tumor, radiation, symptom management	**Red Flags:** **Refer to GP for further assessment**
Hepatomegaly *Condition of enlarged liver* **Ssx:** Yellowing of skin, nausea vomiting, weakness, fatigue, poor appetite, muscle aches. Itching, palpable liver *'Hepato = LR* *megaly + enlargement of'* **TCM Illness:** Jaundice (huang dan)	**Causes:** Excessive alcohol and drug use, congestive HT failure, general hepatic conditions **Diagnosis:** Blood tests to determine liver function, abdominal CT/ultrasound **Tx:** Treatment of underlying cause, lifestyle modifications	**Red Flags:** **Refer to GP for further assessment**
Hiatal Hernia *Herniation of portion of the stomach into the esophagus through an opening in the diaphragm* **Ssx:** Often asymptomatic, heartburn	**Causes:** Weak diaphragm muscles, increase intra abdominal pressure (obesity, pregnancy), heavy lifting **Diagnosis:** Abdominal x-ray	**Red Flags:**

when lying down or after a meal, acid reflux, pain when bending over **TCM Illness: Abdominal mass (ji ju)**	**Tx:** Surgical correction	**Refer to GP for further assessment**
Intestinal Obstruction *Partial or full blockage of a section of the intestines* **Ssx:** Abdominal pain and discomfort, constipation, vomiting, inability to pass gas and stool, swelling of abdomen, firm to touch **TCM Illness: Abdominal mass (ji ju), Abdominal pain (fu tong), Constipation (bian bi)**	**Causes:** Intestinal adhesions, colon cancer, inflammatory bowel disease, chronic constipation **Diagnosis:** Review of symptoms, abdominal x ray **Tx:** Resting the bowel and allow for it to work itself out naturally, worst case scenario surgery to remove blockage and return normal bowel function	**Red Flags:** **Refer to GP ASAP for further assessment or to ER if pain is severe** **NEVER LET THE SUN SET ON AN ACUTE STOMACH**
Irritable Bowel Syndrome*** *Chronic condition affecting the large intestine - does not cause changes in bowel tissue* **Ssx:** Abdominal cramping, bloating, gas, constipation, and diarrhea, mucous in the stool **TCM Illness: Abdominal pain (fu tong)**	**Causes:** Idiopathic however is triggered by common factors - spicy food, illnesses, stress, hormones **Diagnosis:** Review of physical manifestations, colonoscopy, abdominal CT, lactose intolerance test to rule out allergy **Tx:** Strict diet modification - rule out fatty, high sugar foods, medications to manage (usually anti-depressants are given)	**Red Flags:** **Refer to GP for further assessment**
Liver Disease *Broad term for disturbance of the liver that causes illness* **Ssx:** Weakness and fatigue, nausea/vomiting, weight loss, yellowing of the skin **TCM Illness: Jaundice (huang dan)**	**Causes:** Epstein Barr virus, cirrhosis, alcohol abuse hepatitis virus, chronic stress **Diagnosis:** Physical examination, blood tests, abdominal CT **Tx:** Lifestyle changes, reduce alcohol intake, worst case scenario liver transplant	**Red Flags:** **Refer to GP for further assessment**
Malabsorption *Condition in which the intestine cannot absorb nutrients properly* **Ssx:** Weight loss (rapid), light colored stool (white/chalky), fatigue, diarrhea, anemia (low iron levels), hair loss, swollen abdomen	**Causes:** Prolonged antibiotics use, colitis, IBS, parasitic diseases, celiac disease, Crohn's disease **Diagnosis:** Blood tests **Tx:** Nutrient and fluid replacement, treatment of underlying cause (pre	**Red Flags:** **Refer to GP for further**

	existing conditions listed above)	assessment
TCM Illness: Diarrhea (xie xie), possible Abdominal Pain (fu tong)		
Pancreatitis (chronic and acute)* *Inflammation of the pancreas, acute refers to rapid onset of symptoms, chronic = develops over many years* **Ssx:** Upper abdominal pain that radiates to back, nausea, vomiting and/or loss of appetite, abdomen tender to the touch, fever, rapid heart rate, oily and smelly stools, unexplained bruising ACUTE: swollen/tender abd. (gradual or sudden), n/v, fever, rapid pulse, LOOKS very ill *'DON'T TOUCH MY ABDOMEN or I will panker oily stool all over you'* **TCM Illness: Abdominal Pain (fu tong), Epigastric Pain (wei tong)**	**Causes:** Alcoholism, gallstones, high calcium levels in blood (often due to over active parathyroid gland), family history, smoking, infection, injury to abdomen, cystic fibrosis **Diagnosis:** CT scan of abdomen and/or ultrasound, endoscopy, MRI **Tx:** Antibiotics, treatment of gallstones (removal), changes to diet	**Red Flags:** **Refer to GP for further assessment if chronic, and ER if acute and severe**
Pancreatic Cancer *Cancer of the pancreas - very poor prognosis as this cancer spreads extremely fast* **Ssx:** Upper abdominal pain, back pain, loss of appetite, weight loss, yellowing of skin and/or eyes *'Be quick if a yellow person is bent over in pain and is losing weight in front of your eyes'* **TCM Illness: Abdominal Pain (fu tong), Jaundice (huang dan)**	**Causes:** Uncontrolled cell growth (true for ALL cancers), link between poor diet, smoking and alcohol consumption, diabetes **Diagnosis:** Abdominal CT, MRI, or ultrasound, blood tests to detect cancer markers, biopsy of pancreatic tissue **Tx:** Surgical removal (if tumor small enough), radiation, chemotherapy	**Red Flags:** **Refer to GP ASAP for further assessment**
Peptic Ulcer (H.Pylori, Campylobacter) *Achy, gnawing, painful stomach after eating* **Ssx:** Acid/achy/gnawing sensation in upper abdomen after meals, pain may radiate to back, 'empty/all-gone' feeling, nocturnal pain, bloating, steady, well defined pain spot, may be vomiting after eating	Ulceration of mucous membranes and areas exposed to gastric acid and pepsin and having lower mucosal lining (can be duodenal or gastric ulcer) **Causes:** Helicobacter Pylori, NSAID abuse, alcohol, caffeine, tobacco, eating foods that inflame, stress **Diagnosis:** Endoscopy, stool or breath test for	**Red Flags:**

'Eating makes my stomach peppy. In a bad way.' **TCM Illness: Epigastric Pain (wei tong)**	H.Pylori **Tx:** Antibiotics, antacids to reduce acid in stomach, avoiding high acidity food	**Refer to GP for further assessment**
Peritonitis *Inflammation of the peritoneum (membrane that lines the abdominal cavity)* **Ssx:** Abdominal pain, fever, feeling full, loss of appetite, nausea, vomiting, thirst, low urine output, inability to pass stool or gas *'After getting stuck with a dirty sword, I got a fever and couldn't use the washroom! HELP!'* **TCM Illness: Abdominal Pain (fu tong), Vomiting (ou tu)**	**Causes:** Often bacterial cause, a rupture in the abdominal wall (from surgery, or other medical procedures), ruptured appendix, diverticulitis **Diagnosis:** Abdominal CT and/or x-ray, peritoneal fluid analysis (take sample from abdomen) **Tx:** Antibiotics, surgery to remove infected material if necessary	**Red Flags:** **Refer to GP ASAP for further assessment or ER if severe**
Portal Hypertension *Increased blood pressure within the portal venous system (vessels of stomach, intestines, spleen etc.) causing enlargement of the spleen. The portal vein brings blood from the LI to the LR (as well as from the SP/pancreas & GB)* **Ssx:** Increased overall blood pressure, ascites, abdominal pain, low levels of white blood cells, altered level of consciousness, hemefecia or hematemesis *'My portal is tense. I am going to release blood to try to decrease it'* **TCM Illness: Abdominal Pain (fu tong), Edema (shui zhong)**	**Causes:** Chronic heart failure, cirrhosis, chronic Hep C, alcoholism **Diagnosis:** Blood studies, physical examination for esophageal varices **Tx:** No cure, treatment is focused on controlling side effects and symptom management	**Red Flags:** **Refer to GP ASAP for further assessment**
Portal-Systemic Encephalopathy *A neuropsychiatric manifestation of liver damage often found in chronic liver disease, accumulation of ammonia in systemic circulation* **Ssx:** Sleep disturbances, anxiety, irritability, impaired memory, bizarre behaviour *'My LR is mad at my portal causing madness!'*	**Causes:** Chronic liver disease **Diagnosis:** Blood test for liver function and ammonia levels **Tx:** Correction of ammonia levels, antibiotics, improved diet	**Red Flags:** **Call 911 immediately**

TCM Illness: Insomnia (bu mei)		
Proctitis *Inflammation of the lining of the rectum* **Ssx:** Rectal pain, persistent feeling of the need to pass stool, rectal bleeding, passing of mucus stool, lower left abdominal pain *'Sitting in blood is painful and makes me feel like I have to poop!'* TCM Illness: Abdominal Pain (fu tong), Closest is Bleeding Disorders (xue zheng)	**Causes:** Inflammatory bowel disease, infections (particularly STIs), intense antibiotic therapy **Diagnosis:** Lower abdomen CT, colonoscopy, STI tests, stool test to rule out infection **Tx:** Anti-inflammatory medication, antibiotics if needed, stool softeners	**Red Flags:** **Refer to GP for further assessment**
Stomach Cancer *Cancer in the lining of the stomach* **Ssx:** Severe heartburn, upper abdominal pain, prolonged vomiting, feeling bloated after eating, unexplained weight loss TCM Illness: Abdominal Pain (fu tong), Vomiting (ou tu)	**Causes:** Unknown, link between intake of high salt foods, root cause is uncontrolled cell growth (cancer) **Diagnosis:** Review of symptoms, blood tests for cancer markers in the blood, abdominal CT **Tx:** Surgical removal of cancerous material, radiation	**Red Flags:** **Refer to GP ASAP for further assessment**
Ulcerative Colitis*** *Chronic inflammatory bowel disease characterized by ulcers in the rectum and colon* **Ssx:** Bloody diarrhea (sometimes with mucous) and severe abdominal pain, weight loss, loss of appetite, fever, mal absorption TCM Illness: Diarrhea (xie xie), Abdominal Pain, (fu tong), Closest is Bleeding Disorders (xue zheng)	**Causes:** Overactive inflammatory response **Diagnosis:** Blood tests, serum studies (loss of electrolytes), colonoscopy **Tx:** Rest the bowel, control inflammation, manage fluids and nutrition	**Red Flags:** **Toxic megacolon** - bowel expands stopping colon from removing wastes, can cause rupture = life threatening Ssx - rapid heart rate extremely painful and bloody stool, shock **Call 911 if severe. Refer to GP is mild.**

Genito-Urinary Conditions

i. **General Pathophysiology:**
   - Urinary tract infection - can refer to any infection of kidneys, bladder, ureters, or urethra
   - Dysuria - difficulty or pain while urinating
   - Dyspareunia - painful intercourse
   - STIs - sexually transmitted infections

ii. **Common Western Tests:**
   - Cystoscopy - thin tube with camera inserted into urethra, biopsy can be taken or simply visualization of various parts of the urinary tract
   - Blood tests - used to detect markers in the blood (i.e. cancer), test levels of protein, creatine and other solvents
   - Urine culture - sample is obtained and bacterial cultures grown in the lab to determine what type of bacteria is present
   - Urine sample - rapid test used to detect protein, white blood cells, nitrites etc.

iii. **General Red Flags:**
   - Painful urination
   - Blood in urine (hematuria)
   - Lower back pain and/or pelvic pain
   - Urinary frequency/urgency
   - Blood in semen
   - Cloudy/greasy or foul smelling urine or foamy urine

Common Diseases + Specific Red Flags

Condition **Symptoms and signs** Related TCM Illness	**Causes & Diagnostic tests**	Red flags (and what to do about them)
Andropause *Condition of decreased male hormone testosterone, sometimes referred to as 'male menopause'* **Ssx:** Low sex drive, fatigue, depression, irritability, mood swings, loss of muscle mass *'He's become like a depressed android without his testosterone!'* TCM Illness: Depression (yu zheng)	**Causes:** Drop in testosterone hormone levels in the blood **Diagnosis:** Review of physical symptoms, confirmed by a blood test **Tx:** Testosterone replacement therapy	**Red Flags:** **Refer to GP for further assessment**
Bacterial Pyelonephritis (Acute) *Urinary tract infections that extends to the kidneys - bacterial kidney infections* **Ssx:** Nausea, vomiting, fever, chills, frequent painful urination with difficult output, lower back, side and groin pain *'It is shaped like a pylon from the bladder to the kidneys'* TCM Illness: Stranguria (lin zheng)	**Causes:** Bacterial infection, blocked urine flow from kidneys to bladder **Diagnosis:** Urinary analysis, ultrasound **Tx:** Antibiotics to cure infection	**Red Flags:** **Refer to GP ASAP or ER if severe**
BPH (Benign Prostatic Hypertrophy) * *Enlargement of the prostate gland - non cancerous* **Ssx:** Difficulty urinating, urinary frequency, increased urination at night, inability to completely empty bladder, urinary tract infections *'Big Prostate Hinders my urination'* TCM Illness: Ischuria (long bi) + Stranguria (lin zheng)	**Causes:** Generally unknown, normal for prostate to grow throughout life, could be due to hormone imbalances **Diagnosis:** Prostate check (digital rectal exam), blood test, review of symptoms **Tx:** Medications to reduce prostate size, non-invasive procedures preferred before surgery	**Red Flags:** **Refer to GP for further assessment**
Cystitis* *Inflammation of the bladder most often caused by UTI (urinary tract*	**Causes:** Bacterial infection of the urinary tract	**Red Flags:**

infection) **Ssx:** Increased urinary urgency and frequency, discomfort urinating, blood in urine, lower abdominal pain, cloudy, foul smelling urine *'I INCYST that that my bladder is just inflamed'* **TCM Illness: Stranguria (lin zheng), Abdominal Pain (fu tong)**	**Diagnosis:** Urine sample and analysis, cystoscopy (scope into the urethra) **Tx:** Antibiotics to clear bacterial infection	**Refer to GP for further assessment**
Enuresis *Involuntary urination 'bed wetting' most common in children* **Ssx:** Inability to control urination (incontinence) at night **TCM Illness: Enuresis (yi niao)**	**Causes:** UTIs (in adults), bladder infections, severe stress, developmental delays, can be neurological defect **Diagnosis:** Review of physical symptoms, urinary sample and analysis, MRI to rule out neurological deficit **Tx:** Behavioural modification and regular toileting schedule (children), treatment of other causes (UTIs)	**Red Flags:** **Refer to GP for further assessment**
Epididymitis *Inflammation of the epididymis - the small tubes that carry and store sperm from the testicles* **Ssx:** Testicular pain and discomfort, swollen scrotum, lump in the testicles, painful urination or ejaculation, urinary frequency, enlarged lymph nodes in the groin, blood in semen *'It put di-di-di-di pain in my testicles!'* **TCM Illness: Stranguria (lin zheng)**	**Causes:** Bacterial infections, STI's, blockage of urinary tract causing urine to back up into the testicles/epididymis **Diagnosis:** STI testing, urine sample and analysis for infections **Tx:** Antibiotics for bacterial infections, antivirals for STIs if needed	**Red Flags:** **Refer to GP ASAP** **Severe and sudden onset is medical emergency - may be testicular torsion** **Refer to ER**
Erectile Dysfunction (ED)* *Impotence - Inability for men to get and/or maintain erections* **Ssx:** Inability to produce erection during sexual intercourse, reduced sex drive **TCM Illness: None that match**	**Causes:** Age, medications, other medical conditions such as diabetes, heart disease, obesity, stress **Diagnosis:** Review of physical symptoms and various tests (urine test, ultrasound, blood tests) to rule out underlying conditions **Tx:** Medications, lifestyle modifications (healthy diet, exercise, adequate sleep)	**Red Flags:** **Refer to GP for further assessment**
Glomerulonephritis (chronic) *Inflammation of the small filter apparatuses (glomeruli) within the*	**Causes:** Bacterial infections, diabetes (causes damage to the kidneys resulting in scar tissue	**Red Flags:**

kidneys. The glomeruli filter out organic products from the blood to pass to the urine OR retain in the blood. Chronic conditions can eventually lead to renal failure **Ssx:** Blood within the urine, foamy urine (caused by excess protein in urine) lower back pain radiating to the sides, fluid retention - swelling in the face hands, arms or legs *'It looks like something is glommed on to my KI filters causing blood and foam. Yowch!'* **TCM Illness: Stranguria (lin zheng)**	formation = reduced filtering capacity) **Diagnosis:** Review of symptoms, blood and urine tests, lower abdominal ultrasound or CT **Tx:** Goal is to reduce amount of damage to kidneys by controlling condition - improving diabetic control, treating infections, better medication management	**Refer to GP for further assessment**
Incontinence* *Impaired urinary control leading to involuntary urination* **Ssx:** Urinary frequency and urgency, inability to control bladder - leaking when you sneeze, cough, or laugh, stress incontinence **TCM Illness: None that match**	**Causes:** UTIs, constipation - pressure on the rectum squeezes the bladder and urethra, physical changes with pregnancy, childbirth and aging, enlarged prostate **Diagnosis:** Review of symptoms, urine sample and analysis **Tx:** Treatment of underlying cause - antibiotics, laxative, prostate treatment	**Red Flags:** **Incontinence should always be referred to GP**
Kidney Cancer *Cancer originating in the tissue and various cells of the kidneys - most common type is renal cell carcinoma* **Ssx:** Blood in urine, lower back pain either one sided or bilaterally - just below the ribs, fatigue, unexplained weight loss **TCM Illness: Only possible match: Ischuria (long bi) and Abdominal Pain (fu tong)**	**Causes:** Unknown cause, basis is uncontrolled cell multiplication and growth (as is the case with all cancer), link between poor diet, chronic alcohol use, and genetic influences (family members with previous cancers) **Diagnosis:** CT scan of the lower abdomen to detect tumour/abnormal growth **Tx:** Radiation, chemotherapy, surgical removal of cancerous material, comfort care	**Red Flags:** **Refer to GP very soon for further assessment**
Kidney Stones* *Renal lithiasis and/or nephrolithiasis. build-up of hard mineral deposits within the tubes and filtration apparatuses of the kidneys* **Ssx:** Severe pain in back and abdomen just below the ribs, lower abdomen and groin pain, blood in urine, painful urination, cloudy and/or foul smelling urine, nausea	**Causes:** Chronic dehydration (causing concentrated urine), high intake of certain mineral containing foods (high protein, high dose of various vitamins, high calcium) **Diagnosis:** Renal ultrasound, urine testing, examination of passed stones (if occurs) **Tx:** Increase fluid intake to pass	**Red Flags:**

TCM Illness: Ischuria (long bi), Abdominal Pain (fu tong)	stones naturally, if necessary (stones become stuck) surgical removal of stones	**Refer to ER**
Nephritic Syndrome (Acute) *Condition in which the glomeruli in the kidneys are inflamed causing impaired filtration process and water retention* **Ssx:** Blood in the urine, swelling in the feet, ankles and eye sockets, decreased urine output, high blood pressure, shortness of breath/respiratory symptoms (due to build up of fluid in body system and lungs) NEPHRITIC = loss of blood + inflammation of glomeruli **TCM Illness: Stranguria (lin zheng)**	**Causes:** Autoimmune response against the body in reaction to bacterial infection **Diagnosis:** Urine sample and analysis for confirmation, blood test for protein and creatine (materials the kidneys usually excrete) **Tx:** Diuretic medications (cause the body to excrete more water), blood pressure medications, anticoagulant therapy	**Red Flags:** **Refer to GP for further assessment**
Nephrotic Syndrome *Condition in which the kidneys excrete too much protein into the urine causing a fluid imbalance within the body* **Ssx:** Severe swelling in the feet and ankles, occasionally surrounding the eyes, foamy urine (caused by high protein content), weight gain secondary to water retention NEPHROTIC = loss of protein *'He neurotically eats meat because he keeps losing protein'* **TCM Illness: Edema (shui zhong)**	**Causes:** Kidney damage caused by medications, pre existing conditions (diabetes, heart failure), blood clots within the kidneys **Diagnosis:** Urine sample and analysis for confirmation, blood test for protein (will be low levels in the blood), kidney biopsy **Tx:** Diuretic medications (cause the body to excrete more water)	**Red Flags:** **Refer to GP for further assessment**
Prostate Cancer* *Cancer of the tissues and cells of the prostate causing enlarged prostate, urinary symptoms and in the worst case scenario, spread of cancer to other parts of the body (METS)* **Ssx:** Difficult or painful urination, inability to fully empty bladder, erectile dysfunction, blood in the semen, discomfort to the abdominal area, unexplained fatigue/weight loss **TCM Illness: Ischuria (long bi)**	**Causes:** Unknown cause, basis is uncontrolled cell multiplication and growth (as is the case with all cancer, genetic mutation), link between poor diet, chronic alcohol use, and genetic influences (family members with previous cancers) **Diagnosis:** Digital rectal exam to detect enlarged prostate, abdominal CT scan to detect tumour growth, blood tests for cancer markers in the blood **Tx:** Radiation, chemotherapy, surgical removal of cancerous tissues, comfort care	**Red Flags:** **Refer to GP very soon for further assessment**

Prostatitis (Chronic Nonbacterial)* *Generalized condition of swelling and enlargement of the prostate* **Ssx:** Difficulty or painful urination, inability to fully empty bladder, erectile dysfunction, blood in the semen, painful ejaculation, pain to the groin and abdomen, cloudy or bloody urine, frequent nocturnal urination *'An inflamed prostate makes peeing and ejaculation painful*! **TCM Illness: Ischuria (long bi)**	**Causes:** Cause is often unknown, can be nerve damage (trauma to area), age related, history of STIs and frequent UTIs, or simply for no reason at all **Diagnosis:** Digital rectal exam to detect enlarged prostate, abdominal CT scan to detect abnormal growth **Tx:** Anti-inflammatory drugs, medications to relax bladder, natural remedies such as acupuncture	**Red Flags:** **Refer to GP for further assessment**
Renal Failure (chronic) *Gradual decrease and eventually complete loss of kidney function requiring renal dialysis* **Ssx:** General feeling unwell, loss of appetite, nausea and vomiting, muscle cramps and twitching, generalized swelling in feet and ankles, sleep disturbances, chronic itching (body is unable to clear toxins) *'I need to cleanse my kidneys so badly before they fail me!'* **TCM Illness: Ischuria (long bi), Edema (shui zhong)**	**Causes:** Chronic conditions such as diabetes (with poor control, leading to kidney damage), high blood pressure (damages vessels in kidneys), glomerulonephritis, frequent kidney infections **Diagnosis:** Blood tests (checking waste levels in the blood), urine collection and analysis, CT or MRI of kidneys, kidney biopsy **Tx:** Aimed at controlling the underlying cause - proper diabetic control, medication management, reducing blood pressure, dialysis, renal transplant	**Red Flags:** **Refer to GP for further assessment**
Testicular Cancer *Cancer of the cells and tissues within the testicles, usually affects only one testicle* **Ssx:** Palpable lump within the scrotum, dull pain in the groin and lower abdomen, feeling of heaviness in the scrotal area **TCM Illness: Abdominal Pain (fu tong)**	**Causes:** Idiopathic, basis is uncontrolled cell multiplication and growth (as is the case with all cancer, genetic mutation), link between poor diet, obesity, chronic alcohol use, and genetic influences (family members with previous cancers), usually in younger men **Diagnosis:** Ultrasound of testicles, blood test to determine if cancer markers are in the blood **Tx:** Radiation, chemotherapy, surgical removal of cancerous tissues. Testicular cancer is extremely treatable form of cancer - usually good outcome for those affected	**Red Flags:** **Refer to GP for further assessment**
Urethritis *Inflammation of the urethra* **Ssx:** Painful urination, increased	**Causes:** Bacterial infections most common cause, STIs (commonly gonorrhoea and chlamydia)	**Red Flags:**

urge to urinate, difficulty initiating urination, pain or discomfort during sex, blood in semen or urine, discharge from urethra (both sexes) 'Very similar to UTI but more just pain of the 'pee-hole' **TCM Illness: Stranguria (lin zheng)**	**Diagnosis:** Urinary sample and analysis to determine source of infection **Tx:** Antibacterial or antivirals (depending on causative factor) to treat infection	**Refer to GP for further assessment.**
Urinary Bladder Cancer *Cancer of the cells and tissues in the urinary bladder - often starting in the cells lining the inside of the bladder* **Ssx:** Blood in the urine, abdominal discomfort and pain during urination, back pain, pelvic pain, unexplained fatigue or weight loss **TCM Illness: Stranguria (lin zheng)**	**Causes:** Unknown cause, basis is uncontrolled cell multiplication and growth (as is the case with all cancer, genetic mutation), link between poor diet, obesity, chronic alcohol use, and genetic influences (family members with previous cancers) **Diagnosis:** Blood test to determine if cancer markers are in the blood, cystoscopy, bladder biopsy, CT or MRI of bladder **Tx:** Radiation, chemotherapy, surgical removal of cancerous tissues/tumour, entire removal of bladder (cystectomy)	**Red Flags:** **Refer to GP ASAP if suspected.**
Urinary Calculi *Hard deposits of crystallized material in the urinary tract 'bladder stones'* **Ssx:** Painful and burning sensation when urinating, abdominal pain, testicular pain, cloudy or dark urine, frequent urination *'A giant stone in your bladder definitely causes a lot of pain and urine issues!* **TCM Illness: Abdominal Pain (fu tong), Ischuria (lin zheng)**	**Causes:** Inability to fully empty bladder, some infections, kidney stones, damaged nerve function causing impaired bladder function/emptying (neurogenic bladder) **Diagnosis:** Review of physical symptoms, urine sample and tests, X-ray to detect stones **Tx:** Allowing natural passing of stones through the urine, use of ultrasound/laser technology in combination with cystoscope to break up large stones and allow them to pass in the urine	**Red Flags:** **Refer to GP for further assessment.**
Urinary Tract Infection (UTI)* *General term for infection to any part of the urinary tract (kidneys, ureter, bladder, urethra).* *Women have greater chance of suffering from UTI due to the shorter urethra* **Ssx:** Pain and/or burning while	**Causes:** Most often bacterial or viral infections, STIs **Diagnosis:** Urine sample and analysis, STI screening, cystoscope to examine bladder **Tx:** Antibiotics to clear infections	**Red Flags:**

urinating, urinary frequency and urgency - passing frequent small amounts of urine, foul smelling urine, and discomfort around the pelvic bone, back pain **TCM Illness: Stranguria (lin zheng), Abdominal pain (fu tong)**		**Refer to GP for further assessment.**

Gynecological Conditions

i. **General Pathophysiology:**
   - Fibroadenoma - solid non cancerous lump found in breast tissue, common with women under 30
   - HPV - human papillomavirus, sexually transmitted infection linked to cervical cancer
   - Chlamydia - common STI, causes bacterial infection
   - Gonorrhoea - common STI, "the clap", bacterial infection

ii. **Common Western Tests:**
   - PAP test (Papanicolaou test) - procedure that removes small amount of cervical cells by swabbing the area and testing for abnormalities
   - STI Screening - often taken by pap test, or swab of vaginal area
   - Ultrasound - used to identify growths/abnormalities to the uterus
   - Blood tests - to detect hormonal abnormalities or cancer markers

iii. **General Red Flags:**
   - Painful intercourse
   - Pelvic pain
   - Unusual, foul smelling discharge
   - Changes to size/shape of breast and/or nipples
   - Abnormalities to the skin of breast

Common Diseases + Specific Red Flags

Condition Symptoms and signs Related TCM Illness	Causes & Diagnostic tests	Red flags (and what to do about them)
Amenorrhea*** *Abnormal or unknown stop in menses - one or more missed menstrual period. Can be indicative of underlying condition such as polycystic ovaries. Occurs non pathologically in pregnancy and menopause* **Ssx:** Skipping of one or more monthly period for at least 3 months, acne, excessive hair growth, possible pelvic pain *'AMEN I don't have to deal with a period! Just this beard and zits. Hmmmmm....'* **TCM Illness: Amenorrhea (bi jing)**	**Causes:** Contraceptives (birth control), some blood pressure or depression medications, excessive weight loss or gain, hormone imbalances caused by polycystic ovaries, thyroid disorders, or premature menopause **Diagnosis:** Pregnancy test, thyroid function test, male hormone level tests, ultrasound or CT to rule out polycystic **Tx:** Treatment of the underlying cause - hormone replacement, thyroid medication	**Red Flags:** **Refer to GP for further assessment**
Breast Cancer* *Cancer of the cells and tissues within the breast. Most common cancer in women* **Ssx:** Lump in and around the breast area, unusual discharge from nipple, change in size or shape of breast, changes in the skin around the breast (thickening or change or color) **TCM Illness: Breast Stone – ru yan**	**Causes:** Idiopathic, basis is uncontrolled cell multiplication and growth (as is the case with all cancer), strong link between poor diet, chronic alcohol use, and genetic influences (family members with previous cancers), obesity, early menstrual period start **Diagnosis:** Mammogram, CT of breast, blood test to measure cancer markers, review of symptoms **Tx:** Radiation, chemotherapy, removal of tumour, single or double mastectomy, remove lymph nodes	**Red Flags:** **Refer to GP for further assessment**
Breast Mass* *Benign mass found in the breast tissue* **Ssx:** Palpable lump in the breast, changes in shapes and/or size, changes in skin (dry, scaly), persistent pain to the area **TCM Illness: Breast Stone – ru yan + Breast Nodule – ru pi**	**Causes:** Unusual growth of cells (non cancerous), breast or milk duct cysts, fibroadenoma, injury or trauma to the breast **Diagnosis:** Physical examination, breast CT or MRI, biopsy of tissue if necessary **Tx:** Surgical removal of lump (if needed), often will go untreated if not affecting the person	**Red Flags:** **Refer to GP for further assessment**

Cervical Carcinoma *Cancer of the cells in the cervix* **Ssx:** Vaginal bleeding after intercourse, painful intercourse, heavy vaginal discharge with a foul smell *'An very unhappy cervix doesn't allow you to have sex and gushes white discharge to keep men out!'* **TCM Illness: Leukorrhagia (dai xia)**	**Causes:** Exposure to HPV, basis is uncontrolled cell multiplication and growth (as is the case with all cancer), strong link between smoking, genetic influences (family members with previous cancers), obesity, early menstrual period start, multiple sexual partners **Diagnosis:** STI testing, pap test, biopsy of cervical tissue, imaging tests such as MRI or CT **Tx:** Radiation, chemotherapy, removal of cancerous mass, partial or complete hysterectomy	**Red Flags:** **Refer to GP for further assessment**
Dysmenorrhea*** *Painful menstrual periods* **Ssx:** Throbbing or cramping during periods, headache, dizziness or nausea during periods **TCM Illness: Dysmenorrhea (tong jing)**	**Causes:** Endometriosis, inflammatory pelvic disease, cervical stenosis (narrowing of cervical opening) **Diagnosis:** Review of physical symptoms and pelvic examination, Pap test to rule out abnormalities **Tx:** Contraceptives can control symptoms and help regulate menstrual periods, pain killers and anti inflammatory meds	**Red Flags:** **Refer to GP for further assessment**
Ectopic Pregnancy *Pregnancy in which the egg implants outside of the uterus, typically in the fallopian tube - fertilized egg cannot survive and the pregnancy must be terminated.* *Early treatment is imperative to reduce risks or additional pregnancies - if not treated tubes can burst causing severe internal bleeding* **Ssx:** Severe abdominal and pelvic pain, extreme light-headedness or fainting, SHOULDER PAIN (big one) *'EMERGENCY! The fetus got so lost that it ended up in my shoulder!'* **TCM Illness: Abdominal Mass (zheng jia)**	**Causes:** Damaged fallopian tubes (inflammation, scar tissue) hormonal imbalance **Diagnosis:** Abdominal and pelvic exam, ultrasound to confirm **Tx:** In emergency situation surgery is needed to remove fertilized egg and control bleeding	**Red Flags:** **Refer to ER immediately, this is a medical emergency**
Endometriosis*** *Condition in which the tissue normally found in the lining of the uterus grows outside of the uterus.* *Tissue behaves normally (enlarges during menstrual cycle) however*	**Causes:** Exact cause unknown, could be due to scar tissue in the uterus (following surgery like C section), hormonal influences **Diagnosis:** Pelvic examination and	**Red Flags:**

becomes trapped in the tissues with no exit **Ssx:** Sharp and severe abdominal pain, dysmenorrhea, painful intercourse, painful urination or bowel movements **TCM Illness: Dysmenorrhea (tong jing)**	review of physical symptoms, ultrasound to confirm **Tx:** Pain medications to manage, hormone therapy to correct imbalances, in extreme cases hysterectomy	**Refer to GP for further assessment**
Endometrial Carcinoma *Cancer of the endometrial tissues (uterine cancer)* **Ssx:** Unusual vaginal bleeding after menopause, bleeding between periods, pelvic pain, unusual vaginal discharge *'Bleeding after menopause… this is the END'* **TCM Illness: Metrorrhagia and Metrostaxis (beng luo)**	**Causes:** Basis is uncontrolled cell multiplication and growth (as is the case with all cancer), strong link between smoking, genetic influences (family members with previous cancers), obesity, early menstrual period start, multiple sexual partners **Diagnosis:** STI testing, pap test, biopsy of uterine tissue, imaging tests such as MRI or CT **Tx:** Radiation, chemotherapy, removal of cancerous mass, partial or complete hysterectomy	**Red Flags:** **Refer to GP for further assessment**
FBD (Fibrocystic Breast Disease)* *Condition of having multiple cysts within the breast tissue causing lumps throughout. Often not harmful* **Ssx:** Painful or misshapen breast, multiple lumps throughout tissues, monthly swelling during ovulation, lumps that fluctuate **TCM Illness: None that match**	**Causes:** Idiopathic, hormonal influences thought to be the main cause - specifically estrogen **Diagnosis:** Physical examination, ultrasound of breast tissues, mammogram, if needed biopsy of tissue **Tx:** Aspiration of cyst fluid to reduce size of cysts, surgical removal (not common), if non painful often will go untreated	**Red Flags:** **Refer to GP for further assessment**
Infertility – Female & Male* *Difficulty or inability to fertilize/get pregnant* **Ssx:** Unsuccessful attempts to get pregnant, women - missed menstrual periods, obvious signs of hormonal imbalance (hair growth, decreased sex drive) Men - difficulty ejaculating, mechanical problems <u>Primary:</u> Inability for couple to get preg. after one year of unprotected sex <u>Secondary:</u> Inability to become pregnant or carry to term following the birth of one or more children	**Causes:** Abnormally low egg or sperm count, mechanical issues (testicular or penile malformations inhibiting sperm delivery), scar tissue on the uterus/fallopian tubes, overexposure to harmful environmental influences (radiation, chemical) **Diagnosis:** Blood tests, hormone tests, semen analysis, ovulation testing **Tx:** Depends on the underlying cause, could be hormone therapy, lifestyle modifications, self monitoring of ovulation cycle	**Red Flags:** **Refer to GP for further assessment**

TCM Illness: Infertility (bu yun)		
Leiomyoma (Uterine Fibroids) *Non cancerous growths in and around the uterus, can be singular or multiple, range in sizes* **Ssx:** Heavy menstrual bleeding, prolonged periods (longer than 7 days), pelvic discomfort or pain, urinary frequency, back ache or leg pain, constipation *'Hey. Lay off the myomas Body. Yeesh. I have enough!'* **TCM Illness: Abdominal Masses (zheng jia)**	**Causes:** Hormone imbalances, genetic influences (family history) **Diagnosis:** Pelvic exam, Pap test to rule out other conditions, ultrasound of pelvis, biopsy if needed **Tx:** Often not treated, hormone therapy if needed, non invasive procedures such as MRI guided ultrasound to try and reduce size of cysts, hysterectomy	**Red Flags:** **Refer to GP for further assessment**
Mastitis* *Infection of the breast tissue, most common in breast feeding mothers* **Ssx:** Breast pain, swelling and tenderness, fever and chills, redness of breast skin, general feeling unwell **TCM Illness: Acute Mastitis (ru yong)**	**Causes:** Blocked milk duct, bacterial infection that enters breast tissue or milk ducts (through cracks in skin), stagnant breast milk (pregnancy) **Diagnosis:** Physical examination, CT or ultrasound if necessary to rule out other conditions **Tx:** Antibiotics, pain medications, adjustment or breastfeeding technique/education	**Red Flags:** **Refer to GP for further assessment**
Menopause*** *End of a woman's menstrual cycle occurring in 40s/50s, meaning she can no longer reproduce. Characterized by 12 months of no monthly menstrual period* **Ssx:** Hot flashes, prolonged periods and/or missing monthly periods, mood swings, decreased sex drive, vaginal dryness, night sweats, sleep disturbances **TCM Illness: None**	**Causes:** Natural biological process that occurs with the natural decline of estrogen and progesterone **Diagnosis:** Review of physical symptoms and examinations, CBC **Tx:** Lifestyle control of symptoms, antidepressants if needed, HRT	**Red Flags:** **Refer to GP for further assessment**
Menorrhagia*** *Abnormally heavy menstrual periods* **Ssx:** Excessive bleeding during monthly menstrual periods, periods lasting longer than a week, passing large clots during periods *'I bled so heavy that it is the weight of 10 men'* **TCM Illness: None that match!**	**Causes:** Hormone imbalances, cysts on the uterus, non hormonal IUD (intrauterine devices) can occasionally cause heavy bleeding, blood clotting disorders **Diagnosis:** Review of physical symptoms, blood tests to rule out clotting disorders **Tx:** Iron supplements, anti-inflammatories, hormonal IUD (reduces monthly bleeding, ultrasound ablation (reduces size of cysts if present)	**Red Flags:** **Refer to GP for further assessment**

Condition	Causes / Diagnosis / Tx	Red Flags
Osteoporosis*** *Condition in which the bones are extremely brittle, break easily* **Ssx:** Easy fracture, back pain, stooped posture, dowager's hump **TCM Illness: None that match**	**Causes:** Dietary restrictions (calcium), low bone mass/density, sedentary lifestyle, excessive alcohol consumption **Diagnosis:** Bone density test, x-ray **Tx:** Increased calcium intake or supplements, reducing risks of falls, osteoporosis specific medication such as Actonel, Atelvia, weight bearing exercise	**Red Flags:** **Refer to GP for further assessment**
Ovarian Cancer *Cancer originating in the ovaries, very hard to catch early on, often isn't diagnosed until it has spread to other part of the pelvis* **Ssx:** Abdominal bloating and swelling, unexplained weight loss, changes in urination (frequency) or bowel patterns (constipation), weight loss, feeling full quickly when eating *'The ovaries are tricky and sometimes just cause bloating'* **TCM Illness: Abdominal pain (fu tong) is possible**	**Causes:** Basis is uncontrolled cell multiplication and growth (as is the case with all cancer), strong link between smoking, genetic influences (family members with previous cancers), obesity, early menstrual period start, multiple sexual partners **Diagnosis:** STI testing, pap test, biopsy of ovarian tissue, imaging tests such as MRI or CT **Tx:** Radiation, chemotherapy, removal of cancerous mass, partial or complete hysterectomy	**Red Flags:** **Refer to GP for further assessment**
Ovarian Cysts (+ PCOS – Polycystic Ovarian Syndrome***)** *Condition of multiple cysts growing on the ovaries* **Ssx:** Pelvic pain, missed periods or prolonged monthly periods, unusual hair growth, acne, excessive weight gain **TCM Illness: Abdominal Masses (zheng jia)**	**Causes:** Cause is unknown, strong hereditary influence, excessive insulin use (poorly controlled diabetes), hormonal imbalances, obesity **Diagnosis:** Review of physical symptoms, ultrasound of pelvis to confirm **Tx:** Lifestyle changes, reduce weight, birth control pills to regulate hormones	**Red Flags:** **Refer to GP for further assessment**
Pelvic Pain *Pain and discomfort to the pelvic area, can be caused by a variety of things* **Ssx:** Pain to pelvic region, radiating to back or lower abdomen or buttocks **TCM Illness: None that match**	**Causes:** Trauma, cancers, hormonal imbalances, cysts **Diagnosis:** Pelvic exam, review of physical symptoms, imaging (CT or MRI) to rule out existing conditions **Tx:** Treatment of the underlying cause - depends on the diagnosis	**Red Flags:** **Refer to GP if pelvic pain present for unexplained reason**
PMS (Pre-Menstrual Syndrome)*** *A variety of physical and emotional symptoms women experience prior to menstruation*	**Causes:** Natural causes of the changes in hormone levels **Diagnosis:** Review of physical symptoms, pap test to rule out	**Red Flags:**

Ssx: Anxiety, depression, mood swings, abdominal bloating and tenderness, joint and muscle pain, headache, breast tenderness, constipation **TCM Illness:** Severe is Menstrual Mental Disorder (jing xing qing zhi yi chang)	uterine/cervical abnormalities **Tx:** Pain medications to reduce symptoms, hormonal contraceptives to reduce effects of hormone changes	**Refer if emotions are out of control.**
Pregnancy Complications* *Broad category of complications experiences during pregnancy* **Ssx:** Normal symptoms: nausea, loss of appetite, constipation, heartburn, breast tenderness, backache Emergent symptoms: vaginal bleeding, severe abdominal pain, high temperature, sudden cease of fetal movement, foul smelling discharge, shoulder pain **TCM Illness:** Too broad to match – possible Miscarriage (zhui tai xiao chan hua tai) OR Abdominal Pain (fu tong)	**Causes:** Dependent on the case, can be trauma, ectopic pregnancy, viral/bacterial infections, miscarriage, preterm labour **Diagnosis:** Review of symptoms, blood and urine tests, ultrasound **Tx:** Again, dependent on the cause, bed rest if severe complications, worst case scenario pre-term delivery	**Red Flags:** **Refer to ER immediately**
Ovarian Torsion *Condition in which the ovary twists* **Ssx:** Sudden onset (commonly during exercise or other agitating movement) of severe, lower abdominal pain that worsens intermittently over many hours radiating to the back, pelvis, or thigh - usually one sided, nausea and vomiting **TCM Illness:** Abdominal pain (fu tong)	**Causes:** Reduced venous return from the ovary as a result of stromal edema, internal hemorrhage, hyperstimulation, or a mass **Diagnosis:** Ultrasound to confirm **Tx:** Surgical intervention to restore ovary to normal position	**Red Flags:** **Refer to ER or GP or further assessment**
Salpingitis (Acute – PID, Pelvic Inflammatory Disease) *Infection and inflammation of the female reproductive system (fallopian tubes, uterus or ovaries)* **Ssx:** Lower abdomen or pelvic pain, heavy and foul smelling discharge, fever, pain during intercourse, difficulty urinating *'It feels like Sal is stabbing my entire lower abdomen with a pin over and over'*	**Causes:** Often STIs - chlamydia or gonorrhea **Diagnosis:** Ultrasound of pelvis, STI screening, endometrial biopsy **Tx:** Antibiotics for you and your sexual partner	**Red Flags:** **Refer to GP or ER for further assessment**

TCM Illness: Abdominal Pain (fu tong), Leukorrhagia (dai xia)		
Vaginal Bleeding *Abnormal bleeding between menstrual periods* **Ssx:** Bloody discharge, bleeding in between periods TCM Illness: Metrorrhagia and Metrostaxis (beng luo)	**Causes:** Often sign of cancer or other vaginal diseases **Diagnosis:** Review of physical symptoms, STIs testing, CT or ultrasound **Tx:** Treating the underlying cause of the bleeding (depending on diagnosis)	**Red Flags:** **Refer to GP or ER for further assessment if unable to control.**
Vulvo-Vaginitis *Inflammation of the vagina* **Ssx:** Swelling of vagina, itchy and reddened area, pain during intercourse or urination, foul smelling discharge TCM Illness: Leukorrhagia (dai xia)	**Causes:** Bacterial infections, STIs, yeast infections, multiple sexual partners, unprotected sexual intercourse **Diagnosis:** PAP test to rule out cervical abnormalities, STI screening, urine sample and analysis **Tx:** Antibiotics, antifungals, dependent on the cause	**Red Flags:** **Refer to GP for further assessment**

Hematological Conditions

iii. **General Pathophysiology:**

- -EMIA: denoting a substance is present in the blood; especially in excess
- LEUKOPENIA: increase in tendency to infections due to low WBC in blood
- LYMPHOMA: cancer that begins in the lymphocytes
- LYSIS: cell disintegration due to the rupture of the cell wall or membrane
- PENIA: not enough of
- PURPURA: bruising or bruise-like blotches under the skin from tiny blood vessels leaking
- THROMBOCYTOPENIA: bleeding in tissues, bruising and slow blood clotting due to low platelet count

iii. **Common Western Tests:**
- BIOPSY: a sample of bone marrow tissue may be taken to test its function.
- BLOOD SMEAR: tests abnormalities in cell shape and composition
- CBC: Complete blood count – measures composition of blood
- LR FUNCTION TESTS: ALT, AST markers in the blood that indicate function of liver
- URINE CULTURE: analysis of bacteria/composition of urine components

iii. **General Red Flags:**

Depending on the constituent of the blood that is affected, you can see an array of symptoms that would signal a referral to their primary care physician:

- Bleeding that has abnormal flow times
- Unexplained bruising
- Abnormal fatigue that will not abate
- Syncope
- Unexplained rashes under the skin
- Recurrent infections
- Recurrent bleeding from various areas (gums, nose, abnormal menstrual bleeding, etc.)
- Swollen abdomen
- Jaundice
- Persistently swollen lymph nodes

Definitions:

- ADENOIDS/TONSILS: Lymph tissue in back of throat that helps make antibodies against germs breathed in/swallowed.
- B LYMPHOCYTES: protect body from bacteria/viruses by make antibody proteins. The antibodies attach to germs to be marked for destruction.
- BONE MARROW: spongy tissue inside certain bones, where new WBCs, RBC and platelets are made
- CYTO: cells
- HEMATOLOGY: study of the blood in health and disease
- IMMUNOGLOBULIN: proteins in serum of immune system cells – function like antibodies
- LEUKOCYTE: another name for a WBC
- LYMPHOCYTES: a form of WBC mostly found in the lymphatic system
- PLATELETS: helps blood clot
- RBC: red blood cell; carries oxygen from LU to HT and entire body + carries nutrients
- SPLEEN: filters blood where red blood cells are destroyed and platelets and WBCs are stored (fights many invading bacterias)
- STEM CELL: a cell of a multicellular organism that can indefinitely divide to give rise to remain a stem cell or become another type of cell (RBC, muscle cell, you name it). Found in: bone marrow, adipose tissue and blood.
- T LYMPHOCYTES: some destroy bacteria or infected cells (with virus or fungi); some regulate immune system activity

- THROMBO: platelets
- THYMUS GLAND: small organ behind breastbone and in front of HT that helps develop T lymphocytes
- WBC: white blood cell. Circulates in blood and body fluid to counteract foreign substances and disease

Common Diseases + Specific Red Flags

Condition Symptoms and signs Related TCM Illness	Causes & Diagnostic tests	Red flags (and what to do about them)
Anemia (aplastic)** *Body stops producing enough new blood cells due to bone marrow damage* **Symptoms:** Often insidious; fatigue, pallor, dyspnea, tachycardia, hair/skin issues, dizziness, tongue swelling/soreness, paresthesia (esp. in legs), cold hands/feet, headaches, brittle nails (all anemia sxs) + leukopenia, thrombocytopenia (i.e. at higher risk of infections and uncontrolled bleeding) ex) easy bruising, nosebleeds, bruising gums, prolonged bleeding from cuts, skin rash *"A plastic Barbie has no bones, therefore any bone marrow. Poor limp Barbie is always sick and bleeding from everywhere"* **TCM Illness: Bleeding disorders (xue zheng); Consumptive disease (vacuity taxation) (xu lao)**	**Causes:** Depression of bone marrow function decrease stem cells decrease RBC, WBC and platelet production -Above could be caused by: radiation/chemotherapy; exposure to toxic chemicals; certain medications (ex) many RA drugs and some antibiotics; autoimmune disorders that attack bone marrow/stem cells; viral infection; pregnancy **Diagnosis:** CBC **Tx:** Blood transfusions	**Red Flags:** **LOOK FOR: ANEMIA + BLEEDING + EASY INFECTIONS** **Refer to GP for further assessment**
Anemia (Pernicious) *RBC amounts are decreased due to low B12 absorption in intestine. RBCs themselves are enlarged (macrocytes).* **Sxs:** Typical anemia sxs from above (or asymptomatic) +tongue is enlarged, shiny and red (sometimes burning), may be bleeding gums, confusion, depression, loss of balance, paresthesia *"Pernicious was Suspicious that her tongue flames were coming from her ST fire. Too bad B's 12 water hoses were missing!"*	**Causes:** Most common: weak ST lining/chronic gastritis/local inflammation (Intrinsic Factor (IF) is released by cells in the ST, and IF is low, the intestine cannot absorb B12) (do you see why ST36 is so great for anemia?) Autoimmune rxn where body attacks IF -Surgery on ST (parietal cells removed which produce IF, or SI (where absorption happens) -Anything greatly affecting the ST or SI! (H.Pylori, Crohn's, SIBO, leaky gut, you name it) **Diagnosis:** CBC **Tx:** Vitamin B12 injections	**Red Flags:** **LOOK FOR: ANEMIA + ENLARGED, RED, SHINY TONGUE + PARESTHESIA**

TCM Illness: Consumptive disease (vacuity taxation) (xu lao)		Refer to GP if treatment not working.
**Bleeding Disorders**		
Hemophilia (variant: VonWillebrand's Disease) *Easy bleeding and bruising with flow that is difficult to stop.* *There are 3 types (A, B, and C) - A being most common. Mild (trauma excessive bleeding) and severe (spontaneous bleeding) classifications.* **Sxs:** Bleeding from anywhere (hemafecia, hematuria, nose, etc.), deep bruises, pain in the joints, tight joints *von Willebrand's disease is usually less severe unless Type III, then sxs same as haemophilia *'He mo bleedia. He mo bleedia. HE MO BLEEDIA!'* **TCM Illness: Bleeding Disorders (xue zheng)**	**Causes:** Inherited genetic disorder reduces clotting factors VIII, IX, or XI in the blood. Usually passed on by the mother and more common in males. Low levels of von Willebrand factor (VWF) - a clotting protein - results in this hemophilia variation **Diagnosis:** Blood test for clotting factors **Tx:** Desmopressin injection (stimulates clotting factors) (Type A) -Infusing blood with donor clotting factors (Type B) -Plasma infusing (stops profuse bleeding) (Type C)	**Red Flags:** **Refer to GP if severe bleed.**
Hemochromatosis* *Over absorption of iron from the minerals and foods ingested causing the body to store iron in other organs such as the heart, liver and pancreas* **Symptoms:** Fatigue, weakness, pain to the abdomen, joint pain early signs, further on in the disease, loss of sex drive, diabetes, heart and/or liver failure, skin colour changes – yellowish/bronzed, brown patches **TCM Illness: Consumptive Disease (xu lao)**	**Causes:** Gene mutation that alters the amount of iron the body absorbs from food, genetic and can be passed down through generations **Diagnosis:** Blood tests to determine iron overload, liver function tests, genetic testing **Tx:** Phlebotomy routine removal of blood from body (similar to donating blood) to reduce iron levels to normal	**Red Flags:** **Refer to GP for further assessment**
Hemolysis (AKA 'Hemolytic Anemia') *Endogenous breakdown of RBCs (faster breakdown than bone marrow production of RBCs)* *-2 types – intrinsic (RBCs produced are defective) or extrinsic (autoimmune – SP traps and destroys healthy RBCs)* **Sxs:** Anemia sxs + *can be* splenomegaly or hepatomegaly, HT murmur, tachycardia, jaundice, dark urine *'He Lysol-ed his blood. WHAT? Yes! It*	**Causes:** -Hepato- or splenomegaly -Epstein-Barr virus -Typhoid fever -Streptococcus -Leukemia -Lymphoma -SLE -Idiopathic (medication induced) -Blood transfusion of wrong blood type **Diagnosis:** Blood test for bilirubin, hemoglobin -LR function test	**Red Flags:**

disintegrated their walls!!' **TCM Illness:** Consumptive Disease (vacuity taxation) (xu lao); Jaundice (huang dan - if present)	-Reticulocyte count (how many RBCs your body is producing) **Tx:** Blood transfusion -Intravenous immunoglobulin (improves immune function) -Corticosteroids (stops immune system from making antibodies that destroy RBCs) -Surgery (splenectomy)	**Refer to GP ASAP for further assessment**
Hodgkin's Disease (HD) *A lymphoma (cancer that starts in the WBCs - specifically lymphocytes) causing abnormal lymphocyte growth. As the disease progresses, these cells spread outside of the lymphatic system (metastasise). Diagnosed in 4 stages of progression (4th meaning metastases).* **Ssx:** Sore throat, fever, night sweats, cough, itching, unintended weight loss, lymphadenopathy (lymph nodes affected) causing hard, non-painful lumps to form in neck, armpit, groin areas (especially after alcohol) *"To dodge the lumpy hodgey-bumpy, make sure you never don't drink!* **TCM Illness:** Consumptive disease (vacuity taxation) (xu lao)	**Causes:** Idiopathic, but believed that EBV (Epstein Barr Virus – the one which causes mononucleosis) may cause increased risk. -Due to malignant, large B cells. **Diagnosis:** Lymph and bone marrow biopsy; blood panel; urine tests; imaging **Tx:** Chemo/radiation *Very high cure rates with chemo/radiation.*	**Red Flags:** **Refer to GP ASAP for further assessment.**
Leukemia (Acute/Chronic)* *Stems from a defective stem cell in the bone marrow that keeps reproducing abnormal cells in malignant form. Symptoms mostly due to lack of normal blood cells.* <u>Acute:</u> Cells are immature and cannot perform functions. Replicate quickly and is more fatal form. <u>Chronic:</u> Abnormal cells more mature and therefore can perform some normal functions. Decreased multiplication time, better chance of survival. **Sxs:** <u>Acute:</u> Bleeding/bruising, fever, pallor, h/a, vomiting, irritability, bone/joint pain, anemia symptoms from shortage of blood cells, recurring infections <u>Chronic:</u> Fatigue, weakness, anorexia,	**Causes:** Could be combination of genetic or environmental factors. Basically from mutated DNA. Previous cancer tx, smoking, familial. **Diagnosis:** CBC, blood smear **Tx:** Chemo/radiation, corticosteroids, stem cell transplant	**Red Flags:** **Refer to GP for further assessment.**

weight loss, night sweats, fever, enlarged SP (swollen stomach or pain), lymphadenopathy, bleeding, pallor, recurring infections *"Luke. My Stem Cell. I am your Father. Smarten up and start making normal blood cells or I will finish you off."* –Darth Vader. Fed up father. **TCM Illness: Consumptive Disease (vacuity taxation) (xu lao)**		
Leukopenia & Agranulocytosis *Conditions of white blood cell abnormalities* *Leukopenia - low white blood cell count* *Agranulocytosis - acute and life threatening condition of severely low white blood cells* **Symptoms:** Persistent infections/illness (colds, flus, slow healing wounds), any signs of a suppressed immune system, fevers, chills, sore throat *'There is pretty much just one gram of WBCs left. I am exhausted and can't fight anymore.'* **TCM Illness: Consumptive Disease (xu lao)**	**Causes:** Viral infections, certain cancers and cancer treatment (chemotherapy/radiation), HIV/AIDS, and other autoimmune disorders **Diagnosis:** Blood test to measure white blood cell count **Tx:** Medications to increase white blood cell production in the bone marrow, dietary changes, granulocyte transfusion (severe cases)	**Red Flags:** **Refer to GP for further assessment**
Lymphocytopenia *Condition of having abnormally low levels of lymphocytes in circulating blood* **Symptoms:** Enlarged lymph nodes (in neck, armpits or groin), painful swollen joints, constant runny nose/fever (signs of cold) *'The lymph site seems to be missing in the blood. Where did it go?'* **TCM Illness: Consumptive Disease (xu lao), often has a Common Cold (gan mao), Impediment syndrome (bi zheng)**	**Causes:** Recent viral or bacterial infection (common cold), certain cancers and/or cancer treatments (chemotherapy, radiation), HIV/AIDS, other autoimmune disorders **Diagnosis:** CBC - complete blood count **Tx:** Treating the cause - antibiotics/antivirals, medication management	**Red Flags:** **Refer to GP for further assessment**
Lymphoma* *A general term for a form of cancer that affects the lymphocytes (a type of WBC that is part of the immune system).* *-Most often refers to Hodgkin's or Non-Hodgkin's Lymphoma.* **Ssx:** Persistently swollen lymph nodes.	**Causes:** Idiopathic, may be correlation between genetic inheritance **Diagnosis:** Review of physical symptoms, blood test for cancer markers **Tx:** Chemotherapy, radiation, stem cell transplant	**Red Flags:**

Often painless, unless they are pressing on other structures. Fatigue, LOA, itching, unexplained weight loss, night sweats, fever, breathlessness, edema in legs. 'Lymph = lymph Oma = oh my…. Not good' **TCM Illness: Consumptive Disease (xu lao), Edema (shui zhong)**		**Refer to GP for further assessment**
Non-Hodgkin's Lymphoma (NHL) *Same as Hodgkin's disease only this one can be derived from B or T cells in the lymph nodes as well as other organs. Much faster spread of the cancer than HD and lower rates of survival.* **Ssx:** Sore throat, fever, night sweats, cough, itching, unintended weight loss, lymphadenopathy (lymph nodes affected) causing hard, non-painful lumps to form in neck, armpit, groin areas (especially after alcohol) + any other sxs depending on organs affected "This lumpy-Hodgey-bumpy is non-slow". **TCM Illness: Consumptive disease (vacuity taxation) (xu lao)**	**Causes:** Idiopathic, but believed that EBV (Epstein Barr Virus – the one which causes mononucleosis) may cause increased risk. **Diagnosis:** Lymph and bone marrow biopsy; blood panel; urine tests; imaging **Tx:** Chemo/radiation	**Red Flags:** **Refer to GP ASAP for assessment.**
Thrombocytopenia (Thrombocytopenic purpura) *Decreased platelets in the blood* **Ssx:** Bleeding into tissues (petechiae), purpura (bruising/bruise like blotches), and slow blood clotting after trauma *Thrombo = Platelets* *Cyto = Cells* *Penia = Not enough of* **TCM Illness: Consumptive disease (vacuity taxation) (xu lao); bleeding disorders (xue zheng)**	**Causes:** Many: Leukemia, alcoholism, anemia, splenomegaly (platelets 'hide out' in SP), HIV, SLE, lymphoma, cancer, septicemia, etc. **Diagnosis:** CBC, blood smear, bone marrow test (aspiration -fluid sample from needle- or biopsy -tissue sample) **Tx:** Corticosteroids; splenectomy; immunoglobulin; thrombopoietin receptor agonists; immunosuppressants; androgens; avoid aspirin as it thins the blood	**Red Flags:** **Refer to GP ASAP for assessment.**

Infectious Diseases

i. **General Pathophysiology:**
   - Bacterial infection - infections caused by bacterial agents
   - Viral infection - infection caused by virus, often harder to treat, occasionally no cure (herpes, HIV)
   - Fungal infection - infection caused by fungal agent
   - Highly contagious, preventable diseases - Measles, mumps, Rubella, Whooping cough, etc. Vaccinations have been developed and are the only way to prevent re-emergence of these fatal diseases

   Remember that as acupuncturists, we have a duty to report 'certain communicable and reportable diseases (Canada - Health Protection and Promotion Act, report to Health Canada or equivalent provincial offices such as British Columbia Centre for Disease Control, Ontario Agency for Health Protection and Promotion)' Ex) Ebola, Polio

ii. **Common Western Tests:**
   - Blood culture and sensitivity (C&S) - sample taken and analyzed for presence of virus, bacteria or fungi
   - Urine C&S - urine sample taken and analyzed for presence of virus, bacteria or fungi
   - Stool C&S - feces sample taken and analyzed for presence of virus, bacteria or fungi
   - Pap test (Papanicolaou test) - procedure that removes small amount of cervical cells by swabbing the area and testing for abnormalities
   - STI Screening - often taken by pap test, or swab of genital area

iii. **General Red Flags:**
   - Unexplained fever
   - Fatigue
   - Chills
   - Headache
   - Rash on any part of the body
   - Painful urination or intercourse
   - Unusual discharge from genitals
   - Unexplained aches and pains with new onset

Common Diseases + Specific Red Flags

Allergies (4 types) -Over-reaction of the immune system to seemingly harmless proteins and substances Type I: Anaphylactic OR immediate from pollen, food, animals, drugs, etc. ex) hay fever Type II: IgG and IgM antibodies bind to a cell and destroy ex) organ transplant rejection, or Rh incompatibility Type III: Immune complex-mediated reaction Ex) SLE getting flu-like sxs Type IV: Delayed reactions mediated by T-cells. Can take a few hours/days for the allergy to mount. Ex) exposure to poison ivy **Sxs:** Sneezing, SOB, wheezing, runny nose and eyes, sinus pain, coughing, skin rashes, swelling of face or lips, itchy, n/v, abd. cramps/diarrhea ***Anaphylactic: Swelling of throat and mouth clogging airways, rash/itching, weakness and collapse from sudden fall in BP – EMERGENT*** **TCM Illness:** None that match (maybe Dysphagia (ye ge)	**Causes:** Autoimmune reaction to foreign material **Diagnosis:** Review of symptoms and agent of causation **Tx:** Removal of cause, epinephrine shot (emergent situations), anti-histamines	**Red Flags:** **Refer to ER IMMEDIATELY or call 911, medical emergency if anaphylactic**
Bacterial*		
Group A Hemolytic Strep *Infection with Streptococcus pyrogens, a beta-hemolytic bacterium that belongs to the group A streptococci (GAS). It causes a wide variety of diseases in humans.* **Ssx:** Often causes upper respiratory tract infections	**Causes:** Exposure to strep bacteria **Diagnosis:** Blood sampling and cultures to determine bacteria **Tx:** Penicillin medications x 10 days considered standard treatment	**Red Flags:**

such as pharyngitis, **strep throat**, sore throat, cough, fever TCM Illness: Fever (fa re), can start with Common Cold (gan mao), Cough (ke shou)		Refer to GP for further assessment
Bacterial Dysentery *Severe form of shigella infection, a bacterial infection of the intestines often causing severe diarrhea. Most common in children* **Ssx:** Frequent, bloody diarrhea, abdominal and rectal pain, fever, nausea, vomiting *'I have to DYSinfect everything from pooping everywhere. And, blood is so hard to remove!'* TCM Illness: Diarrhea (xie xie), Fever (fa re)	**Causes:** Can be passed through fecal-oral route, coming in contact with infected stool, consuming spoiled food and/or water **Diagnosis:** Stool sample and analysis **Tx:** Antibiotic treatment, oral rehydration	**Red Flags:** Refer to GP ASAP for further assessment.
Cholera *An acute diarrheal conditions caused by an infection of the small intestine by some strains of the bacterium Vibrio cholerae.* **Ssx:** Diarrhea, nausea and vomiting, dehydration (dry mucous membranes, headache, thirst, muscle cramps) *'I am CHOLing out for water. Can you hear me?'* TCM Illness: Diarrhea (xie xie)	**Causes:** Ingestions of contaminated food or water, can be on fresh fruit and vegetables, seafood **Diagnosis:** Rapid cholera testing (first line of defense in high risk areas), additional blood and stool tests **Tx:** Vaccination (preventive), rehydration, antibiotics, zinc supplements	**Red Flags:** Refer to GP ASAP for further assessment – REPORTABLE.
E Coli *Escherichia coli bacteria that is present in the intestines of healthy individuals, normally not harmful but can cause brief, sometimes serious infections* **Ssx:** Mild to severe diarrhea, abdominal	**Causes:** Ingesting undercooked meat, unpasteurized milk, contaminated water, contact with infected person **Diagnosis:** Sample of blood, urine, and/or stool to determine e coli levels **Tx:** No treatment for e coli as it is a normal flora bacteria, rest, oral rehydration if necessary	**Red Flags:**

cramping or pain **TCM Illness: Diarrhea (xie xie), Abdominal Pain (fu tong)**		**Refer to GP for further assessment**
Impetigo *A common and highly contagious skin infection that mainly affects infants and children, often looks like red sores USUALLY surrounding the mouth and nose* **Ssx:** Red sores (usually) around mouth and nose - rupture easy and form scabs, severe cases can manifests as blisters *'The little imps get into everything and get sores all over their mouths'* **TCM Illness: Closest is Sebaceous Cyst (zhi liu)**	**Causes:** Physical contact with infected objects **Diagnosis:** Physical examination - often no tests are performed **Tx:** Antibiotics - ointment or cream applied directly to area	**Red Flags:** **Refer to GP for further assessment**
Meningitis *Inflammation of the meninges caused by viral or bacterial infection and marked by intense headache and fever, sensitivity to light, and muscular rigidity, leading (in severe cases) to convulsions, delirium, and death* **Ssx:** Headache, fever, stiff neck, light sensitivity, sudden confusion or difficulty focusing, vomiting, swollen neck *'If you MENige to live through such a stiff neck, you are a lucky one.'* **TCM Illness: Fever (fa re), Vomiting (ou tu), Headache (tou tong)**	**Causes:** Viral or bacterial infection **Diagnosis:** Blood C&S, spinal puncture for spinal fluid analysis, positive Brudzinki's sign **Tx:** Antiviral or antibiotic - depending on the cause	**Red Flags:** **Refer to ER Immediately.**
MRSA *Methicillin-resistant Staphylococcus aureus (MRSA) infection is caused by a type of staph bacteria that's become resistant to many of the antibiotics used*	**Causes:** Can be hospital acquired or community acquired, affects about 1/3rd of the populations - thought to be caused by overuse of antibiotics leading to antibiotic resistance **Diagnosis:** Swabs of the nares and groin, or infected wound if applicable	**Red Flags:**

to treat ordinary staph infections **Ssx:** Swollen painful red bumps that resemble zits, fever, infected area warm to touch, slow wound healing *'Marissa was of the antibiotic generation. Now she isn't resistant to anything. Poor thing.'* **TCM Illness: Furuncles (jie) or Carbuncles (jie)**	**Tx:** Certain antibiotics currently are still effective	**Refer to GP for further assessment.**
Necrotizing Fasciitis *A rapidly progressive inflammatory infection of the fascia, with secondary necrosis of the subcutaneous tissues* **"Flesh eating disease"** **Ssx:** Rapidly spreading swollen and red skin surrounding wound/lesion, ulcer or blister development, black areas of the skin, often occurs within several hours of injury **TCM Illness: None that match**	**Causes:** Serious bacterial infection, contact with infected material **Diagnosis:** Biopsy of wound/tissue sample, blood tests **Tx:** Prompt treatment is necessary to stop complications, heavy duty antibiotics when necessary surgical removal of infected tissue to stop spread	**Red Flags:** **Refer to ER immediately.**
Staph *Infections caused by staphylococcus bacteria (commonly found on skin, hair, nose, throat), if left untreated can be deadly when it spreads to internal organs* **Ssx:** Present as skin complications - boils, blisters, ulcers in the skin, can cause flare ups of arthritis - painful and swollen joints **TCM Illness: Carbuncles (jie), Furuncles (yong)**	**Causes:** Contact with staphylococcus bacteria **Diagnosis:** Blood test, C&S (culture and sensitivity to test for bacteria) **Tx:** Antibiotics (commonly vancomycin)	**Red Flags:** **Refer to GP for further assessment**
Childhood Infectious Conditions*		
Measles	**Causes:** Contact with the measles virus	**Red Flags:**

Highly contagious infection caused by measles virus **Ssx:** Cough, runny nose, fever, sore throat, swollen eyes, **rash on the skin** TCM Illness: Measles (ma zhen), Fever (fa re)	**Diagnosis:** Blood tests if necessary, review of physical symptoms and immunization records often enough **Tx:** Vaccination for prevention, no treatment is available for existing measles infection	**Refer to GP for further assessment - REPORTABLE.**
Mumps *Viral infection primarily affecting the parotid glands* **Sxs:** Parotitis on one or both sides, fever, h/a, m.aches/pains, weakness, fatigue, LOA, pain w/ chewing and swallowing TCM Illness: Mumps (zha sai)	**Cause:** Breathing in saliva droplets of an infected person **Diagnosis:** Virus culture, blood test **Tx:** Usually it runs it's course in 1-2 weeks	**Red Flags:** **Refer to GP for further assessment.**
Rubella (German Measles) *An infection-causing rash caused by the rubella virus. Similar to measles however not as dangerous, sometimes referred to as 'three days measles"* **Ssx:** Red rash covering the face and body that fluctuates, mild fever, runny nose, aching joints, swollen lymph nodes *'Zi Germans are quick and efficient. In. Rash. Out.'* TCM Illness: Measles (ma zhen)	**Causes:** Contact with infectious virus (different from measles) **Diagnosis:** Review of physical symptoms, blood tests to confirm **Tx:** Measles-mumps-rubella (MMR) vaccine for prevention, no known treatment. Isolation once infected to reduce spread	**Red Flags:** **Refer to GP for further assessment - REPORTABLE.**
Pertussis (Whooping Cough) *A highly contagious respiratory disease caused by the bacteria Bordetella pertussis* **Ssx:** Runny nose, fever, red watery eyes, frequent deep cough attacks (distinct 'whooping sound' as child takes breath after cough) TCM Illness: Whooping Cough (dun ke)	**Cause:** Contact with infected person or Bordetella pertussis bacteria **Diagnosis:** Sputum sample, swab of nose and throat **Tx:** Vaccination for prevention	**Red Flags:** **Refer to GP for further assessment - REPORTABLE.**
Typhoid Fever	**Causes:** Exposure to salmonella bacteria -	**Red Flags:**

An infectious bacterial fever with an eruption of red spots on the chest and abdomen and severe intestinal irritation **Ssx:** Slowly increasing fever, headache, abdominal pain muscle aches and fatigue, sweating, diarrhea, delirium *'Coming back from a tropical vacation sometimes makes you feel like a typhoon hit you!'* **TCM Illness: Fever (fa re), Headache (tou tong), Diarrhea (xie xie)**	contaminated food, water, or contact with infected person **Diagnosis:** Review of physical symptoms, blood C&S **Tx:** Antibiotics - ciprofloxacin and/or ceftriaxone	**Refer to GP for further assessment - REPORTABLE.**
Fever (Pyrexia) *Having a body temperature of over normal body temperature (normal = 37.5 and 38.3 °C (99.5 and 100.9 °F)* **Ssx:** Flushed skin, high temperature, headache, chills, sweating **TCM Illness: Fever (fa re)**	**Causes:** Bacterial or viral infection, flu, common cold **Diagnosis:** Blood tests and review of recent history to determine cause, C&S of wounds if suspected **Tx:** Treatment of the cause - antibiotics or antivirals if necessary, oral rehydration	**Red Flags:** **Unresolved fever for several days, signs of dehydration, fever at or above 104F** **Refer to ER**
Foodborne Illness* *Illness caused by ingesting contaminated food (food poisoning)* **Ssx:** Nausea, vomiting, fever, chills, headache, diarrhea **TCM Illness: Diarrhea (xie xie), Vomiting (ou tu), Fever (fa re)**	**Causes:** Ingesting contaminated food, could be a bacterial cause **Diagnosis:** Review of physical symptoms and exposure, blood C&S if unresolved **Tx:** Symptoms may clear up in a day or two - if not antibiotics for serious infections	**Red Flags:** **Refer to GP for further assessment**
Infection		
Cellulitis *Infection in tissues caused by streptococcus or staphylococcus* **Ssx:** Swollen red area of skin, hot to touch and painful, commonly found on lower legs, fever, headache	**Causes:** Contact with streptococcus and staphylococcus bacteria, or MRSA bacteria entering through a break/lesion in skin **Diagnosis:** Physical examination, blood C&S, wound culture if necessary **Tx:** Antibiotics to treat cause	**Red Flags:**

'My cellulite is so bad that it is RED and SWOLLEN!' **TCM Illness: Phlegmon (fa)**		Refer to GP for further assessment
Lymphadenitis *Swollen lymph glands* **Ssx:** Swollen nodes around the jaw, nape of neck, armpits, and groin, lower right sided abdominal pain 'Add another giant lymph node to the mix!' **TCM Illness: None that match**	**Causes:** Bacterial infection, autoimmune disorders, common illnesses (flu/cold) **Diagnosis:** Physical exam, blood C&S for bacterial/viral infections **Tx:** Dependent on the cause - antibiotics or antivirals, pain killers	**Red Flags:** Refer to GP for further assessment
Lymphangitis *Inflammation and infection of the lymphatic vessels* **Ssx:** Red streaks on surface of skin coming from a lymph gland, swollen lymph nodes around the jaw, nape of neck, armpits, and groin, fever, chills, general feeling unwell 'ANG missed her lips with her lipstick and accidently drew a red streak up her arm' **TCM Illness: Fever (fa re)**	**Causes:** Bacterial or viral infection of lymphatic system (staph infection is common) **Diagnosis:** Blood culture, physical examination **Tx:** Treatment of the causative factor - antibiotics or antivirals	**Red Flags:** Refer to GP for further assessment.
Parasitic*		
Fungal *Primitive organism that lives in the air, soil, plants and water, commonly causes skin infections in warm moist areas - groin, buttocks, mouth, inner thighs, skin folds* **Ssx:** Infections such a jock itch, athletes foot, thrush general - itching, reddened area **TCM Illness: None that match**	**Causes:** Contact with specific fungal parasite, poor hygiene **Diagnosis:** Blood C&S to rule out other infections, sample from affected area (swab collected), review of physical symptoms, wood's lamp **Tx:** Topical creams/ointments	**Red Flags:** Refer to GP for further assessment.
Leptospirosis *A bacterial disease that affects humans and animals caused by corkscrew-shaped bacteria called Leptospira*	**Cause:** Corkscrew-shaped bacteria called Leptospira usually from the urine of infected animals. Can transmit to human through contact with animal fluids; or through soil/food contaminated with urine	**Red Flags:**

Sxs: High fever, h/a, chills, m.ache, n/v, jaundice, red eyes, abd. Pain, diarrhea, rash (can take 2 days to 4 weeks to progress) *'The bacteria LEPT from the animals, right on to me! Now I feel sick'* **TCM Illness:** Fever (fa re), Diarrhea (xie xie), Jaundice (huang dan)	**Diagnosis:** Urine sample; blood sample **Tx:** Antibiotics (doxycycline or penicillin)	Refer to GP for further assessment.
Malaria *A life-threatening disease caused by parasites that are transmitted to people through the bites of infected female Anopheles mosquitoes* **Sxs:** Fever, h/a, chills, vomiting (7-10 days after bite) → if not treated in 24 hours → multi-organ involvement, death *'MAsquitos in the AIRia can kill you in some countries'* **TCM Illness:** Fever (fa re), Night Sweats (dao ban), Vomiting (ou tu)	**Cause:** Bite of infected female Anopheles mosquitoes **Diagnosis:** Microscopy or rapid diagnostic test for parasite **Tx:** Artemisinin-based combination therapy (ACT) (2 drugs w/ diff. actions). Prevention is key through anti-malarial drugs (no current vaccine)	**Red Flags:** Refer to GP for further assessment - REPORTABLE.
Schistosomiasis *An acute and chronic disease caused by parasitic worms from tropical and subtropical areas* **Sxs:** Abdominal pain, diarrhea, hemafecia, ascites, splenomegaly, aortic hypertension (all these if in LI) -If in BL - hematuria, fibrosis of BL and ureter, KI damage, vaginal bleeding, pain with intercourse, can lead to BL cancer, infertility, prostate issues *'This parasite is SCHIZOPHRENIC in the body. Causing a giant belly and so many problems'*	**Cause:** Coming in contact with excrement of a carrier (usually in water) **Diagnosis:** Stool and urine sample to check for eggs **Tx:** Praziquantel	**Red Flags:**

TCM Illness: Diarrhea (xie xie), Intestinal Parasitic Worms (chang dao chong zheng), Abdominal Pain (fu tong), Drum Distension (gu zhang)		**Refer to GP for further assessment.**
Viral**		
Chicken Pox *Common, preventable childhood infection caused by the varicella-zoster virus, highly contagious* **Ssx:** Elevated red bumps across body, itchy, can rupture, fever, general feeling unwell, nausea, loss of appetite **TCM Illness: Chicken Pox (shui du)**	**Causes:** Varicella-zoster virus **Diagnosis:** Review of physical symptoms **Tx:** Vaccinations are now available - if not symptom management to promote comfort - no treatment	**Red Flags:** **Refer to GP for further assessment - REPORTABLE.**
Conjunctivitis **Ssx:** **TCM Illness:**	**Causes:** **Diagnosis:** **Tx:**	**Red Flags:** **Refer to GP for further assessment .**
Epidemic Encephalitis (Encephalitis Lethargica) *Known as 'sleepy sickness', this disease attacks the brain, leaving some victims in a statue-like condition, speechless and motionless.* **Ssx:** High fever, sore throat, confusion or decreased level of consciousness, confusion, muscles stiffness and/or tremors *'Yes, watch out for this 100 year old EPIDEMIC. If zombie*	**Causes:** Cause is unknown **Diagnosis:** Difficult to diagnose, review of physical symptoms **Tx:** Anti-parkinson drugs appear to have good effect if the condition is caught early enough	**Red Flags:**

apocalypse is real, SO IS THIS' **TCM Illness:** Fever (fa re), none other that match		**Refer to ER immediately.**
Hepatitis **Ssx:** **TCM Illness:**	**Causes:** **Diagnosis:** **Tx:**	**Red Flags:** **Refer to GP for further assessment - REPORTABLE.**
Herpes Simplex I & II *Viruses causing skin outbreaks* **Ssx:** Herpes I = cold sores around mouth (oral herpes) Herpes II = STD/genital or rectal sores **TCM Illness: Carbuncles closest (yong)**	**Causes:** Exposure to herpes virus, direct contact - sexual intercourse, skin to skin contact **Diagnosis:** STI tests, swab and culture of wounds, physical examination, blood tests **Tx:** No cure for either strain, once you contract it you will be a carrier for life. Drugs are available to help suppress virus and symptoms	**Red Flags:** **Refer to GP for further assessment.**
HIV (AIDS - Acquired Immune Deficiency Virus) *Immunodeficiency syndrome caused by HIV (Human Immunodeficiency Virus), will eventually develop into AIDS - final stages of disease* **Ssx:** Fever, frequent illness (cold, flu), joint and muscles pain, unexplained weight loss, prolonged wound healing, fatigue, soaking night sweats, chronic diarrhea, white sores on tongue **Flu-like sxs usually show up 2-4 weeks after HIV exposure and may be 2 weeks to 6 months for HIV antibodies to form* **Average incubation period*	**Causes:** Exposure to the HIV virus, spread through bodily fluids - semen, blood, vaginal discharge, breast milk **Diagnosis:** HIV rapid testing and additional blood tests **Tx:** Strict antiretroviral medication schedule	**Red Flags:**

from HIV to AIDS is a few months to 10+ years **TCM Illness: Internal Damage Fever (nei shang fa re), Common Cold (gan mao), Consumptive Disease (xu lao)**		**Refer to GP for further assessment.**
Influenza (A) (Flu) *Infection caused by influenza virus* *-Influenza A = Avian flu* **Ssx:** High fever, chills, headache, nausea, vomiting, muscle aches and pain. diarrhea, dehydration **TCM Illness: Fever (fa re), Diarrhea (xie xie), Headache (tou tong), Vomiting (ou tu)**	**Causes:** Exposure to virus - rapidly evolving and mutating virus so difficult to predict/prevent **Diagnosis:** Review of symptoms, blood test to rule out infection if necessary **Tx:** Painkillers for headache, lots of fluids and rest, no treatment	**Red Flags:** **Refer to GP for further assessment - REPORTABLE.**
Meningitis *Inflammation of the meninges caused by viral or bacterial infection* **Ssx:** **TCM Illness:**	**Causes:** **Diagnosis:** **Tx:**	**Red Flags:** **Refer to ER immediately.**
Mononucleosis (Glandular Fever) *An infection commonly caused by the Epstein–Barr virus (EBV)* *Commonly known as the 'Kissing virus" or "Mono"* **Ssx:** Extreme fatigue and weakness, increased sleepiness, sore throat, swollen tonsils, frequent illness (cough, cold, flu) 'I have mono % energy' **TCM Illness: Can cause Consumptive Disease (xu**	**Causes:** Exposure to infected bodily fluids - kissing, sneezing, sharing utensils **Diagnosis:** Physical examination and review of symptoms, blood test to rule out infection/other conditions **Tx:** No treatment available - treat secondary illnesses (colds, flus, strep throat etc), rest	**Red Flags:** **Refer to GP for further assessment.**

lao)		
Shingles **Ssx:** **TCM Illness:**	**Causes:** **Diagnosis:** **Tx:**	**Red Flags:** **Refer to GP for further assessment if treatment not effective.**
STIs**		
HPV (Human Papillomavirus) *Sexually transmitted virus that causes warts on the skin or mucous membranes strong link between HPV and Cervical Cancer* **Ssx:** Warts on the genitals, anus, mouth/hands feet *'I didn't realize that butterflies laid warty eggs!' (papillon is French for butterfly)* **TCM Illness**: None that match	**Causes:** Exposure to the virus, skin to skin contact, unprotected sexual intercourse **Diagnosis:** Pap test/STI screening **Tx:** No cure for the virus, topical or oral medications to reduce/clear up warts	**Red Flags:** **Refer to GP for further assessment.**
Chlamydia *Sexually transmitted bacterial infection, extremely common and often asymptomatic in the early phases* **Ssx:** Often no symptoms, can have genital pain, lower abdominal pain, painful intercourse, discolored discharge from penis or vagina, ulcers on tongue *'My clam is full of discharge and the clam tongue has went up to my eyes and blindfolded me'* **TCM Illness**: Abdominal	**Causes:** Exposure to bacteria, skin to skin contact, unprotected sexual intercourse **Diagnosis:** Pap test/STI screening **Tx:** Antibiotics to clear up infections	**Red Flags:** ***Can affect eyes and cause blindness** **Refer to GP for further**

Pain (fu tong)		assessment – REPORTABLE.
Gonorrhoea *Sexually transmitted bacterial infection, extremely common and often asymptomatic in the early phases* **Ssx:** Painful urination, pus like discharge from penis, discoloured discharge from vagina, painful intercourse *'When I saw the discharge, I was GONE from that relationship!'* **TCM Illness: Stranguria (lin zheng)**	**Causes:** Exposure to bacteria, skin to skin contact, unprotected sexual intercourse **Diagnosis:** Pap test/STI screening **Tx:** Antibiotics	**Red Flags:** **Refer to GP for further assessment – REPORTABLE.**
Trichomoniasis *STI caused by parasitic infection* **Ssx:** Foul smelling discharge from penis or vagina (white, green or yellow), painful urination, burning during ejaculation *'The parasite tried to trick me by making my discharge stinky and different colours!'* **TCM Illness: None that match (kind of Leukorrhagia – dai xia)**	**Causes:** Exposure to parasite during sexual intercourse **Diagnosis:** PAP test/STI screening **Tx:** Metronidazole	**Red Flags:** **Refer to GP for further assessment.**
Syphilis *Bacterial STI spread through unprotected sexual intercourse, extremely dangerous if left untreated - will develop neurological symptoms and deficits* **Ssx:** Begins as painless sore on genitals, progresses to rash covering body, sores surrounding mouth and nose, fever, sore throat **TCM Illness: Can be Fever (fa re)**	**Causes:** Skin to skin contact with infected person, unprotected sexual intercourse, exposure to bacteria **Diagnosis:** Pap test/STI screening, blood tests, spinal fluid analysis if necessary **Tx:** infections caught early on are treated easily with penicillin	**Red Flags:** **Refer to GP for further assessment – REPORTABLE.**
Public Lice (Crabs) *Small parasitic insects found in genital area* **Ssx:** Itchiness to groin and	**Causes:** Exposure to infected person through unprotected sexual intercourse **Diagnosis:** Physical examination and confirmation of moving lice	**Red Flags:**

genitals, rash development, can spread to armpits, chest, abdomen and head hair **TCM Illness: None that match**	**Tx:** Over the counter lice treatment	**Refer to GP for further assessment.**
PID (Pelvic Inflammatory Disease) **Ssx:** **TCM Illness:**	**Causes:** **Diagnosis:** **Tx:**	**Red Flags:** **Refer to GP for further assessment.**
Tuberculosis** *An infection caused by slow-growing bacteria that grow best in areas of the body that have an abundance blood and oxygen (most often the Lungs)* **Ssx:** Coughing that lasts longer than three weeks, coughing blood, fever, night sweats, unexplained weight loss **TCM Illness: Pulmonary Tuberculosis (fei lao), Cough (ke shou), Night Sweats (dao han), Fever (fa re)**	**Causes:** Spread through droplet contact - sneezing, coughing, saliva of infected person, occurs most often in people with compromised immune systems (HIV/AIDS) **Diagnosis:** Skin test to determine exposure to bacteria, Sputum C&S, blood tests **Tx:** Antibiotics long term - 6 to 9 months	**Red Flags:** **Refer to GP for further assessment – REPORTABLE.**

Mental and Behavioural Conditions

i. **General Pathophysiology:**
   - Mood disorders - Psychological disorder characterized by the elevation or lowering of a person's mood, such as depression or bipolar disorder
   - Hormonal imbalance - Issues with thyroid can cause mental health like symptoms - depression, anxiety, fatigue etc.
   - Addictions - Physical and emotional dependence on substance or activity

ii. **Common Western Tests:**
   - Mental health screening questionnaires
   - Cognitive behavioural therapy - short-term, goal-oriented psychotherapy treatment with a goal to change patterns of thinking that are causing issues so as to change the way they feel
   - DSM 5 - The Diagnostic and Statistical Manual of Mental Disorders, used as gold standard of mental health diagnosis, has various criteria clinicians can review and make appropriate diagnosis

iii. **General Red Flags:**
   - Decreased mood or feelings of depression
   - Changes in personality
   - Feelings of hopelessness
   - Difficulty concentrating
   - Social withdrawal

Common Diseases + Specific Red Flags

Condition Symptoms and signs Related TCM Illness	Causes & Diagnostic tests	Red flags (and what to do about them)
Addiction Disorder*** *Condition of partial or complete dependence on a substance or activity, drugs, alcohol, food, fitness, not eating etc.* **Ssx:** Excessive craving and willingness to do anything to consume addictive material (drugs, alcohol), inability to function without, daily use despite negative consequences **TCM Illness:** None that match	**Causes:** Addictive characteristics of the substances - chemical, physical, mental, lower dopamine receptors in brain **Diagnosis:** Review of physical symptoms/behaviour **Tx:** Rehabilitation for drug dependent individuals, lifestyle modifications, behavioural counselling	**Red Flags:** **Refer to GP/counselling for further assessment.**
Anxiety*** *Excessive, ongoing anxiety and worry that interferes with day-to-day activities* **Ssx:** Persistent worrying and obsessing over small things, distress about making decisions, inability to let go of events or issues	**Causes:** Unknown cause (as with most mental illnesses) **Diagnosis:** Review of physical symptoms and behaviours **Tx:** Behavioural counselling, cognitive behavioural therapy	**Red Flags:** **Refer to GP/counselling for further assessment** **Suicidal thoughts or ideations: Call 911/suicide hotline for advice**

		immediately
TCM Illness: None that match		
ADD/ADHD – Attention Deficit Disorder/Attention Deficit Hyperactivity Disorder *Condition characterized by inability to focus, hyperactivity and impulsive behaviour* **Ssx:** Hyperactivity, inability to focus on one thing for any extended period of time, impulsive behaviour, disorganized thinking and behaviour, frequent mood swings, easily frustrated **TCM Illness: None that match**	**Causes:** Unknown cause, can be genetic, problems during developmental years **Diagnosis:** Physical exam and review of behaviour, various psychological tests **Tx:** Medications (ritalin), psychological counselling	**Red Flags:** **Refer to GP/counsellor for further assessment.**
Autism Spectrum* *Neurodevelopmental disorder that impairs children's ability to communicate and connect with the environment around them* **Ssx:** Repetitive and obsessive actions/behaviours, inability to communicate needs, failure to respond to name, avoidance of physical contact, lack of eye contact, abnormally sensitive to sounds, smells, and light, poor social skills **TCM Illness: None that match**	**Causes:** Unknown cause, can be genetic, problems during developmental years **Diagnosis:** Physical exam and review of behaviour, various psychological tests **Tx:** There is no cure, medications can decrease side effects, psychological counselling, family counselling and support, education	**Red Flags:** **Refer to GP for further assessment.**
Eating Disorders*		
Anorexia Nervosa *Eating disorder characterized by starvation or extreme limited nutritional intake, extremely low body weight* **Ssx:** Extreme weight loss, fatigue, loss of muscle mass, thin hair, thin nails, chronic coldness, absence of menstruation, denial of hunger, social withdraw little or no intake of food, overuse of laxatives, diuretic medications, or enemas **TCM Illness: Anorexia (yan shi) – kind of**	**Causes:** Mental illness in which the person obsesses over weight and body image **Diagnosis:** Review of physical symptoms and behaviours **Tx:** Cognitive behavioural therapy, psychological counselling, rehabilitation and/or hospitalization if necessary	**Red Flags:** **Refer to GP/specialized counsellor for eating disorders for further assessment.**
Bulimia Nervosa *Eating disorder characterized by obsessive purging following intake of food* **Ssx:** Fear of gaining weight, obsession over physical image,	**Causes:** Mental illness in which the person obsesses over weight and body image **Diagnosis:** Review of physical symptoms and behaviours	**Red Flags:**

binge eating followed by forceful purging **TCM Illness:**	**Tx:** Cognitive behavioural therapy, psychological counselling, rehabilitation and/or hospitalization if necessary	**Refer to GP/counsellor for further assessment.**
Mood Disorders***		
Depression *Mood disorder causing persistent feelings of sadness, worthlessness, hopelessness etc., is cyclical and lasts more than several days/weeks* **Ssx:** Feelings of sadness, hopelessness, social withdrawal, sleep disturbances, lowered sex drive, anxiety, difficulty focusing, fatigue, headache **TCM Illness:** Depression (yu zheng)	**Causes:** Imbalance in neurotransmitters in the brain, environmental influences (seasonal depressive disorder), emotional trauma, hormonal imbalance, genetic influence **Diagnosis:** Review of physical symptoms, blood test to rule out hormonal influences **Tx:** Medications - selective serotonin reuptake inhibitors (SSRIs), other general antidepressants, psychological therapy	**Red Flags:** **Suicidal thought or ideations: Call 911 immediately**
Bi-Polar *Mental health condition that causes extreme mood swings* **Ssx:** Extreme moods - intensely happy followed by intensely depressed, irrational thinking, sleep disturbances, poor decision making (spending savings on irrational purchase), euphoria, depression, feelings of worthlessness, suicidal thoughts/actions **TCM Illness:** Mania (dian kuang) and Depression (yu zheng)	**Causes:** Unknown cause, can be genetic, problems during developmental years **Diagnosis:** Physical exam and review of behaviour, various psychological tests, use of DSM 5 **Tx:** There is no cure, medications can decrease side effects (mood stabilizers, lithium), psychological counselling, family counselling and support, education, is a lifelong condition	**Red Flags:** **Call 911 immediately for further support. Refer to GP or counselling.**
PTSD – Post-Traumatic Stress Disorder** *Mental health disorder that develops following a traumatic event/experience such as sexual assault, car accidents, abuse of any kind, watched violence* **Ssx:** Delayed response following traumatic event (months or years after), recurrent bad memories or stress response to certain events/triggers, traumatizing nightmares, avoidance of activities that remind person of events **TCM Illness:** None that match	**Causes:** Exposure/experience of traumatic event - assault, accident, physical, sexual or mental abuse **Diagnosis:** Review of physical symptoms, behaviour, various psychological tests, use of DSM 5 **Tx:** There is no cure, avoidance of traumatic event/trigger, mood stabilizers if necessary, psychological counselling, cognitive behavioural therapy	**Red Flags:** **if not severe, refer to GP/counsellor for assessment**
Suicidality* *Desire or feeling of no other option than to take one's own life* **Ssx:** Feelings of hopelessness,	**Causes:** Largely due to depression, lack of coping mechanisms, personal trauma, stress, financial distress, many different causes	**Red Flags:**

despair, social withdrawal, obtaining means of taking own life (pills, gun, etc.), devising a plan, giving away personal belongings or unnecessary gifts **TCM Illness: None that match (maybe Depression - yu zheng)**	**Diagnosis:** Physical and mental health assessment and review of symptoms **Tx:** Acute event - call 911 antidepressants, cognitive behavioural therapy	**Call 911 or suicide hotline immediately for further support**

Musculo-Skeletal Conditions

i. **General Pathophysiology:**
   - Fracture - Partial or full break in the bone
   - Strain - Stretching or tearing of ligaments
   - Soft tissue injury - Caused by blunt force trauma, bruising from superficial to deep tissue

ii. **Common Western Tests:**
   - X-ray - Electromagnetic tests used to produce images
   - MRI - Magnetic Resonance Imaging is a diagnostic test that uses magnetic fields and radio waves to produce a detailed image of the body's soft tissue and bones.
   - CT Scan - Detailed images of internal organs are obtained by this type of sophisticated X-ray device
   - Antinuclear antibody (ANA) test. A test for specific antibodies that indicates a stimulated immune system. Usually indicates an autoimmune disease.

iii. **General Red Flags:**
   - Painful joints
   - Swelling of joints
   - Loss of function/decreased mobility
   - Fever
   - Unexplained weight loss

Common Diseases + Specific Red Flags

Condition / Symptoms and signs / Related TCM Illness	Causes & Diagnostic tests	Red flags (and what to do about them)
General conditions		
Bacterial Arthritis (Acute) *Also called: Infectious/Septic Arthritis or Osteomyelitis) Bacterial infection of the joints causing arthritis like symptoms* **Ssx:** Painful swollen joints, difficulty moving joint, fever, reddened area **TCM Illness:** Impediment Syndrome (bi zheng)	**Causes:** Bacterial infection from the blood stream that enters fluid and tissues of the joints **Diagnosis:** Blood tests to isolate causative bacteria, joint fluid analysis and sample if necessary **Tx:** Antibiotics to clear infection	**Red Flags:** Refer to GP ASAP or ER for further assessment.
Bursitis *Inflammation of the bursae (fluid filled sacs that cushion the joints), most common in shoulders, elbows and hips* **Ssx:** Achy and stiff joints, swollen joints, difficulty moving said joint **TCM Illness:** Impediment Syndrome (bi zheng)	**Causes:** Repetitive motions that irritate the joints and bursae (throwing a ball, leaning on elbows/knees for extended period of time) **Diagnosis:** X-ray of area, sample of fluid from joint **Tx:** Pain relievers, antibiotics if necessary, drainage of affected area	**Red Flags:** Refer to GP for further assessment if treatment ineffective.
Gout *Sudden and severe from of arthritis*	**Causes:** Build-up of uric acid within the joint forming sharp crystal like	**Red Flags:**

flare up, most commonly affecting the big toe **Ssx:** Extreme pain to joint (base of big toe), swollen and reddened area, limited mobility *'King's disease'* **TCM Illness: Impediment Syndrome (bi zheng)**	substances **Diagnosis:** Review of physical symptoms, blood test if necessary **Tx:** Non steroidal inflammatories, corticosteroids, diet modification	**Refer to GP for further assessment if treatment ineffective.**
Fibromyalgia *Widespread musculoskeletal pain of no obvious cause* **Ssx:** Widespread, generalized pain on both sides of body, above and below waist, fatigue, headaches/migraines **TCM Illness: Impediment Syndrome (bi zheng)**	**Causes:** Unknown, could be related to stress, diet, sleep habits, could be due to repetitive nerve stimulation **Diagnosis:** Hard to diagnose, review of physical symptoms and various imaging tests to rule out other causes. 18 specific body points cause pain **Tx:** A wide variety of pain killers, antidepressants, lifestyle modification (healthy diet, adequate exercise)	**Red Flags:** **Refer to GP for further assessment if treatment ineffective.**
Neoplasms *Abnormal growth of tissues within the body - referred to as a tumour, can be benign (non cancerous), malignant (cancerous), insitu, or of uncertain behaviour* **Ssx:** Depends on where tumour is, can be fatigue, unexplained weight loss, fever, night sweats, unexplainable lump **TCM Illness: None that match**	**Causes:** Genetic mutation in which the control mechanisms for cell division are compromised **Diagnosis:** Ultrasound, MRI or CT scan to locate tumour, biopsy of tissue if needed **Tx:** Surgical removal of tumour, no treatment if not harmful, or cancer treatment if necessary	**Red Flags:** **Refer to GP ASAP for further assessment.**
Osteoarthritis (OA)*** *Most common form of arthritis - condition in which the protective cartilage of the joints is worn down* **Ssx:** Most common in hands, fingers knees and hips, painful swollen joints, limited mobility, sensation of grating (as bones move and catch across each other) **TCM Illness: Impediment Syndrome (bi zheng)**	**Causes:** Occurs overtime from the normal wear and tear of the joints, previous joint surgeries or injuries, repetitive movements over long period of time **Diagnosis:** X-ray of joints, review of physical symptoms and history **Tx:** Tylenol and other over the counter medications for arthritis relief	**Red Flags:** **Refer to GP for further assessment if treatment ineffective.**
Polymyositis (POLIO) *Rare inflammatory disease of the muscle tissue that affects both sides of the body* **Ssx:** Most commonly affecting the	**Causes:** Unknown cause, has similar characteristics to autoimmune diseases **Diagnosis:** Blood tests for specific markers of the disease/excessive	**Red Flags:**

muscles closest to the trunk of the body - shoulders, hips thighs, upper arms and neck, extreme weakness and loss of mobility 'Poly = Many Myo = Muscles -it is = Inflammation' **TCM Illness: Atrophy-Flaccidity (wei zheng)**	inflammation, MRI of muscles to isolate inflammation **Tx:** There is no cure, pain medications to manage, corticosteroids to reduce inflammation	**Refer to GP for further assessment.**
Rheumatoid Arthritis (RA)*** *Chronic inflammatory condition of the joints - autoimmune disorder* **Ssx:** Painful flare ups of arthritis, swollen, deformed and red joints, difficulty or inability to move, in severe cases weight loss, fatigue and fever **TCM Illness: Impediment Syndrome (bi zheng)**	**Causes:** Autoimmune response in which the body attacks the lining of the joints causing inflammation and bone damage **Diagnosis:** X-ray of affected joints, blood tests for specific inflammatory markers **Tx:** Anti-inflammatories, corticosteroids, heat compress, worst case scenario joint replacement (end stage of disease)	**Red Flags:** **Refer to GP for further assessment.**
Scleroderma *Rare disease characterized by tightening and hardening of skin and connective tissues, can cause hardening of lung, heart of digestive tissues* **Ssx:** Hard shiny patches on the skin, acid reflux (if GI is affected), exaggerated response to temperatures in fingers and toes - excessive numbness, pain and/or discoloration 'The skin is stretch-o-derma'd over the bone' **TCM Illness: Impediment Syndrome (bi zheng)**	**Causes:** Excessive amount of collagen circulating within the body causing build-up in tissues **Diagnosis:** Review of physical symptoms, blood tests for certain antibodies (autoimmune markers) **Tx:** No treatment for condition, only can manage the side effects - blood pressure medications, reduce stomach acid, reduce inflammatory response	**Red Flags:** **Refer to GP for further assessment.**
SLE (Systemic Lupus Erythematosus) *Chronic inflammatory disease in which the body attacks its own tissues including joints, skin, kidneys, blood cells, brain and heart* **Ssx:** Fatigue and joint/muscle pain, fever, Butterfly-shaped rash on the face that covers the cheeks and bridge of the nose, Skin lesions that appear or worsen with sun exposure (photosensitivity), unexplained rash to other parts of body	**Causes:** Unknown cause, autoimmune disorder that causes attack on own body tissues and inflammatory response **Diagnosis:** Specialized blood tests to test for autoimmune markers (ANA test) **Tx:** Anti-inflammatories, anti malaria drugs appear to have good effect controlling symptoms of lupus, immunosuppressants	**Red Flags:**

'Lupus = latin for 'wolf'' TCM Illness: Consumptive Disease (xu lao)		Refer to GP for further assessment.
Sprains/Strains *Strains - pulled muscles* *Sprain - pulled tendons/ligaments* **Ssx:** Swelling, pain, and redness to affected area, loss of mobility TCM Illness: Impediment Syndrome (bi zheng) OR Sprained Ankle (huai guan jie niu cuo shang)	**Causes:** Trauma to area (rolling joint, blunt force, falls, accidents, sports) **Diagnosis:** X-ray to rule out bone fracture, MRI or CT to determine ligament or tendon damage **Tx:** Rest, elevation, compression, ice	**Red Flags:** Refer to GP for further assessment if treatment ineffective.
Tendonitis *Chronic inflammation of the tendons causing pain and tenderness outside of the joint, such as:* *Tennis elbow, golfers elbow, swimmer's shoulder, jumpers knee* **Ssx:** Dull achy pain when using joint, tenderness to touch, swelling TCM Illness: Impediment Syndrome (bi zheng) or Achilles Tendon Injury (gen jian sun shang)	**Causes:** Repetitive motions, often sports injury **Diagnosis:** Review of physical symptoms **Tx:** Rest, ice, elevation, compression, anti-inflammatories, pain killers, worst case scenario surgery to repair tendons	**Red Flags:** Refer to GP for further assessment if treatment ineffective.
Axial Structure***		
Disc Herniation *Bulging of soft sacs between the vertebrae causing nerve irritation, pain and loss of mobility* **Ssx:** Severe back pain, arm and/or leg pain, numbness or tingling to limbs, weakness or impaired mobility TCM Illness: Prolapse of lumbar intervertebral disc (yao zhui jian pan tu chu zheng)	**Causes:** Gradual age related wear and tear, previous spinal injuries, excessive weight, occupational hazards **Diagnosis:** X-ray of spine, MRI or CT of spine, review of physical symptoms **Tx:** Narcotic pain killers, anti-inflammatories, muscle relaxants	**Red Flags:** Refer to GP for further assessment if treatment ineffective.
Spinal Stenosis *Narrowing of the open spaces within the spinal cavity putting pressure on the spinal cord* **Ssx:** Often asymptomatic and is only diagnosed by imaging results, others have back/spinal pain radiating down arms and/or legs, issues with balance and walking,	**Causes:** Osteoarthritis, age related changes, thickening of ligaments, tumours within the spinal cavity **Diagnosis:** MRI or x-ray of spine **Tx:** Muscles relaxants, anti seizure medications, physical therapy to improve side effects	**Red Flags:**

'Stenosis = Narrowing' **TCM Illness:** Impediment Syndrome (bi zheng)		**Refer to GP for further assessment.**
Spondylolisthesis *Condition in which one vertebra slides over the vertebra below it causing pinched nerves* **Ssx:** Back pain radiating down gluts and back of legs, muscle weakness, tingling or burning sensation, difficulty walking, loss of bladder or bowel control **TCM Illness:** Impediment Syndrome (bi zheng)	**Causes:** Joint damage from trauma, abnormalities or arthritis **Diagnosis:** MRI or x-ray of spine **Tx:** Muscles relaxants, anti seizure medications, physical therapy to improve side effects, surgery to fuse joint	**Red Flags:** **Refer to GP for further assessment.**
TMJ *Problems with your jaw and the muscles in your face that control it* **Ssx:** Pain and tenderness to the jaw, locking or popping jaw, clicking with chewing swelling to side of the face **TCM Illness:** Impediment Syndrome (bi zheng)	**Causes:** Grinding or clenching of teeth, trauma to the jaw or face, arthritis to the joint **Diagnosis:** Physical examination and review of physical symptoms **Tx:** Mouth guard worn at night to reduce clenching, painkillers, muscle relaxants	**Red Flags:** **Refer to GP for further assessment if treatment ineffective.**
Whiplash *Neck injury caused by forceful and rapid back and forth movement of the head often during car crashes* **Ssx:** Headache, nausea, vomiting, sore stiff neck, inability to move neck, fatigue, dizziness, tenderness to upper shoulders and arms **TCM Illness:** Strained Neck (luo zhen)	**Causes:** Traumatic events such as automotive accidents, physical abuse, contact sports **Diagnosis:** Physical examination, test of motion and reflexes, head CT/MRI to rule out further damage **Tx:** Rest is biggest one, pain medications, muscle relaxants	**Red Flags:** **Call 911 immediately if neurological symptoms.**
Upper Extremities*		
Frozen shoulder *Adhesive capsulitis - gradual stiffness and pain in the shoulder joint* **Ssx:** 'Freezing stage' - Any movement of your shoulder causes pain; range of motion starts to become limited. 'Frozen stage' - Pain may begin to diminish during this stage but joint becomes stiffer, more and more difficult to use. 'Thawing stage'. The range of motion in your shoulder begins to improve. **TCM Illness:** Frozen Shoulder (jian	**Causes:** The joint capsule of the shoulder thickens and tightens around the components of the joint **Diagnosis:** Review of physical symptoms and examination **Tx:** Painkillers, steroid injections to reduce inflammation, physical therapy	**Red Flags:** **Refer to GP for further assessment if treatment**

guan jie zhou wei yan)		ineffective.
Bicipital Tendinitis *Inflammation of the tendon connecting the biceps to the bones of the upper arm* **Ssx:** Shoulder pain, loss of function, dull ache, stiffness **TCM Illness: Impediment Syndrome (bi zheng)**	**Causes:** Repetitive motions of competitive sports, normal aging process/wear and tear **Diagnosis:** Physical examination and review of symptoms **Tx:** Reduce inflammation and pain - rest, ice, compression, anti-inflammatories, over the counter painkillers, worst case scenario surgery to repair tendon	**Red Flags:** **Refer to GP for further assessment if treatment ineffective.**
Carpal Tunnel Syndrome *Pinched median nerve in the wrist causing pain in the wrist and hands (esp. thumb, index and ring finger).* **Ssx:** Pain to hands, wrists and fingers, numbness or tingling, weakness to wrist, worse at night **TCM Illness: Carpal Tunnel Syndrome (wan guan zong he zheng)**	**Causes:** Repetitive motions, wrist injuries **Diagnosis:** Physical examination, review of symptoms, X-ray to rule out bone damage **Tx:** Corticosteroids to reduce inflammation, over the counter pain killers, wrist splints to reduce nerve pinching, carpal tunnel surgery	**Red Flags:** **Refer to GP for further assessment if treatment ineffective.**
Epicondylitis *Tennis elbow - tendons in elbow become irritated and inflamed due to overuse* **Ssx:** Pain to elbow, forearm and wrist, difficulty turning doorknob/opening jars **TCM Illness: Tennis Elbow (hong gu wai shang ke yan)**	**Causes:** Repetitive wrist and hand motions **Diagnosis:** Review of physical symptoms and physical exam **Tx:** Resting the joint, corticosteroid injections, painkillers	**Red Flags:** **Refer to GP for further assessment if treatment ineffective.**
Lower Extremities***		
Meniscal Injury *Injury to the meniscus cartilage in the knee resulting in bone on bone motion* **Ssx:** Pain to outside or inside of knee joint, feeling of joint grinding, difficulties with balancing/stabilizing knee **TCM Illness: Meniscal Injury (ban yue ban sun shang)**	**Causes:** Twisting or turning suddenly, contact sports, trauma to knee **Diagnosis:** Physical tests by physicians, MRI to confirm, McMurray test **Tx:** Rest, ice, compression, elevation, physical therapy, surgery to repair	**Red Flags:** **Refer to GP for further assessment if treatment ineffective.**
Compartment Syndrome *Condition in which excessive pressure builds up inside an enclosed tissue space, stopping the flow of blood to the area and if left untreated leads to death of the tissues*	**Causes:** Crush injuries, burns, too tight of bandages, blood vessel surgery, prolonged compression during period of unconsciousness **Diagnosis:** Review of history and physical symptoms, measurement	**Red Flags:**

Ssx: New onset of dull ache and pain within a muscle group that doesn't go away, numbness/pins and needles to area, swelling, tightness and bruising *'Compartment built in area, not allowing anything in = necrosis'* **TCM Illness: Impediment Syndrome (bi zheng)**	of internal pressure using specialized needle **Tx:** Removal of constricting dressing/splint, most acute cases require emergency surgery to perform fasciotomy (cutting through skin and fascia to release pressure)	**Refer to ER immediately if severe.**
Sciatica *Pain that radiates along the sciatic nerve (lower back through hips and buttock)* **Ssx:** Sharp or radiating pain to lower back, hips, leg and buttocks, typically affects just one side of the body **TCM Illness: Impediment Syndrome (bi zheng), maybe Piriformis Syndrome (li zhuang ji zong he zhang)**	**Causes:** Pinched nerves, bone spurs within the spinal cavity, herniated discs, tight piriformis muscle **Diagnosis:** X-ray, MRI and CT scan to confirm diagnosis, review of symptoms **Tx:** Anti-inflammatories, muscle relaxants, narcotic painkillers, steroid injections, surgery on herniated disc if applicable	**Red Flags:** **Refer to GP for further assessment if treatment ineffective.**
Low Back Pain *Chronic unresolved pain to the lower back* **Ssx:** Dull radiating pain to lower back, can spread to hips and buttocks **TCM Illness: Could be Lumbar Muscle Sprain (yao bu lao sun) or Prolapse of Lumbar Intervertbral Disc (yao zhui jian pan tu chu zheng)**	**Causes:** Innumerable different causes, herniated discs, arthritis, spinal stenosis, trauma, birth abnormalities, soft tissue injuries, nerve damage **Diagnosis:** Review of symptoms, CT, MRI and X-ray to determine cause **Tx:** Dependent on the cause, often painkillers or muscle relaxants	**Red Flags:** **Refer to GP for further assessment if treatment ineffective.**
Bone Disorders *General term for any abnormalities to the bones* **Ssx:** Bone pain, weakness, easily breakable bones, joint pain, visible abnormalities **TCM Illness: Possible Bone Fracture (gu zhe)**	**Causes:** Cancer, decreased density, arthritis, osteoporosis, various other bone diseases **Diagnosis:** X-ray, CT, MRI, blood tests, physical examination **Tx:** Will depend on the cause	**Red Flags:** **Refer to GP for further assessment.**
Fractures *Partial or complete break to the bone* **Ssx:** Pain and large lump to the area, protruding bone (extreme cases), swelling and bruising to the area, inability to bear weight	**Causes:** Trauma such as a fall, accident, contact sports **Diagnosis:** Confirmed by x-ray **Tx:** Cast/splint for 4-6 weeks to immobilize	**Red Flags:**

TCM Illness: Bone Fracture (gu zhe)		**Refer to ER immediately.**
Osteogenic Sarcoma *Cancer of the bones that starts in the end of the bones where new growth starts, common in teenagers* **Ssx:** Bone pain, bone fractures, swelling, redness and loss of function, can be easily confused with 'growing pains' **TCM Illness: Bone Fracture (gu zhe), Impediment Syndrome (bi zheng)**	**Causes:** Unknown cause, as with every cancer. Gene mutation that results in uncontrolled cell growth **Diagnosis:** MRI, CT scan, X-ray, Bone scan to confirm **Tx:** Chemotherapy, radiation, surgery when possible	**Red Flags:** **Refer to GP ASAP for further assessment.**
Osteoporosis*** *Condition in which the bones are extremely brittle, break easily* **Ssx:** Easy fracture, back pain, stooped posture, Dowager's hump **TCM Illness: Bone Fracture (gu zhe)**	**Causes:** Dietary restrictions (calcium), low bone mass/density, sedentary lifestyle, excessive alcohol consumption **Diagnosis:** Bone density test, x-ray **Tx:** Increased calcium intake or supplements, reducing risks of falls, osteoporosis specific medication such as Actonel, Atelvia	**Red Flags:** **Refer to GP for further assessment.**

Neurological Conditions

i. **General Pathophysiology:**

- Tinnitus - ringing in the ears
- Bradykinesia - slowed movement

ii. Common Western Tests:

- Electronystagmography (ENG) - Detect abnormal eye movement, can help determine if dizziness is due to inner ear disease by measuring involuntary eye movements while your head is placed in different positions or your balance organs are stimulated with water or air.

- Electromyogram (EMG) – Needle electrode into various muscles to determine a muscle or nerve condition
- Magnetic Resonance Imaging (MRI) – Uses radio waves and a powerful magnetic field to produce detailed images of brain and spinal cord.
- Muscle Biopsy – A small portion of muscle is removed and sent to a lab for analysis (local anaesthesia used)
- Spinal Tap (Lumbar puncture) – A small needle inserted between 2 vertebrae in low back to remove a sample of cerebrospinal fluid
- Glasgow Coma Scale - 15- point test a doctor or other emergency medical personnel uses to assess the initial severity of a brain injury by checking a person's ability to follow directions and move their eyes and limbs
- Electroencephalogram (EEG) - Electrodes attached to the scalp with a paste-like substance. The electrodes record the electrical activity of your brain.

iii. **General Red Flags:**
- Increased forgetfulness
- Changes in personality
- Loss of memory (short term or long term)
- Depression
- Facial droop or difficulty speaking
- Sudden and severe headache
- Vision changes

Common Diseases + Specific Red Flags

Condition Symptoms and signs Related TCM Illness	Causes & Diagnostic tests	Red flags (and what to do about them)
Alzheimer's* *Degenerative neurological disorder that affects behaviour, thinking, and memory* **Ssx:** Increased forgetfulness, impaired memory, repeating questions, distrust in others, personality changes **TCM Illness:** None that match	**Causes:** Unknown cause, may be environmental and/or genetic influences **Diagnosis:** Review of physical symptoms, head MRI/CT to confirm damage **Tx:** There is no treatment, some drugs slow the progression, family support and education	**Red Flags:** **Refer to GP for further assessment.**

Concussion & Traumatic Brain Injury *An external mechanical force causes brain dysfunction, usually from a violent blow or jolt to the head or body, or object that penetrates the skull.* *Can have lifelong effects to personality, mobility and wellbeing* **Ssx:** LOC, headache, nausea vomiting, seizures, slurred speech, coma, brain death **TCM Illness: Headache (tou tong)**	**Causes:** Violent blow to the head or body, penetration injury, bleeding in or around the brain **Diagnosis:** Head CT/MRI, Glasgow coma scale, intracranial pressure monitoring **Tx:** Dependent on the cause, mild injury is rest and pain medications, moderate to severe focuses on maintaining oxygenation to the body, reducing amount of damage done, preserving life	**Red Flags:** **Any head injury should be referred to ER immediately** **Increased in headache, sudden severe head pain, or changes to consciousness in person suffering from concussion should be referred to ER immediately**
Dementia* *Progressive neurovascular disease characterized by problems with reasoning, planning, judgment, memory and other thought processes caused by brain damage* **Ssx:** Confusion, trouble paying attention and concentrating, reduced ability to organize thoughts or actions, decline in ability to analyze a situation, develop an effective plan and communicate that plan to others, difficulty deciding what to do next, problems with memory, restlessness and agitation, unsteady gait, sudden or frequent urge to urinate or inability to control passing urine **TCM Illness: None that match**	**Causes:** Exact cause unknown, could be due to lack of blood flow to brain, genetic influences, environmental influences **Diagnosis:** No specific tests, confirmation from physical symptoms **Tx:** Some drugs slow the progression, family support and education	**Red Flags:** **Refer to GP for further assessment.**
Epilepsy* *Neurological disorder (central nervous system) where nerve cell activity in the brain becomes disrupted, causing seizures or periods of unusual behaviour, sensations and sometimes loss of consciousness* **Ssx:** Temporary confusion A staring spell, Uncontrollable jerking movements of the arms and legs, Loss of consciousness or awareness, Psychic symptoms **TCM Illness: Epilepsy (xian zheng)**	**Causes:** Genetic influence, brain tumours or conditions, prenatal injuries, infectious diseases **Diagnosis:** EEG, review of physical symptoms, CT/MRI scan **Tx:** Antiepileptic medications (anti seizures), explorative surgery	**Red Flags:** **Call 911 immediately if severe.**

Guillain-Barre Syndrome *Rare autoimmune disorder in which the body attacks normal, healthy nerve cells of the peripheral nervous system, eventually leaving the person paralyzed* **Ssx:** Weakness, numbness and tingling to the extremities, Prickling, "pins and needles" sensations in fingers, toes, ankles or wrists Weakness in legs that spreads to upper body, Unsteady walking or inability to walk or climb stairs, Difficulty with eye or facial movements, including speaking, chewing or swallowing, Severe pain that may feel achy or cramp-like and may be worse at night, Difficulty with bladder control or bowel function, Rapid heart rate **TCM Illness: Atrophy-flaccidity (wei zheng)**	**Causes:** Unknown cause, often precedes an upper respiratory tract or digestive tract infection **Diagnosis:** Can be extremely difficult to diagnose, review of symptoms, Electromyography, Nerve conduction studies **Tx:** There is no cure, immunoglobulin therapy, physical therapy, supportive care	**Red Flags:** **Refer to GP ASAP for further assessment.**
Headaches (cluster, tension, sinus, trauma, migraines)*** **Ssx:** **Cluster** - headaches that occur in a cyclic pattern characterized by extreme and sudden pain, often in the night, chronic and recurrent with periods of remission, unknown cause **Tension** - generally a diffuse, mild to moderate pain in your head that's often described as feeling like a tight band around the head, most common and unknown cause **Sinus** - headaches caused by increased pressure in the sinuses, usually caused by sinus infections **Trauma** - headache caused by trauma to the head and/or neck **Migraine** – photophobia, nausea, sees aura/halo, vomiting, one-sided pain, throbbing/pulsating, phonophobia **TCM Illness: Headache (tou tong)**	**Causes:** See previous column **Diagnosis:** Review of physical symptoms, head CT/MRI to rule out underlying cause **Tx:** Painkillers, migraine medications, avoidance of triggers, unfortunately no cure	**Red Flags:** An abrupt, severe headache, headache with a fever, nausea or vomiting, a stiff neck, mental confusion, seizures, numbness, or speaking difficulties, headache after a head injury, even if it's a minor fall or bump, especially if it worsens **Refer to ER immediately if above symptoms present.**

Meniere's Disease Ssx: TCM Illness:	Causes: Diagnosis: Tx:	Red Flags: Refer to GP for further assessment if treatment ineffective.
Multiple Sclerosis (MS)* Ssx: TCM Illness:	Causes: Diagnosis: Tx:	Red Flags: Refer to GP for further assessment.

Neurosis *A relatively mild mental illness that is not caused by organic disease, involving symptoms of stress (depression, anxiety, obsessive behaviour, hypochondria) but not a radical loss of touch with reality* **Symptoms:** Sadness or depression, anger, irritability, mental confusion, low sense of self-worth, etc., behavioural symptoms such as phobic avoidance, vigilance, impulsive and compulsive acts, lethargy **TCM Illness: May be Depression (yu zheng)**	**Causes:** Unknown cause, as with many mental illnesses **Diagnosis:** Review of physical symptoms, use of DSM5 to confirm **Tx:** Treatment of the effects - is different with every person, avoidance of triggers, cognitive behavioural therapy	**Red Flags:** **Watch for any signs of becoming a danger to themselves or others.** **Refer to GP/counselling if you see these signs.**
Parkinson's Disease** Ssx: TCM Illness:	**Causes:** **Diagnosis:** **Tx:**	**Red Flags:** **Refer to GP for further assessment.**
Radiculopathies (nerve root, sciatica*** *Condition of compressed spinal nerve causing severe back pain* **Ssx:** Pain, numbness, tingling along back and buttocks into legs, weakness and muscle fatigue in the extremities **TCM Illness: May be under Prolapse of Lumbar Intervertebral Disc (yao zhui jian pan tu chu zheng)**	**Causes:** Mechanical compression, build-up of fluid, bone spurs, tumour or infection **Diagnosis:** Spinal MRI/CT **Tx:** Chiropractic treatment, surgical removal of mechanical compression, pain killers, muscle relaxants	**Red Flags:** **Refer to GP for further assessment if treatment ineffective.**
Seizures (4 kinds) **Focal -** Seizure activity is limited to a part of one brain hemisphere. There	**Causes:** Epilepsy genetic influence, brain tumours or conditions, prenatal injuries, infectious diseases	**Red Flags:** **The seizure lasts more than five minutes, Breathing or**

is a site, or a focus, in the brain where the seizure begins and symptoms will depend on which area (twitching, vision changes, emotional distress)

Absence (petit mal) - Epileptic activity occurs throughout the entire brain, milder type of activity that causes unconsciousness without convulsions. After the seizure, the person has no memory of it. Usually lasting only two to 10 seconds. There is no confusion after the seizure

Convulsive (grand mal) - Electric discharges instantaneously involve the entire brain. The person loses consciousness immediately, lasts one to three minutes, but may last up to five minutes muscles will stiffen, Increased pressure on the bladder and bowel may cause incontinence, extremities will then jerk and twitch rhythmically

Atonic - Abruptly loses consciousness, collapses and falls to the floor. There is no convulsion, but may hit their heads as they fall, regains consciousness several seconds after and can stand and walk again.

TCM Illness: Epilepsy (xian zheng) or Convulsive Syndromes (jin zheng)

	Diagnosis: EEG, review of physical symptoms, CT/MRI scan **Tx:** Antiepileptic medications (anti seizures), explorative surgery	consciousness doesn't return after the seizure stops, A second seizure follows immediately **Call 911 immediately if above symptoms present.**

Sleep Disorders*** (3)

Narcolepsy *Chronic sleep disorder characterized by overwhelming daytime drowsiness and sudden attacks of sleep.* **Ssx:** Suddenly falling asleep, difficulty staying awake for long periods of time, sudden loss of muscle tone, extreme daytime sleepiness **TCM Illness: None that match**	**Causes:** Unknown cause, could be due to low levels of the chemical hypocretin - an important neurochemical in your brain that helps regulate wakefulness and REM sleep. **Diagnosis:** Sleep history, sleep record, review of symptoms **Tx:** Stimulants, antidepressants have shown good effects	**Red Flags:** **Refer to GP for further assessment.**
Sleep Apnea *Condition in which a person continually ceases to breath while*	**Causes:** can be: Obstructive - muscles in the throat relax and close off airway	**Red Flags:**

asleep **Ssx:** Loud snoring interrupted by silent spells, abrupt awakening with shortness of breath, waking up with dry mouth and sore throat, morning headache, excessive sleepiness during the day, pauses in breathing during sleep **TCM Illness: None that match**	momentarily Central - brain isn't sending proper signals to muscles that control breathing or Complex - emergent treatment needed as person has combination of two above described conditions Obesity **Diagnosis:** Sleep log/monitoring, Nocturnal polysomnography - monitors heart, lung and brain activity, breathing patterns, arm and leg movements, and blood oxygen levels while you sleep. **Tx:** CPAP - continuous positive airway pressure device keeps airways open overnight, lifestyle changes (improved diet and decreased weight)	**Refer to GP for further assessment.**
Insomnia *Common sleep disorder that makes it difficult to fall, or stay asleep* **Ssx:** Difficulty falling asleep at night, waking up too early, not feeling well-rested after a night's sleep, daytime tiredness or sleepiness, Irritability, depression or anxiety, difficulty paying attention, focusing on tasks or remembering, Increased errors or accidents, ongoing worries about sleep **TCM Illness: Insomnia (bu mei)**	**Causes:** Stress, work or travel schedule, poor sleep habits, side effect of medications, mental illness, caffeine or alcohol dependence **Diagnosis:** Review of symptoms and history, sleep log/monitoring **Tx:** Sleep aids such as zopiclone, melatonin, improve sleep habits (limit caffeine and alcohol consumption, no electronics 1 hour before bed etc.)	**Red Flags:** **Refer to GP for further assessment if treatment ineffective.**
Trigeminal Neuralgia** **Ssx:** **TCM Illness:**	**Causes:** **Diagnosis:** **Tx:**	**Red Flags:** **Refer to GP for further assessment if treatment ineffective.**

| Vertigo**
Sensation of dizziness or falling - loss of balance and can cause motion sickness

Ssx: Dizziness, a sense that you or your surroundings are spinning or moving, loss of balance or unsteadiness, nausea, vomiting

TCM Illness: Vertigo (xuan yin) | **Causes:** Inner ear disorders are the most common cause

Diagnosis: Review of symptoms and triggers, ENG tests, MRI

Tx: Canalith repositioning procedure consists of several simple and slow manoeuvres for positioning your head to move particles from the fluid-filled semicircular canals of the inner ear | **Red Flags:**

Refer to GP for further assessment if treatment ineffective. |

Oncology

i. **General Pathophysiology:**

   Definitions:

   - NEOPLASM: A new and abnormal growth of tissue in some part of the body, especially as a characteristic of cancer
   - NEOPLASTIC: Relating to a neoplasm or neoplasia

ii. **Common Western Tests:**
   - Magnetic Resonance Imaging (MRI) – Uses radio waves and a powerful magnetic field to produce detailed images of brain and spinal cord.
   - Muscle/Tissue Biopsy – A small portion of muscle is removed and sent to a lab for analysis (local anaesthesia used)
   - Ultrasound - High-frequency sound waves to produce images of structures within your body.
   - CT scan - Combines a series of X-ray images taken from different angles and uses computer processing to create cross-sectional images, or slices, of the bones, blood vessels and soft tissues inside your body.
   - Tumour Marker Blood Tests – Tumour markers found in high concentrations when cancer is present. Most are proteins and there is a large variety.

iii. **General Red Flags:**
   - Unexplained weight loss
   - Fatigue
   - Skin discoloration/rash development
   - Difficulty urinating/change in bowel patterns
   - Palpable lumps

Common Diseases + Specific Red Flags

Condition **Symptoms and signs** **Related TCM Illness**	**Causes & Diagnostic tests**	Red flags (and what to do about them)
Breast* Ssx: TCM Illness:	Causes: Diagnosis: Tx:	**Red Flags:** **Refer to GP ASAP for further assessment.**

Bone* Ssx: TCM Illness:	Causes: Diagnosis: Tx:	Red Flags: **Refer to GP ASAP for further assessment.**
Cervical* Ssx: TCM Illness:	Causes: Diagnosis: Tx:	Red Flags: **Refer to GP ASAP for further assessment.**
Colon* Ssx:	Causes: Diagnosis:	Red Flags:

TCM Illness:	Tx:	Refer to GP ASAP for further assessment.
Liver* (Hepatic Carcinoma) Ssx: TCM Illness:	Causes: Diagnosis: Tx:	Red Flags: Refer to GP ASAP for further assessment.
Lung* Ssx: TCM Illness:	Causes: Diagnosis: Tx:	Red Flags: Refer to GP ASAP for further assessment.
Pancreas*	Causes:	Red Flags:

Ssx: **TCM Illness:**	**Diagnosis:** **Tx:**	Refer to GP ASAP for further assessment.
Prostate* **Ssx:** **TCM Illness:**	**Causes:** **Diagnosis:** **Tx:**	**Red Flags:** Refer to GP ASAP for further assessment.
Stomach* **Ssx:**	**Causes:** **Diagnosis:**	**Red Flags:**

TCM Illness:	Tx:	Refer to GP ASAP for further assessment.
Uterine* (Endometrial Carcinoma) Ssx: TCM Illness:	Causes: Diagnosis: Tx:	Red Flags: Refer to GP ASAP for further assessment.

Respiratory Conditions

i. **General Pathophysiology:**

- Emphysema - Lung disease causes destruction of the fragile walls and elastic fibres of the alveoli. Small airways collapse when you exhale, impairing airflow out of your lungs
- Dyspnea - Difficulty breathing
- Tachypnea - Rapid breathing
- Hypopnea - Shallow breathing
- Hyperpnoea - Deep breathing
- Apnea - Absence of breathing
- Orthopnea – Difficulty breathing while lying flat

ii. **Common Western Tests:**

- Spirometry - Estimates the narrowing of your bronchial tubes by checking how much air you can exhale after a deep breath and how fast you can breathe out.
- Peak flow - Simple device that measures how hard you can breathe out. Lower than usual peak flow readings are a sign your lungs may not be working as well and that your asthma may be getting worse.
- Pulmonary function test - Patient blows into a spirometer, which measures how much air the lungs can hold and how quickly you can get air out of your lungs
- Arterial blood gas analysis. This blood test measures how well your lungs are bringing oxygen into your blood and removing carbon dioxide.
- Pulse oximetry - Measures the oxygen level in your blood (clip on finger that shines light through to detect amount of O2 present in blood)

iii. General Red Flags:

- Difficulty breathing
- Prolonged cough/cold like symptoms
- Wheezing
- Chest tightness
- Large amount of secretions/inability to clear respiratory tract

Common Diseases + Specific Red Flags

Condition / Symptoms and signs / Related TCM Illness	Causes & Diagnostic tests	Red flags (and what to do about them)
Allergies*** Ssx: TCM Illness:	Causes: Diagnosis: Tx:	Red Flags: Refer to GP for further assessment if treatment ineffective.
Asthma (Intrinsic/Extrinsic)*** *Marked by spasms in the bronchi of the lungs, causing difficult breathing. Extrinsic = allergic. Intrinsic = non-allergic* Ssx: Cough, increased mucus, hypoxia, tachycardia, restless, tachypnea, SOB, chest tightness, increased CO2 retention, wheezing & prolonged expiration TCM Illness: Asthma (xiao chuan)	Causes: Hypersensitivity, exercise, air pollutants, resp. infections, GERD, familial Diagnosis: Respiratory function tests, peak flow and spirometry Tx: Various inhaled medications - puffers. Routine puffers to control symptoms and 'rescue' puffers for asthma attacks	Red Flags: If patient does not respond to treatment or attack worsens, send to ER.
Bronchitis (Acute/Chronic)*** *Inflammation of the mucous membrane in the bronchial tubes. Often causes bronchospasm,*	Causes: Viral or bacterial infections, smoking, air pollution or other environmental influences	Red Flags:

increased mucous and cough. Chronic bronchitis under the term 'COPD'. **Ssx:** <u>Chronic</u>: 'Blue Bloater' (means more bronchitis underneath): cyanotic, recurrent cough and increased sputum, hypoxia, respiratory acidosis, increased haemoglobin and resp. rate, exertional dyspnea, digital clubbing <u>Acute</u>: Painful cough, coughing up mucous, wheezing, SOB, fever, chest discomfort. Usually lasts a few to 10 days. *'Bronchitis = blue bloater – big sputum and barking cough'* **TCM Illness: Cough (ke shou), Lung Distention (fei zhang)**	**Diagnosis:** Lung function test, sputum sample, chest x ray **Tx:** Antibiotics, cough medicine, inhalers if asthma present	**Refer to GP for further assessment if treatment ineffective.**
Common Cold *Viral infection of nose and throat* **Ssx:** Runny or stuffy nose, sore throat, cough, congestion, Slight body aches or a mild headache, sneezing, low-grade fever, generally feeling unwell **TCM Illness: Common Cold (gan mao)**	**Causes:** Viral infection - constantly mutating so impossible to predict or prevent **Diagnosis:** Review of physical symptoms, possible blood test if persistent to rule out infection **Tx:** No treatment, over the counter pain killers for ease, decongestants, cough medicine	**Red Flags:** **Refer to GP for further assessment if treatment ineffective.**
COPD (Chronic Obstructive Pulmonary Disease)** *Chronic obstruction of LU airflow that interferes with normal breathing and is not fully reversible. Also called a 'Pink Puffer' meaning more emphysema sxs (used to be the same names as chronic bronchitis and emphysema). More destruction of airways distal to terminal bronchioles therefore decreased O2 in blood.* **Ssx**: Easily fatigued, freq. respiratory infections, using accessory muscles to breathe, othopnea, wheezing, pursed-lip breathing, chronic cough, barrel chest, dyspnea, prolonged expiratory time, increased sputum, digital clubbing, cor pulmonale in later stages *'COPD – Pink Puffer – Pretty fatigued*	**Causes:** Most common cause is smoking - upper airway damage, emphysema, chronic bronchitis, environmental factors (inhaled pollutants) **Diagnosis:** Lung function tests, chest CT, x-ray, blood gas analysis, blood tests **Tx:** Quitting smoking, bronchodilators, inhaled or oral steroid to reduce inflammation, oxygen therapy, pulmonary rehab	**Red Flags:**

and poor breathing" **TCM Illness: Cough (ke shou), Consumptive Disease (xu lao), Wheezing Syndrome (xiao zheng), Watery Phlegm/Sputum (tai yin), Lung Distention (fei zhang)**		**Refer to GP for further assessment.**
Flu **Ssx:** **TCM Illness:**	**Causes:** **Diagnosis:** **Tx:**	**Red Flags:** **Refer to GP for further assessment if treatment ineffective.**
Lung Cancer (Primary Broncopulmonary Carcinoma) *Cancer of the tissues and cells of the lung One of the leading causes of cancer related deaths* **Ssx:** New cough that doesn't go away, changes in a chronic cough or "smoker's cough", coughing up blood, even a small amount, shortness of breath, chest pain, wheezing and hoarseness, unexplained weight loss and fatigue, bone pain, headache, finger clubbing **TCM Illness: Consumptive Disease (xu lao), Wheezing Sydrome (xiao zheng)**	**Causes:** Smoking is primary cause of lung cancers, can also occur for no reason (genetic mutation that causes uncontrolled cell growth) **Diagnosis:** Chest x-ray or CT, sputum cytology, lung tissue biopsy **Tx:** Chemotherapy, radiation, surgical removal, lung transplant	**Red Flags:** **Refer to GP ASAP for further assessment.**
Pleurisy *Condition in which the pleura (membrane consisting of a layer of tissue that lines the inner side of the chest cavity and a layer of tissue that surrounds the lungs) becomes inflamed* **Ssx:** Sharp chest pain, difficulty breathing/moving air in and out of lungs, pain to shoulders and upper back *'Think icicle'*	**Causes:** Viral, bacterial or fungal infection, rib fractures, certain medications, side effect of lung cancer **Diagnosis:** Blood tests to determine origin of infection, chest x-ray, ultrasound or CT, electrocardiogram to rule out cardiac conditions **Tx:** Antibiotics/antivirals, treatment of the underlying cause	**Red Flags:**

TCM Illness: Chest Impediment (xiong bi)		Refer to ER for further assessment
Pneumonia*** *Lung inflammation caused by bacterial or viral infection, in which the air sacs fill with pus and may become solid. Inflammation may affect both lungs* **Ssx:** Chest pain when you breathe or cough, confusion or changes in mental awareness (in adults age 65 and older), cough, which may produce phlegm, fatigue, fever, sweating (including night sweats) and shaking chills, nausea, vomiting or diarrhea, SOB **TCM Illness: Chest Impediment (xiong bi), Cough (ke shou)**	**Causes:** Viral - Common cause of pneumonia, caused by viral infections, usually no treatment is necessary Pneumococcal - Streptococcus pneumoniae bacterial infection that enters lungs and causes pneumonia Staphylococcal - Caused by staphylococcal bacteria, can often be antibiotic resistant, making treatment difficult Fungal - People with cancers/HIV (immunocompromised) are at highest risk, least common type of pneumonia -Cold/flu or lying down for long periods **Diagnosis:** Chest x-ray, blood C&S, pulse oximetry, sputum analysis **Tx:** Antibiotics, antifungals, dependent on the cause	**Red Flags:** **Refer to GP ASAP for further assessment (or ER if severe).**
Pneumothorax*** *Collapsed lung occurs when air leaks into the space between the lung and chest wall. This air pushes on the outside of your lung and makes it collapse* **Ssx:** Sudden chest pain and shortness of breath, often following blunt force injury **TCM Illness: Chest Impediment (xiong bi)**	**Causes:** Blunt or penetrating chest injury, certain medical procedures, or damage from underlying lung disease, or no obvious reason. **Diagnosis:** Chest x-ray **Tx:** Aspiration of air using needle or chest tube insertion, in severe cases surgery to correct lung placement	**Red Flags:** **Refer to ER for further assessment**
Strep Throat *Streptococcal pharyngitis, an infection of the back of the throat including the tonsils caused by group A streptococcus* **Ssx:** Fever, sore throat, swollen tonsils with red spots or pus, enlarged lymph nodes, fever, chills, muscle aches, difficulty swallowing	**Causes:** Bacterial infection from group A streptococcus **Diagnosis:** Swabs of throat, physical examination, blood tests **Tx:** Antibiotics, over the counter painkillers for headaches/pain	**Red Flags:** **Refer to GP for further assessment**

TCM Illness: Dysphagia		
TB (Pulmonary Tuberculosis) Ssx: TCM Illness:	Causes: Diagnosis: Tx:	Red Flags: Refer to ER for further assessment – REPORTABLE.

Miscellaneous

i. **General Pathophysiology:**
Too broad to add in

ii. **Common Western Tests:**

- Enzyme-linked immunosorbent assay (ELISA) test - The test used most often to detect Lyme disease, ELISA detects antibodies to B. burgdorferi
- Western blot test - Detects antibodies to antibodies of several chronic conditions (Lyme disease, HIV)
- Erythrocyte sedimentation rate — Commonly referred to as the sed rate. Blood test that measures how quickly red blood cells fall to the bottom of a tube of blood. Red cells that drop rapidly may indicate inflammation in your body

iii. **General Red Flags**
- Unexplained weight loss
- Sudden, severe headache
- Unexplained rash
- General feeling unwell
- Fever

Common Diseases + Specific Red Flags

Condition **Symptoms and signs** Related TCM Illness	**Causes & Diagnostic tests**	**Red flags (and what to do about them)**
Autoimmune Disorders**		
Systemic Lupus Erythematosus, (SLE) **Ssx:** **TCM Illness:**	**Causes:** **Diagnosis:** **Tx:**	**Red Flags:** **Refer to GP for further assessment.**
RA – Rheumatoid Arthritis **Ssx:** **TCM Illness:**	**Causes:** **Diagnosis:** **Tx:**	**Red Flags:** **Refer to GP for further assessment.**
Multi-System Conditions**		
Lyme Disease *An inflammatory disease characterized at first by a rash, headache, fever, and chills, and later by possible arthritis and neurological and cardiac disorders, caused by bacteria that are transmitted by ticks* **Ssx:** Rash following tick bite, flu like symptoms, Erythema-migrans (expanding ring of unraised redness with an outer ring of brighter	**Causes:** Infected by bites from ticks carrying the bacteria Borrelia burgdorferi, Borrelia mayonii, Borrelia afzelii or Borrelia garinii bacteria **Diagnosis:** ELISA test, western blot test **Tx:** Oral antibiotics	**Red Flags:**

redness and a central area of clearing), flu-like sxs (all early stage) *'Kill the tick with a lime and you get a lime-shaped red patch'* **TCM Illness: Consumptive Disease (xu lao)**		**Refer to ER or GP for further assessment.**
Chronic Fatigue Syndrome *Disorder characterized by extreme fatigue that can't be explained by any underlying medical condition. The fatigue may worsen with physical or mental activity, but doesn't improve with rest.* **Ssx:** Fatigue, loss of memory or difficulty concentration, sore throat, enlarged lymph nodes in your neck or armpits, unexplained muscle pain, pain that moves from one joint to another without swelling or redness, headache of a new type, pattern or severity, unrefreshing sleep, extreme exhaustion lasting more than 24 hours after physical or mental exercise **TCM Illness: Consumptive Disease (xu lao)**	**Causes:** Unknown, could be due to viral infections or psychological stress, hormone imbalances **Diagnosis:** No specific test, usually confirmed by presence of previously listed symptoms and various blood/physical tests to rule out different medical causes **Tx:** Antidepressants, sleeping aids, psychological counselling	**Red Flags:** **Refer to GP for further assessment.**
Fibromyalgia **Ssx:** **TCM Illness:**	**Causes:** **Diagnosis:** **Tx:**	**Red Flags:** **Refer to GP for further assessment.**
Temporal Arteritis *"Giant cell arteritis" inflammation of the lining of your arteries. Most often, it affects the arteries in the head, especially those in the temples* **Ssx:** Headaches, scalp tenderness, jaw pain and vision problems, if untreated can lead to stroke and vision loss	**Causes:** Unknown cause, Certain genes and gene variations may increase your susceptibility to the condition **Diagnosis:** Head CT, physical examination, erythrocyte sedimentation rate **Tx:** Heavy and high dosing of corticosteroids to reduce inflammation	**Red Flags:** **Refer to GP ASAP for further**

TCM Illness: Headache (tu tong)		assessment.
Acute poisoning *The negative, adverse effects of a substance that resulted either from a single exposure or from multiple exposures in a short period of time* **Ssx:** Nausea, vomiting, watery diarrhea, abdominal pain and cramps, fever, changes in consciousness, burns or redness around the mouth and lips, Breath that smells like chemicals, such as gasoline or paint thinner *Remember to smell the breath if you suspect poisoning!* **TCM Illness: Vomiting (ou tu), Diarrhea (xie xie), Abdominal Pain (fu tong)**	**Causes:** Chemical, environmental influences, food, ingestion of any harmful substance accidental or purposely **Diagnosis:** Toxicology screen (blood tests) **Tx:** Antidote depending on cause of poisoning	**Red Flags:** If suspected poisoning call poison help line or 911 immediately
Organic Phosphate Insecticide Poisoning *Poisoning due to organophosphates (OPs). -commonly used as insecticides, medications, and nerve agents* **Ssx:** Difficulty breathing or severe respiratory distress, low blood pressure, sweating, incontinence, increased salivation, blurred vision, vomiting **TCM Illness: Vomiting (ou tu), Chest Impediment (xiong bi)**	**Causes:** Ingestion, aspiration or dermal contact of OPs accidentally or purposely (suicidal attempt) **Diagnosis:** Urine and blood toxicology test to confirm **Tx:** Removal of infected clothing, eye irrigation if necessary, atropine to counteract poison, airway management	**Red Flags:** **Difficulty breathing or severe respiratory distress, low blood pressure, sweating, incontinence, increased salivation, blurred vision, vomiting, known or suspected contact with OPs** **Refer to ER or call 911 immediately**

143 TCM Illnesses

Internal Medicine

NOTE: herbal formulas with an Asterix are NOT listed on the CARB-TCMPA exam list, however commonly used none-the-less
*If you are taking your herbal exam as well, please try to fill in the herbal formulas + modifications BEFORE looking to your answer key. This will help you with memorization!

Abdominal Mass (ji ju)

(Note: also known as "aggregation and accumulation" syndrome in some textbooks)

Definition:
Palpable or impalpable abdominal masses accompanied by pain, fullness, or distension. Ji (aggregation) = substantial mass with pain at a fixed location. Disorder of the Blood level and Yin organs. Ju (accumulation) = insubstantial masses with distension greater than pain. Distending pain migrates, and insubstantial mass appears intermittently and unpredictably. Disorder of the Qi level and Yang organs.

Red Flags:
- Western diagnosis is essential for masses. Refer if painful, hard, immoveable, or not improving.
- Presence of jaundice and upper or lower gastrointestinal bleeding indicates worsening of disease.
- Seek emergency help for mass with severe abdominal pain. This could be a sign of a ruptured aortic aneurysm, perforated ulcer, or obstructed bowel.

Western Medicine Relevant Diseases:
- Resembles various benign or malignant abdominal tumors in modern medicine.
- Other relevant diseases: enlarged liver and spleen due to wide range of pathologies, partial bowel obstruction, fecal masses, intestinal disturbances, and cysts.

Etiology and Pathogenesis:
- Emotional stress - constrains liver and disturbs spleen function - impairs blood circulation and transportation and transformation (T&T) fails - blood stasis and phlegm
- Improper diet - greasy, sweet, rich food and alcohol - disturbs spleen and stomach - phlegm forms and obstructs qi and blood (Maciocia says that cold/raw foods may cause contraction, poor Qi and Blood circulation, and can lead to Blood stasis)
- EPI - cold-damp or damp-heat invades and lingers - accumulates as phlegm, forms ju then aggregates to form ji
- Liver pathologies (jaundice, malaria, hypochondriac pain, schistosomiasis/bilharzia) - turbid damp - qi, blood and phlegm accumulate

TCM Differentiation and Treatment:
(Note: based on pathogenesis and clinical manifestations, disease is divided into two types: ji and ju. Stagnant qi forming accumulation, or ju, precedes blood stasis forming aggregation, or ji – Maciocia calls ju "qi masses" and ji "blood masses". Qi masses are much easier to disperse than blood masses. Treatment is always based on moving Qi and Blood; but, in late stage when righteous qi is exhausted, need to primarily focus on supporting righteous qi.

Ju Syndrome

Pattern	Signs and Symptoms	Treatment Principle	Acupuncture	Formula
Liver Qi Stagnation	Movable abdominal masses that come and go, distending abdominal pain, emotional stress aggravates condition, pain or distention in hypochondriac region, alternating constipation and diarrhea. Tongue: thin coat Pulse: wiry	Spread Liver Qi, eliminate stagnation, move Qi and dissolve masses	Principle points:	*You will find all of your formulas in your online course!*
Food Retention and Phlegm Obstruction	Abdominal distension and pain, soft masses (rod-shaped or strip-like prominence), pain with pressure, constipation (or diarrhea), and poor appetite. Tongue: greasy Pulse: wiry and slippery	Guide out accumulation (resolve food retention), regulate bowel, move Qi and transform phlegm	Supplementary:	

© 2017 LIFT Education Academy — www.lifteducation.academy

Ji Syndrome

Pattern	Signs and Symptoms	Treatment Principle	Acupuncture	Formula
Stagnation of Qi and Blood	Abdominal masses, soft and fixed to palpate, distension and pain Tongue: thin coat Pulse: wiry	Move Qi and Blood, reduce aggregation	Principle points:	
Blood Stasis	Substantial abdominal masses, firm and tender/painful on palpation, dusky complexion, emaciation, dry and flaky skin. Tongue: purple with petechiae and thin coat Pulse: thready and choppy	Expel stasis, soften hardness	Supplementary:	
Deficiency of Righteous Qi with pathological aggregation	Chronic, hard masses with excruciating pain, sallow or dark complexion, reduction in food intake, emaciation. Tongue: pale purple without coat Pulse: thready and rapid, or wiry and thready	Strongly tonify Qi and Blood, invigorate Blood, transform stasis		

Abdominal Pain (fu tong)

Definition:
Abdominal (ABD) pain is a common disorder involving unpleasant or painful sensations in the abdominal region (umbilicus to pubic bone). It presents in a wide range of illnesses and does not include surgical or gynecological disorders that might contribute to abdominal pain.

(Note: CTCMA separates into ABD pain/Fu Tong and Epigastric pain/Wei Tong. Also, ABD pain may overlap with other conditions such as diarrhea, constipation, and ABD masses. For Fu Tong, ABD pain is the main presenting symptom. Finally, hypogastric pain is more often of urinary origin, so refer to urinary diseases.)

Red Flags:
Refer immediately in the case of severe ABD pain with shock, collapse (inability to continue with day to day activities), and rigidity, guarding, swelling and rebound tenderness. This may have benign causes, but must rule out serious illnesses such as:

- Acute appendicitis – pain usually starts around umbilicus and goes to right lower abdominal region. Accompanied by nausea and vomiting. Tenderness in the right lower quadrant on McBurney's Point.
- Acute pancreatitis – severe abdominal pain (better with leaning forward) with nausea and vomiting
- Peritonitis -- inflammation of the peritoneal cavity that is very painful and almost always signals a very serious or life-threatening disorder. It can result from any abdominal problem in which the organs are inflamed or infected.
- Bowel obstruction – severe and constant pain in mid-lower abdomen (colicky), swelling/bloating, and inability to pass stool due to intestine partially or fully blocked, vomiting.
- Ruptured ABD aortic aneurism
- Kidney stones (renal calculus) – pain usually starts in one loin and radiates to ABD region/groin. May also radiate to back. Pain is sudden and severe, comes in waves, and may be accompanied by: nausea, vomiting, sweating, even shock.
- Colon cancer - Epigastric pain or dyspepsia for the first time in someone over the age of 50, or resistant to treatment, especially if accompanied by changes in bowel movements, blood, and/or weight loss.
- Helicobacter pylori infection - Epigastric pain or dyspepsia for the first time in someone over the age of 50, or resistant to treatment (requires antibiotic treatment)

Western Medicine Relevant Diseases:
Abdominal pain can arise from many causes, including infection, inflammation, ulcers, perforation or rupture of organs, muscle contractions that are uncoordinated or blocked by an obstruction, and blockage of blood flow to organs. In Western medical diagnosis, the relevant organs involved may be:

- Appendix (see red flags)
- Large intestine
  - Diverticulitis (inflamed protrusions in colon): Pain is unilateral, more often on lower left side, with tenderness, fever, and alternating diarrhea and constipation.
  - Cancer (see red flags)
  - Irritable bowel syndrome: Disorder of the entire digestive tract that causes recurring ABD pain, bloating, gas, constipation or diarrhea. Pain is lateral or diffuse and varies from ache to severe spastic pain. Cause is unclear, but a variety of substances and emotional factors can trigger symptoms.
  - Ulcerative colitis: Chronic, inflammatory bowel disease in which the large intestine becomes inflamed and ulcerated, leading to attacks of bloody diarrhea, ABD cramps, and fever. The exact cause of the disease is unknown.
- Small intestine
  - Crohn's disease: an inflammatory bowel disease, typically involving the small intestine (but may affect any part of the digestive tract). Typical symptoms include chronic diarrhea (sometimes bloody), crampy ABD pain, fever, loss of appetite, and weight loss. The exact cause of the disease is unknown.

Etiology and Pathogenesis:
- EPI invasion – cold, heat or damp-heat can obstruct Qi and Blood flow – this impairs SP T&T function
- Improper diet – overindulgence in greasy, sweet food or raw and cold food causes stagnation and impairs T&T
- Emotions – constrain Liver Qi causing Qi stagnation and blood stasis – Liver Qi can also overact on SP/ST causing pain
- Constitutional Yang Deficiency – internal cold congeals and fails to warm organs – this is a chronic and deficient pain

TCM Differentiation and Treatment:

Pattern	Signs and Symptoms	Treatment Principle	Acupuncture	Formula
	Sudden, urgent onset of severe (usually sharp) pain, better with warmth, no thirst, abundant clear urine, loose stool. Tongue: pale (or light purple) with white coat Pulse: tight	Warm Middle Jiao, disperse cold, stop pain.	REN 8 (shen que), REN 12 (zhong wan) ST34 (liang qiu), ST25 (tian shu), ST36 (ZSL) SP4 (gong sun) P6 (nei guan) (if nausea)	
	Sudden, burning pain, worse with pressure, diarrhea or constipation, irritability, dark scanty urine, thirst, foul breath, sweating/fever. T: yellow greasy coating P: rapid	Clear Heat, harmonize Middle Jiao, stop pain (and drain damp, if needed)	ST25 (tian shu), ST36 (ZSL), ST37 (shang ju xu), ST44 (nei ting) LI4 (he gu), LI11 (qu chi) SP9 (yin ling quan), GB34 (yang ling quan)	
	ABD distention, fullness and pain aggravated by pressure, nausea after meals, loss of appetite, belching, acid regurgitation, diarrhea with undigested food or constipation. Tongue: greasy coat Pulse: slippery	Relieve stagnation/promote digestion. Stop pain.	REN12 (zhong wan) ST25 (tian shu), ST34 (liang qiu), ST36 (ZSL), ST44 (nei ting), LiNeiTing P6 (nei guan) LI4-LV3 (4 gates)	
	Often chronic pain, stabbing and fixed, sharp pain, maybe masses Tongue: purple Pulse: choppy or wiry	Move Qi and Blood. Transform stasis. Stop pain.	ST34 (liang qiu), ST36 (ZSL) REN12 (zhong wan) BL17 (ge shu) SP10 (xue hai) LV3-LI4 (4 gates)	
	Often repeated and chronic, intermittent dull pain, preference for pressure and warmth, aggravated by hunger or exertion, loose stool, tired, cold intolerance, pale complexion Tongue: pale Pulse: deep and thin	Warm and tonify Yang Qi. Stop pain.	ST25 (tian shu), ST36 (ZSL) REN6 (qi hai), REN12 (zhong wan), REN8 (shen que) SP4 (gong sun), SP6 (SYJ) BL20 (pi shu), BL21 (wei shu)	

Atrophy-Flaccidity (wei zheng)

Definition:
Refers to a group of disorders in which the limbs become weak, flaccid, and unresponsive to voluntary motor control. Lower extremities are most often affected resulting in difficult mobility. As the disorder progresses, total loss of mobility may result. Weakness is, generally, without pain.

Red flags:
- Essential for patient to obtain diagnosis from a Western medical specialist to determine type of disease and appropriate treatment. For example,
Guillain-Barré syndrome (see below) can worsen rapidly and is a medical emergency. Establishing the diagnosis is crucial because the sooner appropriate treatment is started, the better the chance of a good outcome.

Western medicine relevant diseases:
Atrophy-Flaccidity patterns may include the following Western medical conditions:
- Guillain-Barré syndrome (acute inflammatory demyelinating polyneuropathy): rapid-onset muscle weakness caused by the immune system damaging the peripheral nervous system. Symptoms usually begin in both legs, and then progress upward to the arms. Occasionally, symptoms begin in the arms or head and progress downward. Symptoms include weakness and a pins-and-needles sensation or loss of sensation. Weakness is more prominent than abnormal sensation. During the acute phase, the disorder can be life-threatening some people developing weakness of the breathing muscles requiring mechanical ventilation.
- Multiple sclerosis: disease resulting in de-mylenation of myelin sheath around spinal cord, brain, and optic nerve. Characterized by remissions and relapse. The cause is unknown but may involve an autoimmune reaction. Symptoms differ based on area affected and range from blurred vision, to limb disorders, problems with urination, etc. In late stages there may be complete paralysis.
- Myasthenia gravis: autoimmune disorder that impairs communication between nerves and muscles, resulting in abnormal fatigue of muscles. First symptoms are weakness when chewing, swallowing, and speaking. People usually have drooping eyelids and double vision, and muscles become unusually tired and weak after exercise.
- Poliomyelitis: highly contagious, sometimes fatal, viral infection that affects nerves and can cause permanent muscle weakness, paralysis, and other symptoms. It is caused by a virus and may be spread by contaminated food, water, or surfaces. Serious symptoms include fever, headache, stiff neck/back, deep muscle pain, respiratory symptoms, and sometimes weakness or paralysis.
- Muscular dystrophy: a group of inherited non-inflammatory, progressive muscle disorders without central or peripheral nerve abnormality. Usually starts within first 3 years of life. The disorders differ in which muscles or organs are affected, the degree of weakness, and how fast they progress. Many people eventually become unable to walk.
- Motor neuron diseases: characterized by progressive deterioration of the nerve cells that initiate muscle movement. Muscles also deteriorate and can no longer function normally, becoming weak and wasting. Movements become stiff, clumsy, and awkward. Amyotrophic lateral sclerosis (Lou Gehrig's disease) is a common form of motor neuron disease.

Etiology and Pathogenesis:
- Lung heat with fluid injury (from exterior attack) – injures fluid and impairs LU dispersing – moisture does not go to sinews and muscles impairing function
- Damp heat invasion (from exterior invasion or improper diet) – accumulation of damp heat obstructs blood and qi flow – weakness and muscle atrophy results
- Spleen and stomach deficiency – impaired T&T function – inadequate Qi and Blood and failure to circulate – lack of nourishment
- Liver and Kidney deficiency (Yin, Marrow, and Qi weak) – LV governs sinews and stores blood, KD governs bones and stores essence that produces marrow to nourish bones – if LV and KD are deficient, sinews and bones cannot be nourished – leads to atrophy syndrome

TCM Differentiation and Treatment:
Note: to treat Wei syndrome, treat yang-ming (brightness) channels and organs (i.e. large intestine and stomach) as they generate and are the source of qi and blood. Also, treat spleen as spleen governs muscles and provides them with nourishment.

Differential DX of similar disorders is important. Atrophy Syndrome, painful obstruction syndrome, and wind-stroke all involve pathologies of the extremities, as follows:
- Atrophy syndrome is characterized by weakness and flaccidity of extremities and atrophy of muscles and leads to loss of function. Pain is not common.
- Painful obstruction syndrome is marked by soreness, pain, heaviness and difficulty moving. Numbness and swelling is also common.

- Wind stroke may involve muscular flaccidity and atrophy; however, these are usually one-sided.

Pattern	Signs and Symptoms	Treatment Principle	Acupuncture	Formula
Lung Heat injuring fluid	Following high fever, acute onset and rapidly developing weakness, flaccidity, and immobility of extremities with muscular atrophy, dry skin, thirst, cough, scanty sputum, scanty urine, dry stool/constipation. T: red with yellow coat P: rapid	Clear heat (clear LU heat), moisten dryness, nourish LU and generate fluid		
Damp-heat invasion	Acute onset, development of heavy limbs, weak and flaccid extremities, possible swelling, lower extremities most affected, may have fever, stifling sensation in chest, decreased appetite, nausea, dark and scanty urination. T: red with greasy coat P: slippery and rapid	Clear heat and drain damp, unblock channels		
Deficiency of Spleen and Stomach	Usually slow onset, flaccidity and weakness of extremities aggravated by exertion, gradual loss of muscle mass, fatigue, SOB, poor appetite, loose stools, sallow complexion. T: pale P: weak	Tonify Spleen and Stomach, nourish Qi and Blood		
Deficiency of Liver and Kidney Yin	Gradual onset, weak and flaccid lower limbs, sore, weak low back, possible tidal fever, night sweats, emaciation, fatigue, dizziness, tinnitus. T: red, scanty coat P: thin and rapid	Tonify Liver and Kidney, nourish Yin and clear heat		

Bleeding Disorders (xue zheng)

Definition:
Bleeding disorders include any bleeding outside proper courses (e.g. from nose, mouth, passed through feces, subcutaneous bleeding). Most common types:
- Hemoptysis (coughing up blood) - (consider LU or LR pathologies)
- Hematemesis (vomiting up blood) (consider SP or ST)
- Hematuria (blood in urine) – (consider KD, SP, HT, BL)
- Hematochezia (fresh) and melena (blood in stool) – (consider SP, ST, intestines)
- Subcutaneous and mucosal hemorrhages including epistaxis, bleeding gums, purpura, and petechiae
    - Epistaxis – (consider LU, ST, SP, or LR)
    - Bleeding gums – (consider ST or KD)
    - Subcutaneous – (consider SP, HT, LR or KD)

Red Flags:
Excessive bleeding can be life threatening if hemorrhagic shock or asphyxia occurs; asphyxia is caused by blood clots obstructing the airway.

Administer first aid and send for emergency care if blood has been lost and the following symptoms and signs have been present for more than a few minutes, or are worsening: Dizziness, fainting and confusion. Rapid pulse of more than 100 per minute. Blood pressure less than 90/60 mmHg. Cold and clammy extremities.

Any excessive bleeding (with the exception of menstruation), especially regular or continuous, should be referred to Western medical assessment and care, including:
- Cough with bloody sputum in patient with respiratory infection
- Painless, frank bloody urination in men over 50
- Vaginal bleeding years after last menses
- Regular blood in stools in patient over 40

Western medicine relevant diseases:

These patterns include a wide range acute and chronic conditions, including: lung cancer, pulmonary abscess or tuberculosis, acute gastritis, peptic ulcer, gastric cancer, liver cirrhosis, kidney stones, bladder or prostate cancer, hemophilia.

The most common conditions to cause blood in stools include: peptic ulcer, diverticulitis, and ulcerative colitis. Typically, the darker the blood is, the higher the site of the bleeding in the alimentary canal. Thus, very dark blood in stools may indicate bleeding from the stomach, while fresh red blood denotes bleeding from intestines.

Etiology and Pathogenesis:

- External Pathogenic Factors – wind-heat, dryness and heat, or fire can injure blood vessels and make blood run recklessly
    - External heat attacking lung – hemoptysis or epistaxsis
    - Fire toxicity trapped in nutritive or blood level – hemorrhages
    - Damp heat in intestines – hematochezia
    - Damp heat in bladder - hematuria
- Improper Diet – hot/spicy/alcohol can cause internal damp-heat accumulation, ST fire, or SP/ST impairment (SP cannot hold)
- Emotional Stress – Qi stagnation turns to fire – fire enters vessels and causes blood to move recklessly (or LV overacts on ST, or LV fire insults LU)
- Overexertion – mental or physical overexertion damages Qi and Yin – deficient Qi cannot control the blood or Yin deficiency creates empty heat
- Chronic illness or late stage febrile disease – empty fire (from insufficient body fluid) – bleeding; also, Qi may be consumed and unable to hold; or, prolonged illness may cause blood stasis in minute collaterals and vessels which will escape into surrounding tissues

TCM Differentiation and Treatment:

1. Epistaxis

Pattern	Signs and Symptoms	Acupuncture	Formula
	Nasal burning, dryness and bleeding, cough with yellow sticky phlegm, fever, thirst. T: red, thin yellow coat P: floating, rapid	Clear heat. Nourish dryness. Release wind (if needed). Stop bleeding. LI20 (ying xiang), DU23 (shang xing) SP1 (yin bai) LI4 (he gu), LI11 (qu chi) LU6 (kong zui), LU9 (tai yuan) SJ5 (wei guan), GB20 (feng chi)	
	Acute, abundant, sudden fresh red bleeding, vertex H/A, dizzy, bitter taste, dry throat, irritable, angry, red eyes. T: red, yellow coat P: rapid, wiry	Clear fire. Cool blood. Stop bleeding. LI20 (ying xiang), DU23 (shang xing) SP1 (yin bai) LV2 (xing jian), GB43 (xia xi) LV14 (qi men), SJ6 (zhi gou) BL40 (wei zhong)	
	Sudden onset, large amount fresh blood, dry mouth, bad breath, constipation, scanty urine. T: red, yellow coat, dry P: rapid	Clear heat. Cool blood. Stop bleeding. LI20 (ying xiang), DU23 (shang xing) SP1 (yin bai) ST44 (nei ting) BL40 (wei zhong)	
	Intermittent, small amount, Yin deficiency signs e.g. dryness, heat, palpitations. T: red, peeled P: thin, rapid	Nourish Liver and Kidney. Clear Heat. Cool Blood. Stop bleeding. LI20 (ying xiang), DU23 (shang xing) SP1 (yin bai) BL23 (shen shu) KD1 (yong quan), KI3 (tai xi) LR3 (tai chong)	
	Light red bleeding, small or big (maybe other bleeding too), pale complexion, tired, other SP T&T issues, possible Blood deficiency signs (insomnia, dizziness). T: pale P: weak	Tonify SP to hold blood. Stop bleeding. LI20 (ying xiang), DU23 (shang xing) SP1 (yin bai) BL20 (pi shu), BL21 (wei shu) SP6 (SYJ), ST36 (ZSL) DU20 (bai hui)	

2. Hemoptysis

Pattern	Signs and Symptoms	Acupuncture	Formula
Dry-heat attacking LU	Cough, itchy throat, blood tinged sputum or coughing up blood, dry mouth and nose, fever, slight aversion to wind. T: dry red, thin yellow coat P: rapid, floating	Clear heat. Moisten lung. Stop bleeding. Use the following primary points and then add auxiliary points based on pattern differentiation: BL13 (fei shu) LU6 (kong zui), LU5 (chi ze), LU10 (yu ji)	
Liver fire	Recurrent cough, blood tinged sputum or coughing up blood, aggravated by emotions, irritable, bitter taste, dry throat,	Clear heat. Cool Blood. Stop bleeding.	

Pattern	Signs and Symptoms	Acupuncture	Formula
	hypochondriac pain. T: red, yellow coat P: wiry, rapid	Use the following primary points and then add auxiliary points based on pattern differentiation: BL13 (fei shu) LU6 (kong zui), LU5 (chi ze), LU10 (yu ji) LV2 (xing jian), GB43 (xia xi) LV14 (qi men), SJ6 (zhi gou)	
LU Yin Deficiency with Empty Fire	Chronic, dry cough with blood tinged sputum or recurring cough with fresh blood, dry mouth/throat, malar flush, tidal fever, night sweats. T: red, scanty coat P: thin, rapid	Nourish yin. Moisten lung. Stop bleeding. Use the following primary points and then add auxiliary points based on pattern differentiation: BL13 (fei shu) LU6 (kong zui), LU5 (chi ze), LU10 (yu ji), SP6 (SYJ)	

3. Hematemesis

Pattern	Signs and Symptoms	Acupuncture	Formula
Stomach Heat	Distending, burning pain in epigastrium, acute vomiting of food and blood, foul breath, constipation or black stools. T: red with yellow greasy coat P: slippery and rapid	Clear heat and drain fire. Stop reversed ST Qi. Stop vomiting. Use the following primary points and then add auxiliary points based on pattern differentiation: SP1 (yin bai) REN12 (zhong wan), PC6 (nei guan) PC7 (da ling), PC4 (xi men)	
Liver Fire	Vomiting red or red-purple (or dry) blood, bitter taste, hypochondriac pain, irritable, insomnia, dark & scanty urine. T: red P: wiry, rapid	Clear liver fire. Cool blood. Stop vomiting. Use the following primary points and then add auxiliary points based on pattern differentiation: SP1 (yin bai) REN12 (zhong wan), PC6 (nei guan) PC7 (da ling), PC4 (xi men)	
Qi Deficiency	Chronic and repeated, light reddish purple blood, pale complexion, SOB, fatigue. T: pale P: weak	Tonify SP Qi and control the blood. Use the following primary points and then add auxiliary points based on pattern differentiation: SP1 (yin bai) REN12 (zhong wan), PC6 (nei guan) PC7 (da ling), PC4 (xi men)	

4. Bleeding gums

Pattern	Signs and Symptoms	Acupuncture	Formula
Stomach fire	Fresh red blood, red swollen painful gums, bad breath, constipation. T: red, yellow coat P: rapid	Clear ST heat and drain fire. Cool Blood. Stop bleeding. DU26 (shui gou), ST6 (jia che), ST7 (xia guan) SP1 (yin bai) LI4 (he gu), ST44 (nei ting)	
Yin deficiency with empty fire	-light red blood, swollen gums, loose teeth -chronic, recurrent bleeding -other Yin xu signs T: red, scanty coat P: thin, rapid	Nourish yin. Clear fire. Cool blood. Stop bleeding. Local + SP1 (yin bai) KD3 (tai xi), KI6 (zhao hai) LR2 (xing jian)	

5. Hematochezia and melena

Pattern	Signs and Symptoms	Acupuncture	Formula
Damp-heat in the intestines	Fresh blood in stool, sensation of incomplete defecation, abdominal distension, loose stool, burning anus, bitter taste. T: yellow, greasy P: slippery, rapid		
Spleen and Stomach Yang Deficiency	Dark red, tarry stool, dull abdominal pain, desire for warm drinks, pale and sallow complexion, fatigue, loose stools. T: pale P: thin, weak	Tonify Yang Qi, nourish blood, stop bleeding. BL20 (pi shu), BL25 (da chang shu) SP4 (gong sun), REN6 (qi hai), ST36 (ZSL)	

6. Hematuria

Pattern	Signs and Symptoms	Acupuncture	Formula
Damp heat in lower jiao	Dark urine with fresh blood, urination is painful, burning and urgent, irritable, thirst, red face, insomnia. T: red with yellow coat P: rapid	Clear heat, drain damp, stop bleeding. REN3 (zhong ji) BL28 (pang guang shu), BL32 (ci liao) SP9 (YLQ) GB34 ((yang ling quan)	
Spleen and Kidney Deficiency	Frequent painless urination, pale red blood in urine, loss of appetite, tired, sallow, low backache, either Yang Xu signs (pale, edema, cold limbs, tired), or Yin Xu signs (night sweats, emaciation).	Tonify SP and KD, stop bleeding. BL20 (pi shu), BL23 (shen shu) ST36 (ZSL) REN4 (guan yuan) SP3 (tai bai)	

Chest Impediment (xiong bi)

Definition:
Group of symptoms caused by obstruction of Qi and Blood in the chest. Condition is characterized by chest oppression and pain that may radiate to left upper back, shoulder and down to the arm. Accompanying respiratory symptoms include: SOB, dyspnea, difficult breathing when lying down. A stuffy sensation and difficult breathing are present in mild cases. Sharp crushing cardiac pain is found in severe cases.

Red Flags:
Seek emergency medical care for:
- Sustained intense chest pain lasting 30 minutes or more, often with feelings of fear or dread, palpitations and breathlessness. These are indications of myocardial infarction. The patient may also vomit or develop a cold sweat. Note: this can present as sudden onset of breathlessness, palpitations or confusion but without pain in the elderly. Women are less likely to experience classic symptoms
- Sudden onset SOB, tearing chest pain radiating to back, and features of shock are indications of pulmonary embolism.

Western Medicine Relevant Diseases:
Chest impediment is observed in numerous Western medical conditions related to the heart and lungs. It is also a common anxiety symptom and feature of peptic ulcer disease, hiatus hernia and oesophagitis. Relevant conditions include:

(table based on Maciocia, *The Practice of Chinese Medicine 1st Ed.*)

Disease	Pathology	Symptoms & signs
	-inflammation of pleura from acute febrile disease affecting chest	-fever, stabbing pain below nipple, worse on inspiration, shallow breathing, constricted chest, hemoptysis
	-embolus detaches from thrombus and occludes a lung artery	-range from severe chest pain and shock, intense breathlessness, pallor, fainting, sweating, drop in blood pressure, collapse to mild constriction in only partial occlusion
	-malignancy more common in men over 40	-dry cough, deep chest pain, loss of appetite, weight loss, hemoptysis, fatigue
	-spasm of coronary artery	-sudden bouts of severe chest pain, may radiate, nausea, possible vomiting -brought on by exercise, cold, excitement, overeating Stable angina: central chest pain related to exertion, eating or the cold lasting less than 30 minutes and which improves with rest and nitroglycerin.
	-blocked coronary artery decreases blood to heart and causes necrosis	-sudden severe, radiating chest pain at rest -see red flags
	-protrusion of upper part of stomach through diaphragm into thoracic cavity	-chest pain on sternum that may radiate -nausea, belching, hiccups, regurgitation, dyspnea
	-malignancy	-retrosternal pain on swallowing, may radiate, tiredness, weight loss, enlarged lymph

Etiology and Pathogenesis:
Note: chest bi is always a combination of excess and deficiency – root is usually a deficiency of SP, HT or KD and branches are related to congealed cold, qi stagnation, phlegm accumulation, and ultimately stasis.
- Cold pathogen w pre-existing Yang deficiency – constricts vessels and blocks Yang – Blood stasis with sharp pain
- Emotional stress – causes SP Qi deficiency and LR Qi stagnation – Blood stasis with pain and distension
- Improper diet – greasy/raw food hinders SP/ST – phlegm blocks circulation of Qi and Blood – Blood stasis
- Aging/deficient constitution – KD Yin or Yang deficiency – Heart Yin & Blood deficiency or Heart Yang deficiency
- EPI damp heat invading – fever, long term heat damage (e.g. rheumatic fever) damages yin and yang

TCM Differentiation and Treatment:

Pattern	Signs and Symptoms	Acupuncture	Formula
Heart Blood Stasis	Fixed, stabbing chest pain, more severe at night, palpitations, restlessness. T: dark purple P: deep, choppy		
Phlegm Stagnation (Turbid Phlegm Accumulation)	Oppressive pressure or pain with sense of suffocation, possibly radiating, obesity, heaviness of limbs, SOB, copious sputum. T: greasy coat P: slippery		
Cold congealed in chest	Acute onset chest pain, radiating, aggravated by cold, SOB, palpitations, difficult respiration, pale complexion, cold limbs. T: white coat P: deep and thready		
Qi and Yin Xu	Intermittent dull and oppressive chest pain, SOB, palpitations, worse with exertion, fatigue, dizziness, vertigo. T: reddish, scalloped P: intermittent, thready and weak		
HT and KD Yin Xu	Congestion and pain in the chest, palpitations, night sweats, insomnia, sore back, dizziness, tinnitus, vertigo. T: red, scanty coat P: thin, rapid or choppy		
Yang Qi Exhaustion	Chest oppression with SOB, dull pain, aggravated by cold, palpitations, sweating, fatigue, cold intolerance, cold limbs, pale complexion, cyanotic lips, nails, tongue. T: pale or purple P: deep, thin or minute		
Emotion/Qi stagnation	Distension, chest pain, worse with emotion, sighing. P: wiry		

Common Cold (gan mao)

Definition:
This is a frequently recurring illness that may occur in any of the seasons, but is most prevalent in winter and spring. It is caused by attacks of exterior pathogenic wind. Key symptoms include: nasal congestion or runny nose, sneezing, aversion to cold, sore throat, and headache. Typically has a short course (approximately 5-7 days) and rapid recovery.

Red Flags:
- Epidemic cold and cold in those with weak constitutions, such as the elderly and infants, may result in complications. Epidemic cold is highly contagious.

Western Medicine Relevant Diseases:
The common cold is a viral infectious disease of the upper respiratory tract that primarily affects the nose. The throat, sinuses, and voice box may also be affected. Other related conditions:
- Flu/influenza
- Upper respiratory infection

Etiology and Pathogenesis:
Note: always consider both the presence of exterior factors and the sufficiency of protective Qi.
1. External factors:
- Six EPI (wind, cold, damp, dry, heat and summer heat) all cause – enter skin, mouth, nose and block Wei Qi – enter LU and prevent descending and dispersing function
- Special high season for each, e.g. cold/winter, summer/heat/damp, fall/dry, wind any season together with EPI, e.g. in spring-winter is often wind-cold
2. Internal causes: extreme environment changes (e.g. high air conditioning), weak resistance (Wei Qi weak)

TCM Differentiation and Treatment:
Note: Review Bootcamp #1 discussion of BEN/BIAO (root/branch)!

1. Excess Patterns

Patterns	Signs and Symptoms	Acupuncture	Formula
Excess	**General signs and symptoms:**	**General acupuncture treatment:**	
	Simultaneous fever and aversion to cold (cardinal sign) Fever/chills, aversion to cold, body pain/headache, nose congestion/runny nose, painful throat, cough T: thin coat P: floating, superficial	• Treatment principle: release the exterior, expel pathogen • LU7 (lie que) and LI4 (he gu) • BL12 (feng men) • SJ5 (wei guan) (more for heat)	
Wind Cold	**Special Symptoms**	**Special points by pattern**	
	• More chills, less or no fever • Aversion to cold • No sweat (re: cold contracting pores) • Clear discharge • Thin, white tongue fur • Superficial tight pulse	• GB20 (Fengchi) • DU16 (Fengfu) • Moxa on BL12 (feng men) and BL13 (fei shu) (smokeless) or barrier method	
Wind Heat	• More fever, less chills • Throat dry, swollen, red • Sweat (slight) • Yellow discharge • Red tongue, thin white/yellow coat • Superficial rapid pulse	• LI11 (qu chi) • LU5 (chi ze) • DU14 (da zhui) (fever) • LU10 (yu ji) or LU11 (shao shang) (throat pain) • Gua sha or cupping on related Shu area/upper back, BL12 (feng men) and BL13 (fei shu)	

Damp	General Signs and Symptoms	General Acupuncture Treatment	
	• General EPI symptoms (above) • Heavy feelings in body/head • Nausea, vomiting, poor appetite, diarrhea • Greasy tongue coating • Superficial and slippery pulse	• ST36 (ZSL), ST40 (feng long) • REN12 (zhong wan)	
Damp Cold	Special Symptoms	Special Points	
	• More common in fall/winter • Similar to wind cold + damp symptoms • Diarrhea watery, not so foul • White greasy coat	• Disperse EPI from exterior: LU7 (lie que), LI4 (he gu), SJ5 (wei guan), BL12 (zhong wan) • Damp points: ST36 (ZSL), ST40 (feng long), REN12 (zhong wan) • For nausea and vomiting: P6 (nei guan) • For Diarrhea: ST25 (tian shu), ST37 (shang ju xu) • Moxa	
Damp Heat	• More common in summer • Fever med-high • Yellow discharge • Red tongue with yellow greasy coat • Foul vomit, yellow sticky stools	• Disperse EPI from exterior: LU7 (lie que), LI4 (he gu), SJ5 (wei guan), BL12 (feng men) • LU6 (kong zui) and SJ6 (Zhigou) • Plus damp points • Plus heat/fever points: LU5 (chi ze) and LI11 (qu chi) • For nausea and vomiting: P6 (nei guan) • For Diarrhea: ST25 (tian shu), ST37 (shang ju xu)	

2. Deficiency patterns

Pattern	Signs and Symptoms	Acupuncture	Formula
Deficiency	General Signs and Symptoms	General Points	
	General EPI symptoms, as above, but often found in seniors or young children, or people with chronic illness.	As above, points to disperse EPI: LU7 (lie que), LI4 (he gu), SJ5 (wei guan), BL12 (feng men)	
Pre-existing Yang Qi Deficiency + EPI (wind cold)	Special Symptoms	Special Points	
	New: EPI wind cold symptoms Plus existing: tired, SOB, pale face, weak pulse, cold, tired, weak vitality	Tx is to disperse wind-cold: LU7 (lie que), LI4 (he gu), SJ5 (wei guan), BL12 (feng men), BL13 (fei shu), LU9 (tai yuan) And tonify Qi: SP3 (tai bai), REN6 (qi hai), ST36 (ZSL), BL13 (fei shu), BL20 (pi shu), REN4 (guan yuan)	
Yin Deficiency + EPI (wind heat)	New: EPI wind heat symptoms Plus existing: poor nutrition, tidal fever, night sweats, red tongue, yellow coat, thin and rapid pulse, fever, dry, tired	Tx is to disperse EPI: LU7 (lie que), LI4 (he gu), SJ5 (wei guan), BL12 (feng men) (also LU9 (tai yuan) or LU5 (chi ze), GB20 (feng chi, LU9 (tai yuan), LU5 (chi ze) Also nourish Yin and disperse heat: KD6 (zhao hai), KD3 (tai xi), SP6 (SYJ), LR2 (xing jian)	

Constipation (bian bi)

Definition:
Refers to difficult or infrequent defecation, hard and dry stools, and sluggish bowel movements. Associated symptoms include: ABD pain, belching, distension, lack of appetite. May result from impairment of LI; also, dysfunction of SP, ST, LU, KD.

Red Flags:
- Not itself a critical disorder.
- Certain accompanying symptoms merit referral for Western medical assessment: prolonged constipation, extreme pain, distended abdomen, vomiting, blood in stool, weight loss, new/worsening constipation in older people.

Western Medicine Discussion:

Common causes of constipation include:
- Changes in diet (such as decreased fluid intake, low-fiber diet, and/or constipating foods)
- Drugs that slow the bowels
- Disordered defecation
- Laxative overuse
- Illness that requires prolonged bed rest

Other disorders and diseases that often cause constipation include: an underactive thyroid gland (hypothyroidism), high blood calcium levels (hypercalcemia), and Parkinson's disease. People with diabetes often develop nerve damage (neuropathy). If the neuropathy affects nerves to the digestive tract, the intestines may slow down, resulting in constipation. Spinal cord injury can also interfere with the nerves to the intestines and cause constipation.

The complications of constipation include:
- Hemorrhoids: Excessive straining during bowel movements increases pressure on the veins around the anus and can lead to hemorrhoids and, rarely, protrusion of the rectum through the anus (rectal prolapse). Passing hard stool can cause a split in the skin of the anus (anal fissure).
- Diverticular disease: Diverticular disease can develop if the walls of the large intestine are damaged by the increased pressure from constipation. Damage to the walls of the large intestine leads to the formation of diverticula, which can become clogged and inflamed (diverticulitis). Diverticula sometimes bleed and **occasionally rupture, causing peritonitis.**
- **Fecal impaction**: stool in the large intestine or rectum completely blocks the passage of other stool, leading to cramps and rectal pain. Sometimes, watery mucus or liquid stool oozes around the blockage, which gives the false impression of diarrhea. Common among older people, particularly those who are bedridden or have decreased physical activity, pregnant women, and people who have been given barium by mouth or as an enema for certain types of x-ray tests.

Etiology and Pathogenesis:
- Constitutional Yang excess and accumulation of heat in ST/intestines, e.g. from diet; residual heat from warm-febrile disease – consumes body fluid
- Qi stagnation – emotions, lack of activity can impair transporting/descending function of Qi – intestinal content is not eliminated
- SP Qi deficiency; improper diet; chronic illness; aging; post-partum -- Qi and blood xu – lack of movement and dryness
- Yang deficiency with internal cold from e.g. chronic illness or aging, too much cold food – cold congeals and flow of Qi becomes sluggish

TCM Differentiation and Treatment:

Pattern	Signs and Symptoms	Treatment Principle	Acupuncture	Formula
	-dry, impacted feces; very dry and difficult defecation, dark scanty urine -heat signs, e.g. fever, red face, irritability, bad breath, mouth sores -possible ABD distension and pain T: red, yellow coat P: strong/rapid	-drain heat, unblock/promote stool, moisten intestine/stool	ST25 (tian shu), ST 28, shui dao), ST29 (gui lai) BL25 (da chang shu) SJ6 (zhi gou) LI4 (he gu) & LI11 (qu chi) for heat DU14 (da zhui) for fever	
	-dry, sluggish bowel movements, aggravated by emotional stress -hypochondriac distension, sighing, belching, ABD fullness/pain better after passing gas (note: this could also cause diarrhea, underlying SP Qi Xu) P: wiry	-move Qi, and promote stool	ST25 (tian shu) SJ6 (zhi gou) LI4-LV3 (4 gates) Yintang, PC6 (nei guan)	
	-desire to defecate, straining, prolonged effort to defecate -pale complexion, tired T: pale P: weak	-strengthen SP and tonify Qi, promote stool	BL20 (pi shu), BL21 (wei shu), BL25 (tian shu) ST36 (ZSL) SJ6 (zhi gou)	
	-very dry little rabbit stools (chronic) -difficult BM, less frequent -ABD distension and pain -low tidal fever, red cheeks, night sweats T: red, yellow coat	-nourish Yin, promote stools, moisten dryness	-ST25 (tian shu) -SJ6 (zhi gou) -KD3 (tai xi), KI6 (zhao hai), SP6 (SYJ), LI4 (he gu)	
	-difficult, dry, infrequent (dry & pebble like) -abdominal distension and pain -pale, dizzy, fatigue, insomnia T: pale P: thin, weak, choppy	-nourish blood and Yin, promote stools, moisten dryness	-ST25 (tian shu) -SJ6 (zhi gou) -ST36 (ZSL), SP6 (SYJ) & SP10 (xue hai)	
	-cold intolerance, cold limbs, poor health -pale, tired, SOB -BM difficult, sluggish, requires great effort -abundant clear urine -ABD distension/pain -pale, dizzy, fatigue T: pale P: weak, deep	-tonify Yang Qi (warm), moisten LI, and promote stool	-ST 25 (tian shu) -SJ 6 (zhi gou – tonify) -ST 36 (ZSL) -REN 4 (guan yuan), Ren6 (qi hai), moxa REN8 (shen que) -SP 4 (gong sun) – for ST pain (or back Shu)	

Consumptive disease (xu lao)

Definition:
Consumptive disease includes various chronic debilitating disorders in which the deficiency of zang-fu organs, and of qi, blood, yin and yang constitute its basic pathogenesis.

Western Medicine Relevant Diseases:
Consumptive disease has a broad range of manifestations may be seen in the disorders of many Western medical conditions, such as auto-immune disorders, endocrine diseases, metabolic disorders, malnutrition, nervous system disorders and other organic degenerative diseases. Therefore, many chronic diseases may be differentiated and treated with the principles of xu lao. Ex) Chronic Fatigue syndrome, cancer, severe anemias, hemochromatosis, TB, thrombocytopenia, SLE, etc.

Etiology and Pathogenesis:
The causes of consumptive disease are:

TCM Differentiation and Treatment:

Pattern	Signs and Symptoms	Treatment Principle	Acupuncture	Formula
Lung Qi Deficiency	Shortness of breath, spontaneous sweating, low voice, alternate feeling of heat and cold, susceptibility to common cold, pale complexion and tongue and feeble pulse.	Benefit Lung Qi	LU9 (tai yuan), BL13 (fei shu), LU7 (lie que), SP6 (SYJ), ST36 (ZSL)	
Deficiency of Spleen Qi	Fatigue, poor appetite, epigastric discomfort after food intake, loose stool, sallow complexion, pale tongue with thin coating and feeble pulse.	Strengthen Spleen Qi	SP3 (tai bai), SP6 (SYJ), ST36 (ZSL), BL20 (pi shu)	
Heart Blood Deficiency	Palpitations, amnesia, dizziness, insomnia, dreamfulness, lusterless complexion, pale tongue, thready or slow and irregular pulse.	Nourish Heart blood and calm the mind	PC6 (nei guan), HT7 (shen men), BL15 (xin shu), BL17 (ge shu), ST36 (ZSL), SP6 (SYJ)	
Liver Blood Deficiency	Dizziness, lusterless complexion, numbness and spasms of extremities, muscular twitching, irregular menstruation or even amenorrhea, pale tongue and thready and wiry or uneven pulse.	Tonify blood and nourish Liver	LR3 (tai chong), BL18 (gan shu), BL17 (ge shu), SP6 (SYJ), ST36 (ZSL)	

Deficiency of Yin	Lung Yin: Dryness of throat, dry cough, hemoptysis, fever, night sweating, flushed cheeks, red and dry tongue with little coating and thready and rapid pulse. Heart Yin: Palpitations, irritability, insomnia, dreamfulness, fever, night sweating, flushed cheeks, dry tongue with little coating and thready and rapid pulse. Stomach Yin: Dryness of mouth and lips, constipation, poor appetite, retching, hiccups, flushed cheeks, dry tongue with little coating and thready and rapid pulse Liver Yin: headache, dizziness, dryness of eyes, tinnitus, blurred vision, irritability, numbness of limbs, muscular twitching and cramps, flushed cheeks, red and dry tongue and thready and wiry, rapid pulse. Kidney Yin: Lumbago, nocturnal emissions, dizziness, tinnitus or even deafness, dryness of mouth, sore threat, weakness of the lower limbs, or hectic fever, flushed cheeks, red and dry tongue and deep and thready pulse.	Nourish Yin	Principle treatment: KD3 (tai xi), SP6 (SYJ), BL23 (shen shu), REN4 (guan yuan) Plus supplement with Source points and Back Shu points according to organ deficiency and points to address specific symptoms.	
Deficiency of Yang	Deficiency of HT Yang: Palpitations, spontaneous sweating, chest upset or pain, fatigue, somnolence, coldness of limbs, pale complexion, pale or dark purplish tongue, thready and weak or slow and irregular or deep and slow pulse. Deficiency of SP Yang: Fatigue, sallow complexion, poor appetite, shortness of breath, loose stool, abdominal pain and creased borborygmus aggravated by improper food intake, cold, pale tongue with white coating and weak pulse. Deficiency of KI Yang: lumbago, backache, nocturnal emissions, impotence, early morning diarrhea, nocturia, pale complexion, aversion to cold, coolness of limbs, pale tongue with teeth marks and deep and slow pulse.	Warm and Support Yang	Principle treatment: DU20 (bai hui), REN8 (shen que), REN4 (guan yuan), REN6 (qi hai) Plus supplement with Source and Back Shu points according to organ deficiency and points to address specific symptoms.	

(Based on http://www.acupuncture.com/Conditions/consumption.htm)

Consumptive Thirst (xiao ke)
(Also called Wasting and Thirsting or TCM Diabetes)

Definition:
Xiao, or wasting, signifies serious depletion of vital substances, despite excessive consumption of food and water. Ke, or thirsting, refers to excessive thirst that is not relieved by drinking. Condition characterized by: "3 UP and 1 DOWN": increased thirst (polydipsia), and increased food intake (polyphagia), urine (polyuria) + emaciation characterized as Xiao Ke. Other symptoms include turbid urine and sugar in the urine (glycosuria).

Note: depending on which of the 3 excesses is dominant, the disorder is subcategorized into: Upper Xiao – intense thirst and drinking frequently; Middle Xiao – excessive hunger and increased food intake; and, Lower Xiao – intense thirst and excess urination.

Red Flags:
- Hypoglycemia (insulin shock) from an excess of insulin causing a deficit of glucose in the blood. The lack of glucose quickly affects the nervous system and can cause a wide range of effects: poor concentration, slurred speech, lack of coordination. A second group of signs relate to stimulation of sympathetic nervous system resulting in increased pulse, pale moist skin, anxiety, tremors. Loss of consciousness, seizures and death may result.
    - Treatment is immediate administration of concentrated carbohydrate, if conscious. Must be treated promptly or can cause brain damage or even death. If unconscious, give nothing by mouth. Intravenous glucose is required.
    - Verify patients have taken appropriate medications to minimize risk.
- Diabetic ketoacidosis (diabetic coma or hyperglycemia) resulting from insufficient insulin leading to high blood glucose levels. Signs are dehydration, rapid pulse, deep respirations, acetone breath, lethargy, nausea, vomiting, loss of consciousness.

Western Medicine Relevant Diseases:
Consumptive thirst patterns have similar manifestations to the Western medical conditions diabetes mellitus and diabetes insipidus.

There are two types of diabetes mellitus, Type 1 and Type 2. Type 1 (formerly called insulin-dependent diabetes or juvenile-onset) is a less common and more severe form where insulin replacement is required because no insulin is being produced by the body. This can be genetic, but the insulin deficit most commonly results from an autoimmune reaction that destroys the pancreatic beta cells, which would normally produce the body's insulin. Type 1 occurs more frequently in children and adolescents, but can develop at any age. The rate of onset is acute. Complications, such as hypoglycemia or ketoacidosis, can be very severe and are more likely to occur in this group.

Type 2 diabetes is a milder form and may be managed (except in severe cases) without taking insulin by making dietary and lifestyle changes. In fact, insulin is often the last resort, after diet/lifestyle therapy and, potentially, oral medications to help reduce insulin resistance. In Type 2 diabetes, there is a decreased effectiveness of insulin due to an increased resistance of body cells to insulin. There may also be a relative deficit of insulin in the body as, over time, the pancreas produces less. Type 2 diabetes often develops gradually in older adults who struggle with obesity. Diet and lifestyle changes early on are critical, as unmanaged Type 2 diabetes can become very serious and, while less common, consequences such as hypoglycemia or ketoacidosis are also possible.

For both types, chronic complications can be very serious, and include a higher risk of stroke, heart attack, and peripheral vascular disease.

Central diabetes insipidus is due to a **lack of vasopressin** (antidiuretic hormone) that causes excessive production of very dilute urine (polyuria).
Central diabetes insipidus has several causes, including a brain tumor, a brain injury, brain surgery, tuberculosis, and some forms of other diseases.
The main symptoms are excessive thirst and excessive urine production.

Etiology and Pathogenesis:
TCM diabetes is always due to heat inside (excess or deficient) – heat damages body Qi/Yin – body weight decreased (and feel tired). Major organs involved are LU, ST, and KI. Causes include:
- Improper diet – too much greasy, rich, sweet food or alcohol – hinders Spleen – food stagnation – generates heat and phlegm inside
- Long term stress, emotion –- stagnant Qi transforms into fire – consumes yin and fluid
- Overexertion – exhausts yin and essence
- Constitutional yin deficiency with fire – consumes yin and fluids

Note: TCM late stage complications:
- LU Yin Xu
- KI Yin Xu leading to night blindness, cataracts, deafness
- Heat dry causing abscesses, sores, gangrene
- Extreme deficient yin not supporting yang – KI & SP cannot metabolize fluids – edema
- Heat dries blood – stasis
- Yin xu and heat dry consume fluid, form phlegm, obstruct channels - wind stroke and hemiplegia
- Yin and Yang collapse

TCM Differentiation and Treatment:
*Note: clinically, the 3 excesses can appear simultaneously; however, a preponderance of 1 symptom can be used to determine organ involvement

Pattern	Signs and Symptoms	Treatment Principle	Acupuncture	Formula
Upper Xiao	-excessive thirst with frequent drinking, dry mouth and tongue -irritability -polyuria and emaciation developing T: red edge, yellow coat P: rapid, flooding	Clear heat, moisten LU, generate fluid and alleviate thirst		
Middle Xiao	-hunger, polyphagia, dry stool -emaciation T: dry yellow coat P: slippery, full, forceful	Clear heat from ST, drain fire, nourish yin/fluid		
Lower Xiao	-Polyuria, turbid, cloudy, sweet urine -dry mouth and lips -five center heat -emaciation T: red P: rapid, deep and thready	Nourish yin and clear heat, tonify KD		

Convulsive Syndromes (jing zheng)

Definition:
Convulsive syndrome patterns manifest in a variety of pathologies and are characterized by rigidity and stiffness of the neck and spine, lockjaw, contractions and tremors of the limbs and, in extreme cases, opisthotonos (arching of head and neck back).

Red flags:
Referral to emergency care is required in cases where there are:
- high fever in adults with other signs of distress
- signs of meningitis/encephalitis: fever, stiff neck, listlessness, confusion, nausea, vomiting, difficult breathing

Western Medicine Relevant Diseases:
- Meningitis: acute inflammation of the meninges (protective membranes covering the brain and spinal cord) and of the fluid filled space between the meninges (subarachnoid space). The most common symptoms are fever, headache and neck stiffness that makes lowering the chin to the chest difficult or impossible. Other symptoms include confusion or altered consciousness, vomiting, and an inability to tolerate light or loud noises. Young children often exhibit only nonspecific symptoms, such as irritability, drowsiness, or poor feeding. The inflammation may be caused by infection with viruses, bacteria, or other microorganisms, and less commonly by certain drugs. Meningitis can be life threatening because of the inflammation's proximity to the brain and spinal cord; therefore, the condition is classified as a medical emergency.
- Encephalitis: Encephalitis is inflammation of the brain that occurs when a virus directly infects the brain or when a virus, vaccine, or something else triggers inflammation. Sign include: fever, headache, or seizures, and they may feel sleepy, numb, or confused. Encephalitis is most commonly due to viruses, such as herpes simplex, herpes zoster, cytomegalovirus, or West Nile virus. Sometimes bacteria cause encephalitis, usually as part of bacterial meningitis (called meningoencephalitis). Protozoa, such as amoebas, those that cause toxoplasmosis (in people who have AIDS), and those that cause malaria, can also infect the brain and cause encephalitis. Rarely, encephalitis develops in people who have cancer; this disorder is called paraneoplastic encephalitis. This type of encephalitis appears to result from the immune system's response to the tumor.
- Febrile convulsions: seizures triggered by fever
- Parkinson's disease: progressive degenerative disease affecting motor function leading to muscle tremors, muscle rigidity, difficulty initiating movement. Primary or idiopathic Parkinson's usually develops after 60. Secondary may follow encephalitis, trauma, or vascular disease.

Etiology and Pathogenesis:
In general, involves pathology of the sinews. Either exterior pathogens invading and obstructing the sinews or malnourishment of the sinews.
- Pathogenic factors accumulating and obstructing channels – block Qi and Blood – sinews are deprived and contract
- Extreme internal heat – consumes body fluid – fails to nourish sinews
- Deficiency of yin and blood (e.g. from constitutional/blood loss/disease) – fails to nourish sinews

DDX of similar disorders:
Convulsive syndromes: primarily stiffness and rigidity of upper back and neck with tremors, contractions, opisthotonos
Wind stroke: contraction of extremities often accompanied by facial paralysis, hemiplegia, and stroke sequelae
Epilepsy: relatively short episodes of unconsciousness, contractions, drooling and foaming of mouth, crying out

TCM Differentiation and Treatment:

Pattern	Signs and Symptoms	Acupuncture	Formula
	-headache, stiffness, rigidity of back and neck -aversion to cold, fever, soreness and heaviness of extremities T: white, greasy coat P: depends on pathogen – superficial and slippery	Dispel EPI, dry dampness, open channels SJ5 (wei guan), GB20 (feng chi) Moxa BL12 (feng men) (if cold/damp) LU7 (lie que) (neck command) LI4 (he gu) BL40 (wei zhong) (open channel)	
	-high fever, stifling sensation, locked jaw, stiffness and rigidity of neck and back -extreme cases delirium, opisthotonos -dry throat, thirst, constipation, irritability T: yellow and greasy P: wiry and rapid	Drain heat, nourish Yin Shixuan DU26 (shui gu), P6 (nei guan) (open orifices) LI4 (he gu), LI11 (qu chi) DU14 (da zhui) BL40 (wei zhong)	
	-repeated muscle spasms (worse with cold, often at night) -often seen after excessive blood loss, sweating, or in seniors -dizzy, vertigo, fatigue -night sweats P: thin and weak	Replenish Yin and nourish Blood BL18 (gan shu), BL23 (shen shu), BL20 (pi shu) KD3 (tai xi), DU4 (ming men) SP6 (SYJ), ST36 (ZSL) GB34 (yang ling quan), GB39 (xuan zhong)	

Cough (ke shou)

Definition:
Function of Lung Qi fails to disperse and descend. Cough may be silent or audible, productive sputum or dry. Ke means coughing with sound but without sputum, Shou means productive cough with sputum. In clinic, just called Ke Shou, as these are difficult to separate.

Red Flags:
Refer the following for Western medical assessment and treatment:

Western Medicine Relevant Diseases:
- **Bronchitis**: acute bronchitis is inflammation of the windpipe (trachea) and the airways that branch off the trachea (bronchi) caused by infection. Acute bronchitis is usually caused by viral infections. Symptoms of the common cold that are followed by a cough with sputum usually indicate acute bronchitis. Acute bronchitis usually lasts days to a few weeks. (for chronic bronchitis, see below)
- **Pneumonia**: an inflammation of the lung alveoli and surrounding tissues. Pneumonia is not a single illness but rather many different ones, each caused by a different organism: either **bacterium, virus, fungus, or parasite**. Bacterial and viral pneumonias are much more common than fungal or parasitic pneumonias. The most common symptom of pneumonia is cough that produces sputum (thick or discolored mucus). Other symptoms include: chest pain, chills, fever, and shortness of breath. Pneumonia is a common cause of death worldwide and is often the final illness that causes death in people who have other serious, chronic diseases.
- Chronic obstructive pulmonary disease (COPD): is persistent narrowing of the airways. Cigarette smoking is the most significant cause of COPD. COPD leads to a persistent decrease in the rate of airflow from the lungs when the person exhales. This is called chronic airflow obstruction. COPD includes the diagnoses of chronic obstructive bronchitis (blue bloater) and emphysema (pink puffer). Chronic bronchitis is defined as cough that produces sputum repeatedly during two successive years. When chronic bronchitis involves airflow obstruction, it qualifies as chronic obstructive bronchitis. Emphysema is defined as widespread and irreversible destruction of the alveolar walls and enlargement of many of the alveoli.
- Carcinoma of the bronchi: common type of cancer; symptoms include: dry cough, breathlessness, deep-seated thoracic pain, weak appetite, and general fatigue and weakness
- Tuberculosis: a contagious infection caused by the airborne bacteria Mycobacterium tuberculosis. It is spread when people breathe air contaminated by a person who has the active disease. Cough is the most common symptom, and is often dry or with scanty, blood specked sputum. Other symptoms are fatigue, low-grade fever, night sweats, and weight loss.

Etiology and Pathogenesis:
- EPI attacking LU – obstructs LU D&D – LU qi reversal – cough
- Disharmony among interior organs, particularly Liver and Spleen
    - Liver Qi stagnation or LR fire, caused by emotional stress, may attack the LU
    - Impaired Spleen function of T&T, caused by improper diet, may generate phlegm and disturb LU
    - LU pathologies (chronic disease, weak constitution) exhaust LU qi and injure LU yin impairing D&D functions and causing cough

TCM Differentiation and Treatment:
Note: Exterior condition is early stage with acute onset, short course, presence of EPI; Interior condition is chronic, intermittent, long course with presence of excess pathogenic factor and/or deficient right Qi.

Pattern	Signs and Symptoms	Acupuncture	Formula
Wind Cold	-acute cough -thin clear or white sputum easily expectorated -itchy throat -aversion to cold, no sweating, H/A, body ache, watery nasal discharge T: thin white coat P: floating and tight	Release exterior. Expel wind-cold. Descend LU Qi. Stop cough. LU7 (lie que)-LI4 (he gu), UB12 (feng men) DU16 (feng fu) LU6 (kong qui), REN22 (tian tu)	
Wind Heat	-acute cough, dry sore throat, thirst -sticky yellow sputum/nasal discharge hard to expectorate -aversion to wind, fever, sweating, H/A T: red w yellow coat P: floating and rapid	Release exterior. Expel wind-heat. Descend LU Qi. Stop cough. LU7 (lie que)-LI4 (he gu), SJ5 (wei guan) LU1 (zhong fu)-UB13 (fei shu) LU5 (chi ze), LI11 (qu chi) DU14 (da zhui) LU6 (kong qui), REN22 (tian tu)	
Wind Dry	-dryness combined with wind-heat -dry cough, maybe scanty or blood-tinged sputum, dry nose, dry lips, dry sore throat -slight aversion to cold, fever, nasal congestion T: red with thin yellow coat P: floating and rapid	Release exterior. Release heat. Moisten dryness. Stop cough. LU7 (lie que)-LI4 (he gu), LU9 (tai yuan), KD3 (tai xi), KI6 (zhao hai) to moisten UB12 (feng men), BL13 (fei shu)	
Phlegm Damp (heat or cold)	-recurrent cough with rattling sound, copious thin watery/white sticky(cold) or thick sticky & yellow sputum (hot) -chest oppression, bloating, nausea, poor appetite, fatigue T: greasy coat P: slippery	Transform phlegm and stop cough. (if cold, warm; if heat, clear heat). Strengthen spleen. BL13 (fei shu)-LU1 (zhong fu) REN22 (tian tu), REN17 (dan zhong) ST20 (cheng man), REN12 (zhong wan) SP3 (tai bai), SP6 (SYJ), ST36 (ZSL), BL20 (pi shu) (LU5 (chi ze), LI11 (quchi) to clear heat)	
Liver attacking LU	-paroxysmal coughing attacks due to emotional stress -dry throat, scanty sputum -chest and hypochondriac pain/distension -red face, dry throat, bitter taste, irritability T: thin yellow coat P: rapid, wiry	Drain liver fire, smooth LU Qi, stop cough. BL13 (fei shu), BL18 (gan shu) LU7 (lie que) LR2 (xing jian), LR3 (tai chong) LI4 (he gu)	
Lung Yin Deficiency	-chronic dry cough -scanty or blood tinged sputum -dry throat and mouth, tidal fever, red cheeks, five center heat, night sweats, insomnia T: red, scanty coat P: thready, rapid	Nourish Yin. Moisten LU. Clear heat. Stop cough. BL13 (fei shu) LU7 (lie que) BL23 (shen shu), KD 3 (tai xi), KI6 (zhao hai), KI7 (fu liu), SP6 (SYJ) LI4 (he gu), LI11 (qu chi)	

Depression (yu zheng)

Definition:
Yu zheng refers to a class of patterns stemming from emotional disturbance that are characterized by a stagnation and obstruction in the flow of Qi. Clinical manifestations include: despondence, depression, irritability, moodiness, anxiety, melancholy, bouts of crying, or a combination of those. Stagnant Qi can, over time, give rise to stagnation of blood, phlegm, damp, or heat.

Red Flags:
- Refer for psychiatric or psychological support and care if patient is experiencing symptoms that are seriously affecting quality of life, including:
    - Intense sadness and hopeless nearly every day, for most of the day (especially with history of depression) and/or feelings of extreme fatigue nearly every day, for most of the day;
    - Difficulty concentrating, remembering details, or making decisions;
    - Loss of interest or pleasure in things they enjoy (i.e. hobbies, sex, going out with friends etc.;
    - Feelings of guilty, helpless, or worthless;
    - Thoughts about death, self-harm or suicide;
    - Hallucinations, delusions or other evidence of thought disorder together with evidence of deteriorating self-care and personality change. These are all features of a psychosis such as schizophrenia. Suicide risk is high.
    - Increasing agitation, grandiosity, pressure of speech and sleeplessness with delusional thinking (mania). Mania is a feature of bipolar disorder, and is a form of psychosis that carries a high risk of behavior that can be socially and physically damaging to the patient. Suicide risk is high.
    - Confusion, deterioration in intellectual skills, loss of ability to care for self.
    - Depression developing in the post-natal period which lasts for more than three weeks, and which does not respond to your treatment. Refer straight away if the woman is experiencing suicidal ideation, or if you believe the health of the baby is at risk.
    - Severe disturbance of body image: if not responding to your treatment, and resulting in features of progressive anorexia nervosa or bulimia nervosa (e.g. progressive weight loss, secondary amenorrhea, or repeated compulsion to bring about vomiting).

Western Medicine Relevant Diseases:
The scope of these patterns includes a wide range of mental health conditions, such as: somatic symptom disorders, mood disorders (depression, bipolar, anxiety), obsessive-compulsive disorders, suicidality and menopausal conditions.

Etiology and Pathogenesis:
- Early stages tend to be excess: Emotional stress (frustration or anger) – leads to LR Qi stagnation – prolonged Qi stag leads to other accumulation pathologies (blood stasis, phlegm/damp) – these remain dormant and eventually turn into fire (which is another source of stagnation)
- Late stages tend to be deficiency. Constrained LR inhibits SP – SP not capable of generating sufficient qi and blood – HT and KD malnourished (Yin xu with empty fire)

TCM Differentiation and Treatment:

Pattern	Signs and Symptoms	Acupuncture	Formula
	-despondence, depression, mood swings, distension and migrating pain in hypochondriac/chest/abd region -repressed anger and frustration -sighing, crying, poor appetite, irregular menstruation -epigastric fullness, belching, may even vomit P: wiry	Soothe Liver and release constrained Qi. Relieve depression. Local head (can be used for all patterns): -sishenchong, yintang LI-4, LV3 (4 gates) BL18 (gan shu)-LV14 (qi men) REN17 (dan zhong)	
	-irritable, short temper, distending & burning pain -H/A, tinnitus, red face/eyes, dry mouth, bitter taste, upset stomach, acid regurgitation, restlessness, constipation T: red, thin yellow coat P: wiry, rapid	Clear and drain liver fire. Release constrained Qi. Harmonize ST. LI4 (he gu), LR2 (xing jian), LR3 (tai chong) HT7 (shen men), PC6 (nei guan) PC8 (lao gong)	
	-discomfort/foreign body sensation in throat (plum pit) -suffocating sensation in chest, distension/pain in hypochondriac/chest regions T: greasy P: wiry, slippery	Resolve phlegm. Regulate Qi movement. Release constraint. Relieve depression. REN17 (dan zhong), REN22 (tian tu) PC6 (nei guan) ST40 (feng long) (often combined with LR5 (li gou) for plum-pit qi) LV3 (tai chong)	
	-over thinking, palpitations, insomnia, poor memory -pale complexion, dizziness, fatigue, poor appetite T: pale P: weak	Benefit Qi and replenish blood. Nourish heart and calm spirit. SP6 (SYJ), ST36 (ZSL) HT7 (shen men), BL15 (xin shu), BL20 (pi shu) LI4-LV3 (4 gates)	
	-depression, trance-like mental state, poor memory, easily irritated, agitation, suspiciousness, spells of grief and crying -hot flashes, menstrual disorders, impotence, night sweats, low tidal fever T: narrow red P: thin, weak	Nourish yin. Clear heat. Calm mind. Relieve depression. PC6 (nei guan), HT7 (shen men) LI4-LV3 (4 gates) KD3 (tai xi) SP6 (SY)	

Diarrhea (xie xie)

Definition:
Frequent passage of semi-formed, loose, or watery stool that may or may not contain undigested food.

Red flags:

Western Medicine Relevant Diseases:
In Western medicine, diarrhea is defined as an increase in the volume, wateriness, or frequency of bowel movements. However, the frequency of bowel movements alone is not the defining feature of diarrhea. Some people normally move their bowels 3 to 5 times a day. Diarrhea is often accompanied by gas, cramping, an urgency to defecate, and, if the diarrhea is caused by an infectious organism or a toxic substance, nausea and vomiting.

Diarrhea can lead to dehydration and a loss of electrolytes, such as sodium, potassium, magnesium, chloride, and bicarbonate, from the blood. If large amounts of fluid and electrolytes are lost, the person feels weak, and blood pressure can drop enough to cause syncope, arrhythmias, and other serious disorders. At particular risk are the very young, the very old, the debilitated, and people with very severe diarrhea.

There are many different causes, depending on how long the diarrhea has lasted. The most common causes of acute diarrhea (lasting less than a week) are
- Infection with viruses, bacteria, or parasites (gastroenteritis)
- Food poisoning
- Drug side effects

The most common causes of chronic diarrhea (lasting more than 4 weeks) are
- Irritable bowel syndrome
- Inflammatory bowel disease
- Drug side effects
- Malabsorption

Diarrhea that has been present for more than 4 weeks may be a lingering case of acute diarrhea or the early stage of a disorder that causes chronic diarrhea.

Etiology/pathology:
- EPI (esp. cold, damp, summer heat, fire) – disrupts SP T&T function (note: cold can invade the Intestines directly, by passing the body's defensive Qi)
- Improper diet – overeating or consumption of too much cold/raw food or spoiled food – injures SP T&T function
- Emotional stress – LV Qi stag – overacts on SP – impairs T&T function
- Deficiency of SP/ST – overexertion, irregular diet, chronic illness - SP unable to T&T – pure and turbid combine and drain out as diarrhea
- KD (SP) yang deficiency – chronic illness, elderly, constitutional weakness – fail to warm SP Yang and hinder KD function of controlling bowel

Diagnosis notes:
- Excess patterns have acute onset and short course; ABD pain worse w pressure; may have fever, chills, nausea, vomit, heaviness
- Deficient patterns have chronic onset and prolonged course; intermittent episodes, moderate ABD pain better w pressure; fatigue, lack of appetite, lassitude

TCM Differentiation and Treatment:

Pattern	Signs and Symptoms	Acupuncture	Formula
Cold Damp Invading	-acute onset -thin clear or loose watery stools, not foul -often severe ABD pain, poor appetite, nausea, and borborygmus -maybe cold EPI signs -feeling of heaviness T: thin white greasy coat P: tight, superficial (slippery)	Disperse cold, drain damp, harmonize MJ and stop diarrhea. ST25 (tian shu), ST36 (ZSL), ST37 (shang ju xu), ST40 (feng long) SP9 (yin ling quan), SP6 (SYJ) REN12 (zhong wan), moxa REN8 (shen que) LI4 (he gu), LU7 (lie sue), SJ5 (wei guan) If vomit/nausea PC6 (nei guan)	
Damp Heat Invading	-acute, urgent defecation, sticky, foul smelling stool, hot pain around anus -irritability, thirst, dark scanty urine -often ABD pain, poor appetite, nausea -maybe hot EPI signs T: red w yellow greasy coat P: rapid, slippery	Clear heat, drain damp, harmonize MJ and stop diarrhea. ST25 (tian shu), ST36 (ZSL), ST37 (shang ju xu), ST40 (feng long) SP9 (yin ling quan), LI4 (he gu), LI11 (qu chi), ST44 (nei ting) DU14 (da zhui) if fever; PC 6 (nei guan) nausea	
Food Stagnation	-acute diarrhea after heavy meals, contains undigested food and has foul smell -ABD pain relieved by bowel movement, borborygmi, bad digestion -ABD distension, poor appetite, nausea, belching, vomiting, bad breath T: greasy P: slippery	Promote digestion. Eliminate stagnation. Harmonize MJ. Stop diarrhea. REN10 (xia wan), REN12 (zhong wan) ST21 (liang men), ST25 (tian shu), ST36 (ZSL), ST44 (nei ting) REN12 (zhong wan) LI4 (he gu), SJ5 (wei guan) Inner Neiting	
Liver attacking Spleen	-recurring painful diarrhea induced by emotional strain (or diarrhea alternating with constipation), temporarily relieved after BM and recurring quickly -rib distension, sighing, mental depression/irritability -poor appetite, poor digestion, pale, tired P: wiry	Pacify Liver. Tonify Spleen. Stop diarrhea. ST25 (tian shu), 36 (ZSL) REN6 (qi hai), REN12 (zhong wan) LV3-LI4 (he gu) BL18 (gan shu), BL20 (pi shu) PC6 (nei guan), Yintang	
Spleen Yang Qi Weak	-chronic diarrhea, loose and watery, may contain undigested food; may be triggered by cold food -poor appetite, nausea, vomit, ABD fullness -pale, tired, SOB, emaciated T: pale P: weak	Tonify Spleen, warm MJ, harmonize MJ, stop diarrhea. ST25 (tian shu), ST36 (ZSL) REN 4 (guan yuan), REN6 (qi hai), REN12 (zhong wan) SP3 (tai bai), SP4 (gong sun) BL20 (pi shu), BL25 (da chang shu)	
KD (and SP) Yang Qi Weak	-chronic early morning diarrhea, ABD pain, cold intolerance, weak knees, poor digestion, pale, tired, SOB T: pale P: weak	Warm and tonify SP and KD, harmonize MJ, stop diarrhea. ST25 (tian shu), ST36 (ZSL) REN4 (guan yuan), REN12 (zhong wan) SP3 (tai bai), SP4 (gong sun) BL20 (pi shu), BL23 (shen shu) Moxa REN8 (shen que), DU4 (ming men)	

Drum Distension (gu zhang)

(also called Tympanic Abdominal Distension)

Definition:
Characterized by drum-like abdominal distension, pale sallow skin tone, distended veins on the abdominal wall, hypochondriac or abdominal masses, and thin limbs. Results from dysfunctions of the Liver, Spleen and Kidney. This is a chronic disorder, lingering, and intractable.

Red Flags:
- Severe pattern requiring Western medical primary care.
- Critical symptoms at end phase include: hematemesis, hematochezia or melena, and comatose.

Western Medicine Relevant Diseases:

Etiology and pathogenesis:
- Improper diet – especially alcohol and irregular eating – damages SP/ST – damp accumulates impeding Qi and affecting liver – Qi and blood stasis result – further injure liver and kidney – clear and turbid fuse and linger internally – pathological water retention develops
- Emotional stress – affects liver causing qi stagnation – leads to blood stasis – LV overacts on SP/ST causing dampness – water, damp, stagnant Qi and blood stasis fuse together and linger in abdomen – KD ability to eliminate water impaired – pathological accumulation of water results
- Chronic jaundice and abdominal masses – damp heat or damp cold in middle burner – damages LV, SP, KD – Qi and blood stagnate – phlegm accumulates
- Infection of schistosomiasis – disharmony between liver and SP by obstructing vessels and channels – Qi stasis, phlegm accumulates, and Blood stasis forms

Differential diagnosis with edema:

	Drum distension	Edema
Areas affected	Abdomen only	Face, four extremities, entire body
Symptoms	Distended veins on ABD, spider angiomas, hematemesis, hematochezia or melena, jaundice, fever, agitation, possible coma.	Stifling chest, palps, dyspnea, nausea, vomiting, lethargy, irritability.

TCM Differentiation and Treatment:

Pattern	Signs and Symptoms	Treatment Principle	Acupuncture	Formula
Qi stagnation and retention of damp	-ABD distension that is soft when pressed -hypochondriac distension, sighing, belching, poor appetite, heaviness T: white, greasy coat P: wiry, slippery	Initial stage or excess: Depending on preponderance of Qi, Blood, Cold, Damp, etc., the treatment should regulate the pathogen and facilitate the movement of qi and blood, strengthen the spleen Late state or deficiency: Strengthen spleen, warm kidney or nourish and replenish liver and kidney yin	Qi stag: REN17 (shan zhong), REN12 (zhong wan), REN6 (qi hai), REN9 (shui fen), LR3 (tai chong), ST25 (tian shu), ST36 (ZSL) Damp: BL20 (pi shu), BL23 (shen shu), REN9 (shui fen), KD7 (fu liu), SP4 (gong sun), LR13 (Zhang men), REN12 (zhong wan), SP9 (yin ling quan) Stasis: LR14 (qi men), LR13 (zhang men), REN5 (shi men), SP6 (SYJ), ST36 (ZSL) SP and KI Yang deficiency: BL20 (pi shu), BL23 (shen shu), REN9 (shui fen), KD7 (fu liu), REN4 (guan yuan), REN6 (qi hai), ST36 (ZSL) LR and KI Yin deficiency: BL18 (gan shu), BL23 (shen shu), REN5 (shi men), REN9 (shui fen), SP 6 (SYJ), KD7 (fu liu), KI3 (tai xi) Plus other symptoms: Cold: moxibustion of REN6 (qi hai) Costal pain: GB34 (yang ling quan), SJ6 (zhi gou) Severe heat: DU14 (da zhui) Jaundice: SI4 (wan gu) + DU9 (zhi yang)	
Retention of cold damp	-ABD distension, enlargement and fullness of the ABD, epigastric fullness -symptoms alleviated with heat -swollen face and lower extremities -lassitude, cold intolerance, scanty urine, watery stool T: white, greasy coat P: slow			
Damp heat accumulation	-ABD distension, tense and firm on palpation, fullness limits flexion at waste -irritable, fever, bitter taste, thirst without desire to drink, dark urine, constipation or loose sticky stools, possible jaundice T: red, yellow greasy coat P: wiry and rapid			
Spleen and Kidney Yang deficiency	-ABD distension better in morning and worse in evening -pale complexion, fullness in epigastrium, poor appetite, cold intolerance T: flabby P: deep, forceless			
Liver and Kidney Yin deficiency	-ABD distension, possibly distended veins on ABD -dusky complexion, purplish lips, dry throat, irritable, insomnia, scanty urine T: dark red with scanty coat P: wiry, thready, rapid			
Blood stasis	-ADB distension that is tight and firm on palpation, veins on ABD, stabbing pain in hypochondriac and ABD regions -tarry stool, dark lips, dull complexion -spider veins on face, neck, arms, chest T: dark purplish with petechiae P: thready, choppy			

Dysentery (li ji)

Definition:
Characterized by abdominal pain, tenesmus (subjective urgency and heavy sensation of the rectum), diarrhea with passage of blood, pus (from decomposed tissues due to blood stasis and heat), or mucous. Often occurs in the summer of fall season. Damp-heat in the Large Intestine is the major predisposing factor. Both sporadic and pandemic occurrences are possible.

Red Flags:
- See diarrhea.
- Dysentery is managed by maintaining fluids by using oral rehydration therapy. If this treatment cannot be adequately maintained due to vomiting or the profuseness of diarrhea, hospital admission may be required for intravenous fluid replacement.

Western Medicine Relevant Diseases:
- Includes conditions such as: bacillary dysentery, amoebic dysentery, viral dysentery, and food poisoning
- In general, dysentery is an inflammation of the intestine that causes diarrhea with blood. Other symptoms may include fever, abdominal pain, and rectal tenesmus. It is caused by a number of types of infection such as bacteria, viruses, parasitic worms, or protozoa. These pathogens typically reach the large intestine after entering orally, through ingestion of contaminated food or water, oral contact with contaminated objects or hands.
- Each specific pathogen has its own mechanism, but in general, the result is damage to the intestinal lining, leading to the inflammatory immune response. This can cause fever, severe cramping, and further tissue damage by the body's immune cells and cytokines, which are released to fight the infection. The result can be impaired nutrient absorption, excessive water and mineral loss through the stools.
- *Shigella* bacteria are a common cause of dysentery throughout the world. The bacteria are excreted in stool and can be easily spread when hygiene or sanitation is inadequate. People may have watery diarrhea, sometimes leading to severe dehydration. Identifying the bacteria in a sample of stool can confirm the diagnosis. Meticulous hygiene is necessary to avoid spreading the infection. Fluids are given by mouth or, if the infection is severe, intravenously. Antibiotics are used.

Etiology and pathogenesis:
- Seasonal epidemic pathogens – especially summer heat-dampness – attack ST and intestines – impair Qi and Blood flow – decompose tissues – cause dysentery
- Improper diet – contaminated food – generates damp heat; or, diet of cold raw food leads to cold damp – obstructs flow of Qi and Blood – stagnant Qi and Blood and digested waste fuse – transform into pus and blood as tissue decomposes

Diagnosis notes:

Diarrhea	-both have tendency to occur in summer and fall seasons -both affect the stomach and intestines	-characterized by increased frequencies of unformed bowel movements	-tenesmus not evident
Dysentery	-both are related to seasonal pathogens and improper diet -both may have ABD pain	-characterized by passage of pus, blood, or mucous stool	-tenesmus -severe ABD pain

TCM Differentiation and Treatment:

Pattern	Signs and Symptoms	Treatment Principle	Acupuncture	Formula
Damp Heat	-ABD pain, tenesmus, diarrhea with blood and pus + heat signs T: yellow, greasy P: slippery, rapid	Clear pathogens, warm or release heat, unblock obstructions during early/excess stage. Tonify insufficiency in chronic/deficiency cases.		
Damp Cold	-ABD pain, tenesmus, diarrhea with more pus and mucus than blood + cold signs T: white, greasy			
Epidemic	-acute onset, fresh blood and pus, excruciating pain in ABD, tenesmus, high fever, thirst, possible loss of consciousness or convulsions T: red, dry yellow coat P: slippery, rapid			
Deficient Cold	-chronic diarrhea with blood and pus + SP Qi weak signs T: pale P: deep, thready, weak			

Dysphagia Occlusion Syndrome (ye ge)

Definition:
In TCM, esophageal constriction is known as ye ge. Ye, or dysphagia, is the inability to swallow or difficulty swallowing. Ge, or gagging, implies the involuntary resistance to food and water after swallowing.

Red Flags:
Any dysphagia is of concern and should be referred for Western medical assessment, but certain findings require emergency care:

Western Medicine Relevant Diseases:
In Western medicine, dysphagia is a disorder where foods and/or liquids do not move normally from the pharynx to the stomach. People feel as though food or liquids become stuck in the esophagus. Dysphagia can cause people to aspirate mouth secretions and/or material they eat or drink. Aspiration can cause acute pneumonia. If aspiration occurs over a long period of time, people may develop chronic lung disease. People who have had dysphagia for a long time are often inadequately nourished and lose weight.

Swallowing requires the brain to unconsciously coordinate the activity of numerous small muscles of the throat and the esophagus. These muscles must contract strongly and in the proper sequence to push food from the mouth to the back of the throat and then down the esophagus. Finally, the lower part of the esophagus must relax to allow food to enter the stomach. Thus, swallowing difficulty can result from the following:
- Disorders of the brain or nervous system
- Disorders of the muscles in general
- Disorders of the esophagus (a physical blockage or a motility [movement] disorder)

Brain and nervous system disorders that cause difficulty swallowing include stroke, Parkinson disease, multiple sclerosis, and amyotrophic lateral sclerosis (ALS). People with these disorders typically have other symptoms in addition to difficulty swallowing. Many have already been diagnosed with these disorders.

General muscle disorders that cause difficulty swallowing include myasthenia gravis, dermatomyositis (inflammation of muscles and skin), and muscular dystrophy.

A physical blockage can result from cancer of the esophagus, webs of tissue across the inside of the esophagus, and scarring of the esophagus from chronic acid reflux or from swallowing a caustic liquid. Sometimes, the esophagus is compressed by a structure such as an enlarged thyroid gland, or a tumor in the middle of the chest.

Esophageal motility disorders include achalasia (in which the rhythmic contractions of the esophagus are greatly decreased and the lower esophageal muscle does not relax normally to allow food to pass into the stomach) and esophageal spasm. Systemic sclerosis (scleroderma) may also cause a motility disorder.

Etiology and Pathogenesis:
- Emotional stress – worry and over-thinking injure the spleen and anger injures the liver – qi stagnates and turns into blood stasis, and phlegm is generated – blood stasis, stagnant and rebellious Qi, and phlegm obstruct the passage and entrance of the stomach

- Improper diet – to much greasy, sweet, spicy food and alcohol – generates heat and phlegm – can injure yin and result in depletion of fluids – lack of lubrication makes it difficult for food to pass
- Aging – SP Qi deficiency and phlegm

TCM Differentiation and Treatment:
(note: to prevent ye ge, the ST, SP, LR, and KI must remain in harmony)

Pattern	Signs and Symptoms	Treatment Principle	Acupuncture	Formula
Constraint of Phlegm and Qi	Sensation of obstruction in throat when swallowing, difficult swallowing, focal distention in chest and diaphragm, aggravation by emotional stress, dry mouth and stool. T: red, greasy coat P: wiry, slippery	Transform phlegm, moisten dryness, relieve constraint	Main Points: REN22 (tian tu), REN13 (shang wan), REN17 (shan zhong), LR3-LI4 (4 gates), PC6 (nei guan) Supplementary: Phlegm and Qi constraint + REN14 (ju que) Fluid depletion and heat + ST36 (ZSL), SP6 (SYJ) Blood stasis + BL17 (ge shu), BL21 (wei shu) Qi deficiency and Yang devastation + BL20 (pi shu), BL21 (wei shu), BL23 (shen shu), REN4 (guan yuan), REN6 (qi hai)	
Fluid Depletion and Heat Accumulation	Difficult and painful swallowing, feeling of obstruction, unable to ingest solid food, emaciation, dry mouth and throat, constipation, five center heat. T: Dry red, cracks P: wiry thready and rapid	Nourish yin, clear heat, generate fluid		
Internal Accumulation of Blood Stasis	Stabbing pain in center of chest, inability to swallow food and drink, immediate vomiting after ingestion, creamy dark emesis with undigested food, pebble like stools, dusky completion, severe emaciation, dark purple tongue. T: dry red or dark purple P: thready, choppy	Nourish Yin and Blood, moisten dryness, break up stasis, invigorate Blood		
Qi Deficiency and Yang Devastation	Longstanding inability of ingestion, and vomiting clear liquid, pale, lassitude, cold intolerance, edema, ABD distension. T: pale P: thready and weak	Warm and tonify SP and KD		

Dyspnea (chuan zheng)

Definition:
Dyspnea, or breathlessness, is a common respiratory condition that is characterized by: labored breathing that is rapid and shallow, breathing with an open mouth, lifted shoulders and dilated nostrils. Symptoms are aggravated by physical exertion. Severe cases may result in orthopnea (difficult breathing while lying down) and prostration. This may be acute or chronic.

Red Flags:
The following symptoms are of particular concern and merit referral for Western medical assessment:
- Shortness of breath at rest
- A decreased level of consciousness, agitation, or confusion
- Chest discomfort or pain
- Feeling the heart is pounding or racing or has skipped a beat
- Weight loss
- Night sweats

Emergency care is required for people feeling: shortness of breath at rest, chest pain, palpitations, a decreased level of consciousness, agitation, or confusion or having difficulty moving air in or out of their lungs. Stridor breathing suggests upper airway obstruction. This is a serious condition and could be due to laryngotracheitis, quinsy, or epiglottitis. It is important not to ask to see the tongue as this can affect the position of the epiglottis and may worsen the obstruction.

Western Medicine Relevant Diseases:
In Western medicine, dyspnea is described as the unpleasant sensation of having difficulty breathing accompanied by the sensation of running out of air. People feel as if they cannot breathe fast enough or deeply enough. They may notice that more effort is needed to expand the chest when breathing in or to expel air when breathing out. They may also have the uncomfortable sensation inspiration is urgently needed before expiration is completed and have various sensations often described as tightness in the chest. Other symptoms, such as cough or chest pain, may be present depending on the cause of dyspnea.

Dyspnea is usually caused by disorders of the lungs or heart. The most common causes include: asthma, bronchitis, pneumonia, COPD, heart attack or angina, and physical deconditioning (weakening of muscles and the heart due to inactivity). Pulmonary embolism (sudden blockage of an artery of the lung, usually by a blood clot) is a less common, but serious cause.

Other causes include:
- Heart failure: With heart failure, fluid may accumulate in the lungs (pulmonary edema). This disorder causes dyspnea that is often accompanied by a feeling of smothering or heaviness in the chest. The fluid accumulation in the lungs may also narrow the airways and cause wheezing (cardiac asthma). Some people with heart failure have orthopnea, paroxysmal nocturnal dyspnea, or both.
- Anemia: anemia, or severe blood loss from injury results in fewer red blood cells to carry oxygen. Thus, people with anemia will breathe rapidly and deeply in a reflex effort to try to increase the amount of oxygen in the blood.
- Metabolic acidosis: if a large amount of acid accumulates in the blood (metabolic acidosis), people may feel out of breath and begin to pant quickly. Severe kidney failure, sudden worsening of diabetes mellitus, and ingestion of certain drugs or poisons can cause metabolic acidosis.
- Hyperventilation syndrome: in hyperventilation syndrome, people feel that they cannot get enough air, and they breathe heavily and rapidly. This syndrome is commonly caused by anxiety rather than a physical problem. Many people who experience it are frightened, may have chest pain, and may believe they are having a heart attack. They may have a change in consciousness, usually described as feeling that events occurring around them are far away, and they may feel tingling in their hands and feet and around their mouth.

Etiology and pathogenesis:
In TCM, dyspnea is due to a failure of LU Qi to descend due to either excess or deficiency.
- EPI (wind heat, wind cold) – obstructs LU function – inhibits LU Qi dispersion
- Improper diet – injures middle burner – SP cannot T&T – phlegm accumulates – blocks descent of LU Qi
- Emotional stress – Qi stagnation – LU Qi cannot D&D
- Chronic illness – LU Qi and Yin become deficient – KD essence deficiency – LU function is weakened and deficient KD cannot grasp qi

TCM Differentiation and Treatment:

Pattern	Signs and Symptoms	Treatment Principle	Acupuncture	Formula
	Aversion to cold, shivering, fever, cough, breathlessness, feeling of chest oppression, thin white mucus, headache, no sweating. P: floating tight	Release exterior, restore dispersing and descending of LU, expel Wind-Cold	LU7 (lie que), LU6 (zong kui), BL12 (feng men), BL13 (fei shu), Dingchuan	
	Aversion to cold, fever, shivering, headache, no sweating breathlessness, cough with profuse white watery sputum, difficulty lying down, swelling of limbs. T: sticky white coat P: floating	Release exterior, expel Wind-Cold, restore LU Qi descending, resolve phlegm	LU7 (lie que), LU6 (kong zui), LU5 (chi ze), BL12 (fen men), BL13 (fei shu), Dingchuan, PC6 (nei guan), ST40 (feng long), REN22 (tian tu)	
	Breathlessness, distension or pain in chest, coarse breathing, runny nose, cough, vomiting of sticky phlegm, feel heat, cold limbs, irritable, aches, thirst. T: red, white or yellow coat P: slippery, rapid	Clear heat, restore LU Qi descending	LU6 (kong zui), LU7 (lie que), LU10 (yu ji), LU1 (zhong fu), LI11 (qu chi)	
	Cough, breathlessness, chest pain, profuse yellow or blood tinged sputum, irritable, chest discomfort, feel heat, sweat, thirst, red face, dry throat, dark urine, constipation. T: red, sticky yellow P: slippery rapid	Clear heat, resolve phlegm, clear LU	LU5 (chi ze), LU1 (zhong fu), LI11 (qu chi), ST40 (feng long), DU14 (da zhui)	
	Sudden attacks of breathlessness worse with emotional stress, suffocating sensation or constriction of throat, chest oppression and pain, insomnia, palpitations. P: wiry	Soothe LR, activate Qi flow, restore LU Qi descending	LR3 (tai chong), LR14 (qi men), SP6 (SYJ), LU1 (zhong fun), REN17 (shan zhong), LU7 (lie que), HT7 (shen men)	
	SOB, weak lung sounds, slight rattling sound in throat, possible low/weak voice, scanty phlegm, spontaneous sweat, pale complexion, lassitude. T: pale or read P: thready weak or rapid	Tonify LU, strengthen Qi, restore LU function	LU7 (lie que), LU9 (tai yuan), BL13 (fei shu), DU12 (shen zhu), REN6 (qi hai), ST36 (ZSL), REN17 (shan zhong)	
	Chronic breathlessness, worse with exertion, difficult inhalation, weight loss, depression, cold limbs, sore back, dizziness, weak knees. T: pale P: deep, weak, slow	Warm and tonify KD, stimulate LU descending	BL23 (shen men), BL13 (fei shu), DU4 (ming men), KI7 (fu liu), KI25 (shen cang), KI3, (tai xi) LU7 (lie que)	

*Diagnosis note: the heart may be involved during critical phase of breathlessness. Manifestations would include: cyanotic lips, tongue and nails, palps...this could result from either a) LU qi xu and failure of heart qi to circulate or b) KD yang xu failing to warm the heart, fluids not transformed and accumulate in heart and lung "kidney yang xu with water overflowing towards the lung and heart"

Edema (shui zhong)

Definition:
Edema refers to the abnormal retention of fluid in the body. Fluid can be retained and result in puffiness around the eyelids, face and limbs. Excess fluid can also be retained systemically leading to swelling of the entire body. In severe cases, edema can develop in the thoracic or abdominal cavities.

Red Flags:
The following signs suggest a more serious etiology of edema and merit referral for Western medical assessment:

Western Medicine Relevant Diseases:
Edema results from increased movement of fluid from the intravascular to the interstitial space or decreased movement of water from the interstitium into the capillaries or lymphatic vessels. The mechanism involves one or more of the following:
- Increased capillary hydrostatic pressure
- Decreased plasma oncotic pressure (POP pulls water into the circulatory system)
- Increased capillary permeability
- Obstruction of the lymphatic system

As fluid shifts into the interstitial space, intravascular volume is depleted. Intravascular volume depletion activates the renin-angiotensin-aldosterone- vasopressin (ADH) system, resulting in renal Na retention. By increasing osmolality, renal Na retention triggers water retention by the kidneys and helps maintain plasma volume. Increased renal Na retention also may be a primary cause of fluid overload and edema. Excessive exogenous Na intake may also contribute. Less often, edema results from decreased movement of fluid out of the interstitial space into the capillaries due to lack of adequate plasma oncotic pressure as in nephrotic syndrome, protein-losing enteropathy, or starvation. Increased capillary permeability occurs in infections or as the result of toxin or inflammatory damage to the capillary walls. The lymphatic system is responsible for removing protein and WBCs (along with some water) from the interstitium. Lymphatic obstruction allows these substances to accumulate in the interstitium.

Generalized edema is most commonly caused by:
- Congestive heart failure
- Liver failure (e.g. due to cirrhosis)
- Kidney disorders (e.g. acute and chronic nephritis)

Localized edema is most commonly caused by
- Deep vein thrombosis or another venous disorder or venous obstruction (e.g. by tumor)
- Infection
- Angioedema
- Lymphatic obstruction

Etiology and pathogenesis:
Water metabolism depends on the movement of Qi. Three organs account for water metabolism in TCM: LU, SP, KI; the Triple Burner is also important as a passageway for Qi flow. Causes of edema include:
- Exterior wind attacking lung or damp attacking spleen (cold or heat)
- Exterior dampness (cold or heat) impairing SP
- Improper diet – SP deficiency then KI deficiency
- Overwork, chronic illness and aging – KI deficiency
- Fire poisons from sores of carbuncles – impedes the space between the skin and muscles

TCM Differentiation and Treatment:
Edema can be divided into Yang and Yin edema on the basis of etiology, pathogenesis, and manifestations.

Yang edema	Yin edema
-begins from upper body (can spread, but usually starts on head/face)	-starts from lower body
-caused by exterior pathogens	-caused my diet, overexertion, too many babies, etc.
-acute and fast developing, short duration	-chronic, slow onset (but could also be fast)
-excess, exterior condition	-interior, deficient (often KI yang xu)
-not usually pitting	-often darker skin and pitting

Pattern, Signs and Symptoms, Treatment Principle, Acupuncture	Formula

Yang Edema Patterns
    o Wind-water attacking: edema of eyes and face with sudden onset, aversion to cold, fever, aches in muscles, retention of urine. P: floating, slow
        ▪ Treatment: release exterior, expel wind, open water passages, stimulate LU dispersing fluids: LI4 (he gu), LU7 (lie que), SJ5 (wei guan), BL12 (feng men), BL13 (fei shu), LI6 (pian li), LI10 (shou san li) (lips), DU26 (shui gou), REN17 (shan zhong), ST36 (ZSL) (harmonizes nutritive and defensive qi and the space between the skin and muscles)
    o Damp invading middle jiao (may be cold or heat): edema of whole body or legs, decreased urine, dizziness, heaviness, nausea, poor appetite. T: swollen, sticky coat, P: slippery
        ▪ Treatment: Strengthen SP, resolve dampness, reduce swelling: BL20 (pi shu), BL21 (wei shu), ST36 (ZSL), REN 5 (shi men), REN9 (shui fen), ST28 (shui dao), BL22 (san jiao shu), SP9 (yin ling quan)
    o Fire poisons: edema of any part of the body, sores, carbuncles or furuncles
        ▪ Treatment: Drain damp, clear heat, resolve fire toxin, tonify lungs and spleen: REN12 (zhong wan), BL20 (pi shu), REN9 (shui fen), ST28 (shui dao), BL22 (san jiao shu), SP9 (yin ling quan), LU7 (lie que), BL13 (fei shu), LI11 (qu chi)	

Yin Edema Patterns
    o Spleen Yang Xu: chronic whole body edema often from lower limbs, pitting on pressure, with SP Qi weak signs (poor appetite, nausea). T: pale, swollen, P: weak
        ▪ Tonify and warm SP and resolve edema: REN12 (zhong wan), ST36 (zu san li), BL20 (pi shu), BL21 (wei shu), SP6 (SYJ), REN6 (qi hai), REN9 (shui fen), ST28 (shui dao), BL22 (san jiao shu)
    o KD Yang Xu: more severe than SP Yang Xu, pitting on pressure, sore back/knees, feel cold, pale, tired, bright white complexion. T: Pale, swollen, P: deep, weak
        ▪ Tonify and warm the KD, resolve edema: REN4 (guan yuan), BL23 (shen shu), KD7 (fu liu), BL20 (pi shu), ST36 (ZSL), BL22 (san jiao shu), ST28 (shui dao)	

Epigastric Pain (wei tong)

Epigastric Pain

Definition:
Painful sensation located between lower margin of sternum and the infra-costal margins. Varies in severity. Accompanied by focal distention in epigastrium, belching, acid regurgitation, lack of appetite, hypochondriac and abdominal distension. Pain is often recurrent.

Red Flags:
- Gastric bleeding and gastric cancer – protracted pain, irregular pain, distention, fullness, nausea, dizziness, possible hematemesis; prompt referral is needed to rule out gastric bleeding. For middle age patients with irregular pain plus emaciation, low-grade fever and intermittent unexplained black stool/vomiting that looks like coffee grinds, refer to rule out gastric cancer.
- Acute pancreatitis – more common over 40; sudden onset and severe pain, increasing; may radiate to back; also nausea, vomiting relieved by sitting up and bending forward.
- Perforated gastric ulcer – severe epigastric pain spreading over abdomen, aggravated on coughing and deep breathing; shock, reluctance to move; rigid abdomen.

Western medicine:
In Western medicine, epigastric pain may result from:

(Above list based on Maciocia, G. *The Practise of Chinese Medicine*)

Etiology and Pathogenesis:
- EPIs attacking the ST – especially cold and damp – obstructs flow of ST Qi preventing it from descending
- Poor diet – too little or too much, excessive alcohol, greasy diet, eating too fast or late at night, eating irregular amounts, working while eating – impairs descending of ST and leads to food retention and stagnation of ST Qi
- Emotional problems – anger and worry – impairs function of LR – LR overacts on ST and obstructs movement of Qi
- Overexertion, overwork, chronic illness, constitutional weakness – cause SP/ST deficiency

TCM Differentiation and Treatment:

Pattern	Signs and Symptoms	Treatment Principle	Acupuncture	Formula
Cold invading Stomach	Sudden onset, severe pain, better with warmth, worse with cold/pressure. P: wiry, tight	Disperse cold, warm ST, alleviate pain	Principle points: REN12 (zhong wan), ST36 (ZSL), PC6 (nei guan), SP4 (gong sun) Stomach cold + REN6 (qi hai), REN8 (shen que), ST21 (liang men), ST34 (liang qiu) Food retention + inner neiting, ST44 (nei ting), ST25 (tian shu) Stomach heat or fire + ST44 (nei ting), ST45 (li dui), ST21 (liang men), SP6 (SYJ) (with phlegm + ST40 (feng long), PC7 (da ling)) LR invading + LR14 (qi men), LR3 (tai chong) Blood stasis + BL17 (ge shu), SP10 (xue hai) Yin deficiency + REN12 (zhong wan), ST36 (zu san li), SP6 (SYJ), REN4 (guan yuan) Yang deficiency + REN12 (zhong wan), ST36 (ZSL), BL20 (pi shu), BL21 (wei shu), PC6 (nei guan), REN6 (qi hai)	
Food retention	Dull pain with fullness and distension, belching, acid regurgitation, foul breath, nausea, vomit undigested food, pain better with passing gas. T: thick, greasy coat P: slippery	Eliminate food retention, promote digestion, relieve pain		
Stomach heat	Burning epigastric pain, thirst, irritable, sour regurgitation. T: dry, yellow coat P: rapid	Clear heat, restore descending of ST Qi, relieve pain		
Stomach Fire (or Phlegm Fire)	Burning pain, thirst, severe irritability, bleeding gums, vomit blood, red face, constipation (plus may be phlegm signs) T: red, yellow coat P: rapid	Clear fire, protect ST Yin, restore descending of ST Qi, relieve pain		
Liver Invading Stomach	Distending pain that radiates to hypochondriac region, worse with emotions, poor appetite, belching, sighing. P: wiry	Soothe liver and regulate Qi, relieve pain		
Blood stasis	Stabbing epigastric pain in fixed location, worse with pressure, pain worse at night, possible hematemesis. T: dark purple P: choppy	Invigorate blood and transform stasis, relieve pain		
Stomach Yin deficiency	Vague, burning epigastric pain, hunger without desire to eat, dry mouth and throat, dry stool. T: dry red P: thready, rapid	Nourish ST Yin, resolve pain		
Spleen and Stomach Yang deficiency	Vague, dull pain, better with warmth and pressure, worse with hunger, vomiting clear fluids, poor appetite, fatigue, cold limbs, loose stool. T: pale P: weak, slow	Warm middle burner, strengthen SP, relieve pain.		

Epilepsy (xian zheng)

Definition:
A recurrent neurological disorder characterized by a sudden, brief episode of altered consciousness. In more severe cases, there may be loss of consciousness, foaming at the mouth, bleating sounds, rolling back of the eyes, and violent involuntary movements of the limbs followed by regained consciousness and no lingering symptoms. These symptoms are the result of liver wind triggering turbid phlegm, which mists the clear orifices and obstructs the channels.

Red Flags:
A seizure is a medical emergency if:
- It is the person's first seizure
- Seizures of any kind go on longer than five minutes
- Multiple seizures occur in a short period of time
- The person stops breathing
- A seizure occurs in water
- The person hits his or her head during a seizure and becomes difficult to rouse, is vomiting, or complains of blurry vision

Follow first aid protocol.

Western medicine:
Normal brain function requires an orderly, organized, coordinated discharge of electrical impulses. Electrical impulses enable the brain to communicate with the spinal cord, nerves, and muscles as well as within itself. Seizures may result when the brain's electrical activity is disrupted.

There are two basic types of seizures:
- Epileptic: These seizures have no apparent cause (or trigger) and occur repeatedly. These seizures are called a seizure disorder or epilepsy.
- Non-epileptic: These seizures are triggered by a disorder or another condition that irritates the brain. For example, a head injury, stroke, or tumor may damage the brain and cause a seizure. Alcohol withdrawal can also cause of seizures.

Conditions that irritate the brain can trigger a single seizure whether a person has a seizure disorder or not, for example: injuries, certain drugs, sleep deprivation, infections, fever; or, conditions that deprive the brain of oxygen or fuel, e.g. abnormal heart rhythms, a low level of oxygen in the blood, or a very low level of sugar in the blood. A single seizure that results from such a stimulus is called a provoked seizure. People with a seizure disorder are more likely to have a seizure when they are under excess physical or emotional stress, when they are intoxicated or deprived of sleep, or when they have suddenly stopped drinking or using sedatives. Rarely, seizures may be triggered by repetitive sounds, flashing lights, video games, or touching certain parts of the body. In such cases, the disorder is called reflex epilepsy.

Etiology and Pathogenesis:
Major factors include: constitutional factors, emotional disturbances, improper diet, stress, overstrain, and trauma. These cause disharmony of yin and yang of the organs and disturb normal Qi movement, allowing phlegm to obstruct the channels and obscure the orifices. Injury to liver, kidney, heart, and spleen is common in the pathogenesis of epilepsy. Epilepsy can also be caused by stagnant Qi and Blood from traumatic injury.

TCM Patterns and Treatment:

Pattern	Signs and Symptoms	Treatment Principle	Acupuncture	Formula
Yang Pattern	Aura with dizziness, headache, stifling chest, sudden fall with a cry, LOC, eyes fixed upward, locked jaw, dark lips, contractions, drooling, gurgling sounds in throat, possible incontinence, exhaustion after. T: greasy coat P: wiry, slippery, rapid	Treatment should be developed based on phase of episode or remission. During or immediately following a seizure, treatment should focus on the branch by, e.g. strongly expelling phlegm, wind, opening orifices. During remission, treatment should focus on the root by strengthening the relevant organ, resolving phlegm, nourishing the heart and calming the spirit.		
Yin Pattern	Pale, sallow, cold limbs, LOC with eys partially open, contraction of body in fetal position or clonic contractions of extremities, drooling, no cry, possible LOC, trance, weakness and quiet/still after. T: pale, greasy P: deep thready, or slippery			
Remission				
Spleen deficiency and phlegm	Fatigue, lassitude, sallow, lack of appetite, ABD distension, loose stool, nausea, coughing white sputum. T: pale, greasy P: soft, slippery			

Fainting (jue zheng)

Definition:
Jue refers to a condition of fainting with cold limbs. Syncope, or jue syndrome, refers to a group of disorders in which sudden and transient loss of consciousness is accompanied by frigid extremities. In mild cases there is spontaneous recovery without any sequelae. Delayed recovery may indicate a life threatening condition (separation of yin and yang).

Red flags:
In people who have fainted, certain symptoms and characteristics are cause for concern. They include:
- Fainting during exercise
- Several episodes within a short time
- Sudden fainting without any warning symptoms or any apparent trigger
- Fainting preceded or followed by possible heart symptoms such as chest pain, palpitations, or shortness of breath
- Older age
- Significant injury as a result of fainting

Transient Ischemic Attack (TIA) is a medical emergency. A TIA is a transient stroke that lasts only a few minutes. It occurs when the blood supply to part of the brain is briefly interrupted. TIA symptoms, which usually occur suddenly, are similar to those of stroke but do not last as long. Most symptoms of a TIA disappear within an hour, although they may persist for up to 24 hours. Symptoms can include: numbness or weakness in the face, arm, or leg, especially on one side of the body; confusion or difficulty in talking or understanding speech; trouble seeing in one or both eyes; and difficulty with walking, dizziness, or loss of balance and coordination.

Relevant Western Medical Diseases:
In Western medicine, fainting is called syncope. It is a sudden, brief loss of consciousness, followed by a complete return to consciousness. Other symptoms include: cool legs and arms, a weak pulse, and shallow breathing. Some people feel light-headed or dizzy before they faint. Others may have nausea, sweating, blurred vision or tunnel vision, tingling of lips or fingertips, chest pain, or palpitations.

A person cannot lose consciousness unless brain function is disturbed. This disturbance usually occurs because overall blood flow to the brain is reduced. Sometimes, however, blood flow is adequate but the blood does not contain sufficient oxygen or glucose, which the brain needs to function.

The most common causes are:
- Strong emotion (such as fear, pain, or sight of blood) - activates vagus nerve and widens blood vessels, reducing blood flow to the heart and slowing heart rate
- Coughing or straining to pass stool or urine - increases chest pressure and can activate the vagus nerve
- Prolonged standing or standing up suddenly - leg muscles have to be active to help return blood to the heart. Sitting or standing up too quickly can cause fainting, because the change in position causes blood to pool in the legs, resulting in a fall in blood pressure
- Pregnancy -- hormonal changes and changes in blood pressure can lead to fainting
- Use of certain drugs
- Idiopathic
- Hypoglycemia, if is severe or prolonged, can also cause fainting.

Less common but more serious causes include
- Heart valve disorders (most commonly, the aortic valve)
- A heart rate that is too fast or too slow
- Pulmonary embolism
- Heart attack or other heart muscle disorders

Although most strokes do not cause fainting, a stroke or transient ischemic attack (TIA) that involves certain blood vessels at the base of the brain (posterior circulation stroke) can cause fainting. Similarly, a migraine that involves these blood vessels sometimes causes fainting.

Etiology and Pathogenesis:

TCM Differentiation and Treatment:

Pattern & Signs and Symptoms	Treatment Principle & Acupuncture	Formula
Excess Qi syncope: strong emotions followed by sudden LOC, rapid and heavy respiration, locked jaws, clenched fists Excess Blood Syncope: sudden LOC after extreme emotional stimulation, red face, locked jaws Phlegm syncope: sudden LOC with gurgling/rattling sounds, often overweight, heavy breathing, may vomit white mucus Qi deficiency syncope: LOC after dizziness, vertigo, weak respiration, pale and clammy cold skin Deficient blood syncope: sudden LOC, pale face and lips, tremors, open mouth, cold skin, weak breathing	Principle points for fainting: DU26 (shui gou), PC6 (nei guan), Five heart point: DU20 (bai hui), KI1 (yong quan), PC8 (lao gong) Excess treatment: open orifices and awake consciousness: DU26 (shui gou), PC6 (nei guan) Plus points according to pattern: Qi syncope: LR3-LI4 (4 gates) Blood syncope: LR2 (xing jian), KD1 (yong quan) Phlegm syncope: ST40 (feng long) Deficiency treatment: Support Qi, restore and rescue yang + tonify: DU20 (bai hui), REN6 (qi hai) Deficient Qi syncope + ST36 (ZSL) Deficient Blood syncope + REN4 (guan yuan) In remission: treat according to root	

Goitre (ying bing)

Definition:
Disorder manifested with enlargement or nodules by thyroid cartilage in the neck.

Western Medicine Relevant Diseases:
The most common cause of goiters is insufficient dietary iodine. The thyroid gland uses iodine to make thyroid hormone. When there is not enough iodine, the thyroid gland grows larger to compensate. Other causes of goiter include: using certain drugs and eating certain foods in unusually large amounts (such as cassava, broccoli, cauliflower, and cabbage). Sometimes goiters form temporarily during puberty, pregnancy, or menopause.

The patterns of goiters in TCM also correspond to thyroid diseases in Western medicine, including hyperthyroidism and thyroid tumor. Hyperthyroidism is over-activity of the thyroid gland that leads to high levels of thyroid hormones and speeding up of vital body functions. Graves disease is the most common cause of hyperthyroidism. It is an autoimmune disorder where antibodies stimulate the thyroid to produce and secrete excess thyroid hormones into the blood. This cause of hyperthyroidism is often hereditary and almost always leads to enlargement of the thyroid. In addition, the thyroid can be swollen with hypothyroid as well.

(For a more detailed discussion, see discussion of goiter in External Medicine section)

Etiology and pathogenesis:
The basic pathogenesis of goiter is Qi stagnation and phlegm accumulation. In chronic cases, these can lead to blood stasis.
- Emotional stress – LV qi stagnates – phlegm forms – Qi accumulation plus phlegm results in goiter
- Improper diet and environment – SP&ST fail to T&T – phlegm accumulates and forms goiter; dietary insufficiencies can also lead to deficiency
- Constitutional factors – Yin deficiency – vulnerable to pathogenic fire from stagnant Qi and accumulated phlegm

TCM Differentiation and Treatment:

Pattern	Signs and Symptoms	Treatment Principle	Acupuncture	Formula
Qi Stagnation and Phlegm Accumulation	Swelling that is soft and without pain, distending sensation, stuffy chest, migrating distending sensation in chest, sighing, worse with emotions. P: wiry	Facilitate Qi flow, relieve constraint, resolve goiter		
Phlegm Accumulation and Blood Stasis	Mass that is hard or nodular, gradual onset and slow progress, stuffy chest, poor appetite. T: greasy P: wiry or choppy	Invigorate blood, resolve phlegm, reduce goiter		
Liver Fire Blazing Upwards	Swelling, soft and smooth on palpation, irritable, hot sensations, profuse perspiration, bitter taste in mouth. T: red, yellow coat P: wiry and rapid	Clear and drain liver fire, reduce goiter		
Yin Deficiency	Soft swelling, gradual onset, slow progression, palpitations, irritability, insomnia, easily sweat, tremors, blurred vision, fatigue. T: red P: wiry, thready, rapid	Nourish yin, reduce goiter (may also need to clear heat or fire if prevalent)		

Headache (tou tong)

Definition:
Headache is a symptom common in clinic presenting as various types of pain in different areas of the head. The head is the merging area for the clear Yang of the body, as well as the Sea of Marrow. Pain results when clear Yang is obstructed or nourishment fails to reach the head (Qi, blood, essence).

Red Flags:
The following symptoms are of particular concern and should be referred for Western medical treatment:
- Evidence of a slow increase in intracranial pressure: Progressive headaches and vomiting over a few weeks to months. Headaches are worse in the morning and the vomiting may be effortless. Blurring of vision may be an additional symptom. Intracranial pressure will slowly increase if there is a gradual development of a "space occupying lesion" such as a brain tumor, abscess in the brain, extra-dural hemorrhage or accumulation of poorly draining cerebrospinal fluid. The pressure will be worse when the patient has been lying down, so the symptoms are characteristically worse in the morning. These include blurring of vision (especially after coughing or leaning forward), "effortless vomiting" (i.e. not much preceding nausea) and headache.
- A sudden onset, very severe headache: The patient needs to lie down and may vomit. There may be neck stiffness (reluctance to move the head) and dislike of bright light. The sudden very severe headache (like a hit to the back of the head) is a cardinal symptom of the potentially devastating subarachnoid hemorrhage. This is a bleed from an area of weakness in one of the arterial branches in the base of the brain (The "circle of Willis"). Subarachnoid hemorrhage may result from an inherited malformation and so may develop in a seemingly fit person.
- A severe headache that develops over the course of a few hours to days with fever, vomiting and neck stiffness. This suggests acute meningitis or encephalitis. Meningitis and encephalitis are infections of the meninges and brain tissue respectively. They can be caused by a wide range of infectious organisms. Although headache and fever are common co-symptoms in benign infections such as tonsillitis, the triad of headache, vomiting and fever is more suggestive of brain infections. Additional symptoms such as reluctance to move the head, arching back of the neck and dislike of bright lights, and a purpuric rash may also be present.
- A severe headache that develops over the course of a few hours to days with fever and with a bruising and non-blanching rash suggests meningococcal meningitis. See notes above. This is an emergency situation.
- A severe one-sided headache over the temple occurring for the first time in an elderly person: An unusual severe, persistent one-sided headache in an elderly person should be taken seriously as this could reflect the inflammatory condition of temporal arteritis. In this condition, which is a form of vasculitis, inflammation of the arteries supplying the head can become inflamed and thickened carrying the risk of obstruction by blood clot. There is a significant risk of thrombosis of a cerebral artery or retinal artery in temporal arteritis.
- A long history of worsening (progressive) headaches, with generalized symptoms such as fever, loss of appetite and exhaustion: Consider referral if there is a progression in severity of the headaches or if there are other symptoms not usually associated with benign headache such as fever, loss of appetite, weight loss or other neurological symptoms. Benign headaches should respond significantly to treatment, so also consider referral of recurrent headaches if no improvement within 1-2 months.

Western Medicine Relevant Diseases:
In Western medicine, a headache is pain in any part of the head, including the scalp, upper neck, face, and interior of the head. Although headaches can be painful and distressing, they are rarely due to a serious condition. There are two types of headaches:
- Primary headaches (i.e. not caused by another disorder), including: migraine, cluster headache, and tension-type headache.
- Secondary headaches (i.e. caused by another disorder) may result from disorders of the brain, eyes, nose, throat, sinuses, teeth, jaws, ears, or neck or from a systemic disorder.

The two most common causes of headache are primary headaches:
- Tension-type: Tension-type headaches feel like tightening of a band around the head. These headaches may be episodic or chronic. Tension-type headaches are rarely severe and usually do not interfere with daily activities. Unlike migraine headaches, tension-type headaches are not accompanied by nausea and vomiting and are not made worse by physical activity, light, sounds, or odors.
- Migraine: In a migraine, pulsating or throbbing pain is usually felt on one side of the head, but it may occur on both sides. The pain may be moderate but is often severe and incapacitating. Physical activity, bright light, loud noises, and certain odors may make the headache worse. The headache is frequently accompanied by nausea, sometimes with vomiting and sensitivity to light, sounds, and/or odors. Severe attacks can be incapacitating, disrupting daily routines and work.

Other causes:
Headaches may also be due to a less common primary headache disorder called cluster headaches, or to one of the many secondary headache disorders. Some secondary headache disorders are serious, particularly those that involve the brain, such as meningitis, a brain tumor, or intra-cerebral hemorrhage (see red flags). Fever can cause headaches, as can many infections that do not specifically involve

the brain (e.g. Lyme disease and influenza). Headaches also commonly occur when people stop consuming caffeine or stop taking pain relievers after using them for a long time (called medication overuse headache).

Etiology and Pathogenesis:
- EPI – wind in primary pathogenic factor, as it affects the upper body first
    - Wind cold can congeal Qi and blood, obstructing channels
    - Wind heat can flare up, disrupting clear orifices
    - Wind damp can injur Yang qi and block Qi, preventing clear Yang rising
- Interior organ dysfunction – brain relies on nourishment from Spleen, Liver and Kidney – dysfunction of these organs leads to malnourishment of head; also, dysfunction of Spleen and lead to phlegm can inhibit clear Yang
- Trauma – accidents can disturb flow of Qi and Blood – Blood stasis
- Overwork (especially excessive mental work) and stress – weakens organs – e.g. overwork weakens SP Qi and in the long term KD Yin, or will lead to LR Yang rising and causing headaches
- Poor diet & dietary irregularities, e.g.
    - Excessive damp producing foods may weaken SP and ST – dull and heavy headaches
    - Excessive hot energy foods can lead to LR Fire and/or ST heat – lateral and frontal headaches sharp in character
    - Too much salt will cause KI deficiency – dull headaches

TCM Differentiation and Treatment:
(Note: basic patterns are covered below. See Maciocia, G, *The Practice of Chinese Medicine,* for a broad discussion on headaches and additional patterns.)

For all H/A patterns, add points by location, for example:

Pattern	Signs and Symptoms	Treatment Principle	Acupuncture	Formula
Wind Cold	H/A with stiffness and radiating pain to neck/back, aggravated by windy weather, aversion to wind or cold, no thirst. P: floating, tight	Disperse and expel wind-cold, remove obstruction from channels	For Exterior, expel pathogen: Wind cold + LU7 (lie que), GB20 (feng shi), DU16 (feng fu), BL10 (tian zhu) Wind heat + LI4 (he gu), GB20 (feng chi), DU16 (feng fu), DU14 (da zhui), SJ5 (wei guan) Wind damp + LU7 (lie que), LI6 (pian li), SP6 (SYJ), ST8 (tou wei), DU23 (shang xing) LR Yang Rising + LR3 (tai chong), LR8 (qu quan), SP6 (SYJ), SJ5 (wei guan), GB20 (feng chi), Taiyang For interior conditions, tonify the deficiency, or determine the root and branch and treat accordingly. KI deficiency + KI3 (tai xi), ST36 (ZSL), SP6 (SYJ), DU20 (bai hui), REN4 (guan yuan), BL23 (shen shu) Phlegm blocking + ST40 (feng long), LI4 (he gu), LU7 (lie que), ST8 (tou wei), DU20 (bai hui) Blood deficiency + ST36 (ZSL), SP6 (SYJ), BL20 (pi shu), LR8 (qu quan), REN4 (guan yuan), DU20 (bai hui), BL15 (xin shu) Blood Stasis + LI4 (he gu), BL17 (ge shu), SP6 (SYJ), LR3 (tai chong), Ah Shi points	
Wind Heat	H/A with distending pain, can be very severe (like head splitting), aversion to wind/cold, fever, red face and eyes, thirst, swollen sore throat. T: red, yellow coat P: floating, rapid	Disperse wind, clear heat, remove obstruction from channels		
Wind Damp	H/A with heaviness (like wrapped in a cloth), worse in cloudy/rainy weather, heavy body, stuffy chest, poor appetite. T: greasy coat P: floating, slippery	Expel wind and damp, remove obstruction from channels		
Liver Yang Rising	H/A with throbbing or distending pain, dizziness, red eyes, unilateral or bilateral pain, aggravated by emotions, hypochondriac distension, irritability, insomnia, red face, bitter taste. P: wiry	*must determine underlying cause of LR Yang Rising (e.g. LR Blood xu, LR Yin xu) Pacify LR, subdue Yang, + treat underlying (e.g. nourish LR blood)		
Kidney Deficiency	H/A with dizziness, sensation of emptiness in head, sore back/knees, lack of strength, insomnia, tinnitus, may be KD Yin or Yang deficiency specific signs.	Tonify Kidneys, replenish Essence		
Phlegm Blocking	H/A with dizziness, cloudy head, stuffy chest, nausea, vomiting phlegm, blurred vision. T: greasy P: slippery	Resolve Phlegm, unblock orifices		
Blood deficiency	H/A with dizziness, worse in afternoon/evening, poor memory, palpitations, restlessness, fatigue, lack of strength, pale complexion. T: pale P: thready, weak	Nourish Blood, tonify and raise Qi		
Blood Stasis	Chronic H/A, severe and intense (stabbing, boring), fixed location, history of injury, possible dark complexion. T: purple P: wiry, choppy	Move blood, transform stasis		

Hiccoughing and belching (e ni)

Definition:
Hiccoughing and belching are caused by stomach Qi rebelling upward to disturb the diaphragm. May cause mild discomfort of short duration or a critical symptom of disease.

Red Flags:
- Neurological signs or symptoms

Western Medicine Relevant Diseases:
In Western medicine, hiccups are repeated involuntary spasms of the diaphragm followed by sudden closure of the glottis, which checks the inflow of air and causes the characteristic sound. Transient episodes are very common. Persistent (> 2 days) and intractable (> 1 mo) hiccups are uncommon but quite distressing.
Hiccups follow irritation of afferent or efferent diaphragmatic nerves or of medullary centers that control the respiratory muscles, particularly the diaphragm. Hiccups are more common among men.

Transient hiccups may be caused by:
- Gastric distention
- Alcohol consumption
- Swallowing hot or irritating substances

Persistent and intractable hiccups have myriad causes, including: indigestion, hiatal hernia, post-gastric surgery, gastro-esophageal reflux disease, other esophageal disorders, bowel diseases, gallbladder disease, hepatic metastases, hepatitis, pancreatitis, pregnancy.

Etiology and Pathogenesis:
The pathogenesis of *e ni* involves the LU, ST and diaphragm; when ST qi rebels upward, it disturbs the diaphragm and attacks the LU
- Improper diet – heat or cold accumulating – obstruct ST Qi & fails to descend
- Emotional stress – liver Qi stagnates – overacts on ST – ST Qi rebels
- Insufficient righteous Qi from chronic disorders or misuse of purgatives or diuretics – KI Qi xu – KI fails to receive

TCM Differentiation and Treatment:

Pattern	Signs and Symptoms	Treatment Principle	Acupuncture	Formula
Cold in Stomach	Deep, slow hiccough relieved by warmth, cold pain in epigastic region, decreased appetite, no thirst. P: slow, tight	Primary principle: Harmonize the stomach, descend rebellious Qi, and calm e ni. Modify strategy according to pattern differentiation.	Principle points: REN12 (zhong wan), PC6 (nei guan), ST36 (ZSL), BL17 (ge shu)	
Stomach Fire Blazing	Sudden loud rigorous hiccough/belching with bad breath and intense thirst, desire for cold drinks. T: yellow coat P: rapid		Cold in ST + ST21 (liang men) ST fire + ST43 (xian gu)	
Liver Qi Stagnation	Persistent hiccough and belching worse with emotions, stifling sensation in chest/hypochondriac regions. P: wiry		LR Qi stagnation + LR14 (qi men), LR3 (tai chong)	
Spleen and Stomach Qi deficiency	Low pitch and weak hiccough, SOB, pale, cold limbs, poor appetite. T: pale P: deep, weak		SP & ST deficiency + REN6 (qi hai)	
Stomach Yin deficiency	Abrupt, intermittent hiccough, dry mouth and throat, irritable, hunger without desire to eat, dry stool. T: red P: thready, rapid		ST Yin deficiency + SP6 (SYJ)	

Hypochondrial Pain (xie tong)

Definition:
Hypochondriac pain is unilateral or bilateral pain in infracostal region. It is a subjective symptom, usually associated with dysfunction of the Liver and Gallbladder, and often accompanied by distention and pain in the epigastrium or by palpable masses in the infracostal regions.

Red Flags:
Hypochondriac pain with the following symptoms merits referral:
- Jaundice: results from a problem in the production of the bile by the liver or an obstruction to its outflow via the gall bladder into the duodenum. Jaundice may result from inflammation of the liver (hepatitis) or from liver cancer. Hepatitis can be a result of infection (for example Hepatitis A, B and C and glandular fever) but can also result from the negative effects of certain prescription medications and excess alcohol on the liver tissue. Jaundice always merits referral for investigation of its cause.
- Prolonged right hypochondriac pain with malaise: This suggests liver or gallbladder pathology and should be investigated even in the absence of jaundice.
- Vomiting of fresh or altered blood: There can be profuse bleeding from the base of the oesophagus in chronic liver disease as distended varicose veins (varices) can rupture in this site. The patient in this situation can easily go into shock - needs to be handled as an emergency.
- Edema, bruising and confusion: Liver disease may remain in a stable state for months to years, but the patient may become suddenly much more unwell once a certain point of progression of the disease has passed. This is the point at which the liver is no longer able to perform its function of manufacture of blood proteins and detoxification. Bruising, oedema and confusion can result. This syndrome requires urgent medical management.
- Right hypochondriac pain which is very intense and comes in waves (may also be fever, vomiting, jaundice) – may indicate obstruction of bile ducts by gallstones

Western Medicine Relevant Diseases:

Etiology and Pathogenesis:
- Liver Qi stagnation – emotional stress interferes with Liver's free flow of Qi function
- Blood stasis – prolonged Qi stagnation or injury to hypochondriac region can develop into Blood stasis
- Liver and gallbladder damp heat – damp-heat from exterior and interior – obstructs flow of LR Qi
- Liver Yin deficiency – chronic illness exhausts essence and blood – fail to nourish LR and its channels

TCM Differentiation and Treatment:

Pattern	Signs and Symptoms	Treatment Principle	Acupuncture	Formula
Liver Qi Stagnation	Distending and migrating pain, aggravated by emotional stress.	Soothe LR and regulate Qi	Principle Points: LR14 (qi men), BL18 (gan shu), (or BL19 (dan shu)-GB24 (ri yue)), GB34 (yang ling quan), GB43 (xia xi), SJ5 (wei guan), SJ6 (zhi gou), ST36 (ZSL), LV3-LI4 (4 gates), PC6 (nei guan) + relevant points depending on pattern Qi Stagnation + LR3 (tai chong), LI4 (he gu) Blood Stasis + BL17 (ge shu), SP10 (xue hai) Damp heat + GB24 (ri yue), GB34 (yang ling quan), LR3 (tai chong) Deficiency + LR14 (qi men), BL18 (gan shu), SP6 (SYJ), BL23 (shen shu)	
Blood Stasis	Stabbing pain with fixed location, worse at night.	Dispel stasis and unblock channels		
Damp-heat in LR and GB	Stuffy sensation and pain, bitter taste, chest distension, poor appetite.	Clear heat and drain damp		
Liver Yin deficiency	Persistent vague pain, worse with exertion, dry mouth, five center heat, tidal fever, night sweats, dizziness.	Nourish Yin and soothe LR		

Impediment Syndrome (bi zheng)

(also called Painful Obstructive Syndrome)

Definition:
Impediment syndrome indicates pain, soreness, numbness, and/or difficulty in movement of muscles, tendons, and joints from invasion of exterior pathogenic factors. In some cases, deformity of the joints may present.

Red Flags:
- If joints are red, hot, and swollen, evaluated by a Western medical doctor is recommended, as these episodes may result from an infection.

Relevant Western Medical Diseases:
Impediment syndrome patterns include several disorders in Western medicine, such as:
- Rheumatoid arthritis (RA): RA is considered an autoimmune disease. Components of the immune system attack the synovial tissue and can also attack connective tissue in many other parts of the body, such as the blood vessels and lungs. Eventually, the cartilage, bone, and ligaments of the joint erode, causing deformity, instability, and scarring within the joint. The joints deteriorate at a variable rate. Many factors, including genetic predisposition, may influence the pattern of the disease. Unknown environmental factors (such as viral infections and cigarette smoking) are thought to play a role.

  RA may start suddenly, with many joints becoming inflamed at the same time. More often, it starts subtly, gradually affecting different joints. Usually, the inflammation is symmetric, with joints on both sides of the body affected about equally. RA can affect any joint, but most often the first inflamed are the small joints. Other commonly affected joints include the: knees, shoulders, elbows, ankles, and hips. The inflamed joints are usually painful and often stiff, especially just after awakening or after prolonged inactivity. Some people feel tired and weak, especially in the early afternoon. RA may cause a loss of appetite with weight loss and a low-grade fever.

  Affected joints are often tender, warm, red, and enlarged because of swelling of the soft tissue lining the joint. Joints can become deformed, which leads to a limited range of motion. Swollen wrists can pinch a nerve and result in numbness or tingling due to carpal tunnel syndrome. Cysts, which may develop behind affected knees, can rupture, causing pain and swelling in the lower legs. Some people with rheumatoid arthritis have hard bumps (called rheumatoid nodules) just under the skin.

- Osteoarthritis (OA): OA is a chronic disorder associated with damage to the cartilage and surrounding tissues and characterized by pain, stiffness, and loss of function. In primary (or idiopathic) OA, the cause is not known. Primary OA may affect only certain joints, such as the knee, or many joints. In secondary OA, the cause is another disease or condition, such as: an infection, a joint abnormality that appeared at birth, an injury, or a metabolic disorder. Some people who repetitively stress one joint or a group of joints are particularly at risk.

  Usually, OA symptoms develop gradually and affect only one or a few joints at first. Joints of the fingers, base of the thumbs, neck, lower back, big toes, hips, and knees are commonly affected. Pain, often described as a deep ache, is the first symptom and is usually made worse by activities that involve weight bearing. As the condition causes more symptoms, the joint may become less movable and eventually may not be able to fully straighten or bend. New growth of cartilage, bone, and other tissue can enlarge the joints. The irregular cartilage surfaces cause joints to grind, grate, or crackle when they are moved and tenderness develops. Bony growths commonly develop in the joints closest to the fingertips (called Heberden nodes) or middle of the fingers (called Bouchard nodes).

- Gout: Gout causes severe pain that occurs suddenly in one or more joints, often at night. The pain becomes progressively worse and is often excruciating, particularly when the joint is moved or touched. The joint becomes inflamed and the skin over the joint may appear red or purplish, tight, and shiny. Other symptoms of an attack sometimes include fever, tachycardia, general sick feeling, and chills.

  The first few attacks usually affect only one joint and last for a few days. The symptoms gradually disappear, joint function returns, and no symptoms appear until the next attack. However, if the disorder progresses, untreated attacks last longer, occur more frequently, and affect several joints. If left untreated, later attacks can last up to 3 weeks. After repeated attacks, gout can become severe and chronic and may lead to joint deformity.

  Gout results from deposits of uric acid crystals, which accumulate in the joints because of high blood levels of uric acid (hyperuricemia). Abnormally high uric acid levels in the blood result from: decreased elimination of uric acid by the kidneys, consumption of too much purine-rich food (e.g. liver, kidneys, sardines) and/or alcohol, and production of too much uric acid.

- **Sciatica**: Sciatica is pain along the sciatic nerve. It usually results from compression of nerve roots in the lower back. Common causes include intervertebral disk herniation, osteophytes, and narrowing of the spinal canal (spinal stenosis). Symptoms include pain radiating from the buttocks down the leg.

- **Bursitis**: painful inflammation of a bursa (a flat, fluid-filled sac that provides cushioning where skin, muscles, tendons, and ligaments rub over bones).
  Movement is painful, and bursae near the skin may become swollen and tender.

- **Fibromyalgia**: a common disorder of unknown cause characterized by generalized aching (sometimes severe); widespread tenderness of muscles, areas around tendon insertions, and adjacent soft tissues; muscle stiffness; fatigue; mental cloudiness; poor sleep; and a variety of other somatic symptoms.

Etiology and pathogenesis:
Deficiency of righteous Qi is the underlying etiology of this syndrome.
- EPI invading, blocking channels – wind, cold, damp, heat – obstruct the muscles, joints, and channels
- Heat – invasion of heat, other pathogens transforming to heat, or constitutional heat tendencies – lead to heat toxin accumulation and Bi syndrome
- Aging, overwork – deficiency of Yin or Blood – malnourishment of channels – prone to EPI invasion

TCM Differentiation and Treatment:
Note: watch for differences between Impediment Syndrome and Atrophy Syndrome. Impediment Syndrome is marked by soreness, pain, heaviness, and difficult movement. Atrophy Syndrome is characterized by weakness and flaccidity of the limbs and atrophy of the muscles. Pain is not common.

Pattern, Signs and Symptoms	Treatment Principle and Acupuncture	Formula
Acute conditions: - Wind bi: soreness and pain that migrates from joint to joint, often multiple joints affected, aversion to wind, limited ROM, P: floating - Cold bi: severe, excruciating pain, limited range of motion, pain worse with cold, stiffness of joints, P: floating, tight - Damp bi: swollen, numb, painful joints, general damp signs (heaviness, fatigue), T: greasy, P: slippery - Hot bi: red, hot, burning pain, swelling, fever, sweating, thirst, irritability, T: red, yellow coat, P: rapid	For all patterns, open channels and stop pain using local points (do not needle into swelling): - Hand: baxie - Wrist: LI4 (he gu), LI5 (yang xi), SJ4 (yang chi), SJ5 (wei guan) - Elbow: LI10 (shou san li), LI11 (qu chi), LU5 (chi ze), SJ10 (tian jing) - Neck: GB20 (feng chi), BL10 (tian zhu), BL11 (da zhu), - Hib: GB30 (huan tiao), BL32 (ci liao), Ashi - Knee: ST34 (liang qiu), ST35 (du bi), ST36 (ZSL), heding, etc - Ankle: BL60 (kun lun), ST41 (jie xi), etc Plus add treatment principle and points according to pattern: Wind bi + BL12 (feng men), GB31 (feng shi) Cold bi + REN4 (guan yuan), REN6 (qi hai) Damp bi + BL20 (pi shu), SP9 (yin ling quan), SP6 (SYJ) Heat bi + DU14 (da zhui), LI11 (qu chi), LI4 (he gu)	
Chronic conditions:	For all patterns, open channels and stop pain using local points (see above). Plus add points according to pattern: Phlegm and Stasis + ST40 (feng long), SP9 (yin ling quan), SP10 (xue hai), BL17 (ge shu) Bone bi + BL11 (da zhu), GB39 (xuan zhong) Kidney deficiency + KI3 (tai xi), SP6 (SYJ), GB39 (xuan zhong), ST36 (ZSL)	

Impotence (yang wei)

Definition:
Impotence is a male reproductive disorder manifesting with inability to achieve or maintain an erection. Clinically, this is often seen with seminal emission or premature ejaculation.

Red Flags:
Certain symptoms and characteristics are cause for concern. They include:
- Absence of erections during the night or upon awakening in the morning
- Numbness in the area between and around the buttocks and genital area (may indicate spinal cord damage)
- Painful cramping in the muscles of the legs that occurs during physical activity but is relieved promptly by rest (claudication)

Western Medicine Relevant Diseases:
In Western medicine, impotence is referred to as erectile dysfunction (ED). ED is the inability to attain or sustain an erection satisfactory for sexual intercourse. ED is called primary if the man has never been able to attain or sustain an erection. ED is called secondary if it is acquired later in life by a man who was previously able to attain erections.

To achieve an erection, the penis needs an adequate amount of blood flowing in, a slowing of blood flowing out, proper function of nerves leading to and from the penis, adequate amounts of the male sex hormone testosterone, and sufficient sex drive (libido), so a disorder of any of these systems may lead to ED. Abnormalities of the blood vessels or nerves of the penis cause most cases of ED. Other possible causes include hormonal disorders, structural disorders of the penis, use of certain drugs, and psychological problems. The most common specific causes are:
- Hardening of the arteries (atherosclerosis) that affects the arteries to the penis
- Diabetes mellitus
- Complications of prostate surgery
- Certain drugs such as those used to treat high blood pressure or an enlarged prostate

Etiology and Pathologenesis:
Impotence is generally caused by:

TCM Differentiation and Treatment:

Pattern	Signs and Symptoms	Treatment Principle	Acupuncture	Formula
Failure of Fire in Gate of Vitality	Complete or partial impotence, spontaneous seminal discharge, dizziness, vertigo, tinnitus, sore and weak low back/knees, pale complexion, cold, frequent urination. T: pale P: deep, thready	Supplement KD, invigorate Yang	REN6 (qi hai), DU4 (ming men), BL23 (shen shu), KI3 (tai xi), DU20 (bai hui), liao points	
Downpour of Damp Heat into lower burner	Flaccidity of penis with inability to achieve or sustain erection, premature ejaculation, sweatiness, heavy & aching lower limbs, dark burning urination. T: yellow, greasy P: slippery, rapid	Clear heat, drain damp	REN4 (guan yuan), DU4 (ming men), SP6 (SYJ), SP9 (yin ling quan), ST36 (ZSL), LR5 (li gou)	
Deficiency of Heart and Spleen	Excessive pensiveness, worry, impotence, insomnia, lassitude, dull complexion. T: pale P: thready	Tonify Heart and Spleen	HT7 (shen men), BL15 (xin shu), SP6 (SYJ), ST36 (ZSL)	
Shock and Fear injuring the Kidney	Impotence, timidity, palpitations, insomnia. T: slightly cyanotic P: wiry, thready	Tonify Kidney and quiet the mind	KI3 (tai xi), SP6 (SYJ), DU4 (ming men), Yintang	

Insomnia (bu mei)

Definition:
Insomnia is defined as an inability to experience normal sleep, e.g. difficulty falling asleep, early waking, waking during night, restless sleep, dream-disturbed sleep, sleeplessness.

Red Flags:
Certain symptoms are cause for concern and merit referral:
- Falling asleep while driving or during other potentially dangerous situations
- Frequently falling asleep without warning
- Stopping breathing during sleep or waking up with gasping or choking
- Moving violently or injuring self or others during sleep
- Sleepwalking
- A heart or lung disorder that is constantly changing
- Continuous attacks of muscle weakness
- A recent stroke

Western Medicine Relevant Diseases:
In Western medicine, insomnia may be caused by:
- Consumption of caffeine or other stimulant drugs (typically near bedtime, but even in the afternoon for people who are particularly sensitive)
- Exercise or excitement late in the evening
- An irregular sleep-wake schedule
- Acute emotional stressors (e.g. job loss, hospitalization) can also cause insomnia
- Physical disorders that cause pain or discomfort (e.g. arthritis, cancer, herniated disks)
- Mental disorders such as depression may cause insomnia.

Etiology and Pathogenesis:
Amount and quality of sleep depend on the state of mind, which is rooted in the heart and nourished by heart blood and yin. Insomnia is induced by pathogenic factors agitating the heart or by malnourishment of the mind, including:
- Emotional stress/anxiety
    - Injures Liver – leads to Liver Qi stagnation and liver fire disturbing mind
    - Over-thinking - injures Spleen leading to deficient Qi and blood failing to nurture heart
    - Overexertion and over-thinking - exhausts Heart blood, fails to nourish spirit

- Prolonged illness -- weakens the constitution and exhausts KI Yin – deficient yin fails to nourish Heart yin, Heart yang becomes hyperactive and empty fire agitates mind
- Qi deficiency of Heart and GB – constitutional weakness – timid, fearful – sleep is light with frequent awakenings and dreams
- Improper diet – overeating or poor eating – leads to food stagnation and phlegm heat harassing mind

TCM Differentiation and Treatment:

Pattern	Signs and Symptoms	Treatment Principle	Acupuncture	Formula
	Restless sleep, unpleasant dreams, irritable, bitter taste, red eyes, H/A, thirst, dark urine, dry stool. T: red P: wiry, rapid	Soothe liver, drain fire, calm spirit	LR2 (xing jian), LR3 (tai chong), GB44 (zu qiao yin), GB20 (feng chi), SP6 (SYJ), BL18 (gan shu), anmian	
	Difficulty falling asleep, restless sleep, irritable, profuse sputum, chest stuffy, heavy head, nausea, bitter taste, dizziness, no appetite. T: red, sticky yellow coat P: slippery, rapid	Resolve phlegm, clear heat, calm spirit	ST40 (feng long), SP9 (yin ling quan), LI11 (qu chi), ST8 (tou wei), GB12 (wan gu), SP1 (yin bai), anmian	
	Insomnia, irritability, palpitations, anxiety, dizziness, tinnitus, forgetfulness, sore back, nocturnal emissions, night sweats, five center heat. T: red, scanty coat P: rapid, thready	Nourish Yin, drain fire, nourish heart and calm spirit	HT7 (shen men), HT6 (yin xi), PC7 (da ling), REN4 (guan yuan), KI3 (tai xi), KI6, (zhao hai) REN15 (jiu wei), BL15 (xin shu), BL23 (shen shu)	
	Insomnia, excessive dreaming, easily awakened, palpitations, forgetfulness, dizziness, fatigue, poor appetite, dull or pale complexion. T: pale P: weak	Tonify Heart and Spleen, generate Qi and Blood, calm spirit	SP6 (SYJ), ST36 (ZSL), HT7 (shen men), BL20 (pi shu), BL15 (xin shu), yintang	
	Waking early in morning & unable to fall asleep again, light sleep, dream disturbed, easily startled, timid, lack initiative, palpitations, fatigue. T: pale, heart crack P: empty	Tonify Heart and GB, calm the mind	HT7 (shen men), GB40 (qiu xu)	

Internal damage fever (FID) (nei shang fa re)

Definition:
Subjective sensations of heat in body, or objective rise in body temperature due to malfunction of internal organs and deficiency of vital substances. Onset is slow and gradual, and the course is prolonged. FID refers to fevers caused by internal problems, not exterior pathogens.

Red Flags:
In people with an acute fever, the following signs and characteristics are cause for concern:
- A change in mental function, such as confusion
- A headache, stiff neck, or both
- Flat, small, purplish red spots on the skin (petechiae), which indicate bleeding under the skin
- Low blood pressure
- Rapid heart rate or rapid breathing
- Dyspnea
- A temperature that is higher than 104° F (40° C) or lower than 95° F (35° C)
- Recent travel to an area where a serious infectious disease such as malaria is common (endemic)
- Recent use of drugs that suppress the immune system (immuno-suppressants)

Western Medicine Relevant Diseases:
Fever is elevated body temperature (> 37.8° C (or 100.4 F) orally or > 38.2° C rectally) or an elevation above a person's known normal daily value. Fever occurs when the body's thermostat (located in the hypothalamus) resets at a higher temperature, primarily in response to an infection. Many patients use "fever" very loosely, often meaning that they feel too warm, too cold, or sweaty, but they have not actually measured their temperature. Symptoms are due mainly to the condition causing the fever, although fever itself can cause chills, sweats, and discomfort and make patients feel flushed and warm.

Many disorders can cause fever. They are broadly categorized as:
- Infectious (most common, but not related to the TCM syndrome of FID)
- Neoplastic (cancer)
- Inflammatory

Many cancers (such as leukemia) and inflammatory disorders cause fever. Inflammatory disorders that might cause fever include joint, connective tissue, and blood vessel disorders such as rheumatoid arthritis, systemic lupus erythematosus (lupus), and giant cell arteritis. Rheumatic fever, TB, and other chronic infections can also cause fever.

Etiology and Pathogenesis:
- Emotional stress – Liver constraint – Liver Qi stagnation – Liver fire - fever
- Blood stasis – from trauma, emotional stress/Qi stagnation – obstructs flow in channels – produces heat/fever
- Damp accumulation – internal damp transforms to heat – damp-heat fever
- Spleen Qi deficiency – from overexertion, improper diet, chronic illness – Qi or Yang lose connection with Yin and float up and out to body surface - fever
- Blood deficiency – due to SP deficiency, trauma, surgery, childbirth – deficiency Blood and Yin fail to bind Yang – Yang floats up and out - fever
- Essence and yin deficiency – constitutional or due to Yin exhaustion from, e.g. warm febrile disease – excess Yang generates deficiency Yin fire

TCM Differentiation and Treatment:

Pattern	Signs and Symptoms	Treatment Principle	Acupuncture	Formula
Liver stagnation fever	Subjective, low-grade fever, irritability, fluctuates with emotional state, agitation, bitter taste. T: yellow coat P: wiry	Spread Liver Qi, relieve constraint, drain heat		
Blood stasis fever	Fever in afternoon or at night, possible masses, dry skin, dusky completion. T: purple P: choppy	Invigorate Blood, transform stasis		
Damp accumulation fever	Slow onset low grade fever worse in afternoon, stifling sensation, fullness, thirst with no desire to drink, poor appetite, body heavy, loose stool. T: greasy coat P: slippery	Drain damp, clear heat		
Qi Deficiency fever	Fever aggravated by exertion, lack of strength, spontaneous sweat, reluctance to speak, easily catch colds, poor appetite. T: pale P: weak	Augment Qi, Strengthen Spleen		
Blood Deficiency Fever	Low-grade fever, pale lips and nails, pale complexion, dizzy, blurred vision, fatigue. T: pale P: thready and weak			
Yin Deficiency Fever	Fever in afternoon or at night, five center heat, tidal fever, malar flush, irritable, insomnia, night sweats. T: red, scanty coat P: thready, rapid	Nourish Yin, clear heat		

Ischuria (long bi)

Definition:
Ischuria refers to conditions characterized by diminished volume of urine, dribbling urination and, in extreme cases, complete cessation of urine passage. It may be due to a failure of urine formation or to obstruction

Red Flags:
- Acute urinary retention with the inability to pass any urine is a medical emergency.
- Difficulty urinating and nocturia may have many causes. Benign prostatic enlargement is common and the symptoms can respond to acupuncture treatment. However, the same symptoms can be caused by a prostatic tumor, and so referral for further investigations is warranted.

Western Medicine Relevant Diseases:
In Western medicine, urinary retention may result from urinary tract obstruction. This is a blockage that inhibits the flow of urine through the urinary tract, including the kidneys, ureters, bladder, and urethra. The blockage can be complete or partial and can lead to kidney damage, kidney stones, and infection.

An obstruction may occur suddenly or develop slowly. The most common causes in adults are: benign prostatic hyperplasia (BPH), prostate cancer, tumors, and stones. Other common causes of obstruction include strictures (narrowing caused by scar tissue) of the ureter or urethra that develop after radiation therapy, surgery, or procedures done on the urinary tract.

The many other possible causes of urinary tract obstruction include: polyps, blood clots in the ureter, disorders of the muscles or nerves in the ureter or bladder, birth defects, spinal cord injury, certain drugs, abscesses, and cysts of the bladder, cervix, uterus, prostate, or other pelvic organs, or a large mass of feces stuck in the rectum (rectal impaction).

Etiology and Pathogenesis:
Formation and elimination of urine depend on proper functioning of organs involved in water metabolism: Lung, Spleen, Kidney and Triple Burner.

TCM Differentiation and Treatment:

Note: In ischuria, urination is **difficult and inadequate**. Total daily output of urine is less than normal **and** anuresis (or no urine output) is possible. It is important to differentiate with Stranguria (Lin Zheng) (aka Painful Urinary Syndrome), which involves pricking pain during urination and increased frequency with a decreased amount each time, but total daily urine output is adequate.

Pattern	Signs and Symptoms	Treatment Principle	Acupuncture	Formula
Lung Heat Accumulation	Difficult, dribbling, dark urine, rapid shallow respiration, dry throat, short rapid breathing, possible cough, heat signs. T: thin yellow coat P: rapid	Clear Lung heat, unblock urinary passage	LU5 (chi ze), LI4 (he gu), REN3 (zhong ji), BL28 (pang guang shu)	
Damp Heat Accumulation	Dribbling or extremely small volume of hot, dark urine, burning sensation on urination, sticky/bitter taste, heat signs. T: red, yellow greasy coat P: rapid, slippery	Clear heat, drain damp, unblock urinary passage	BL23 (shen shu), REN3 (zhong ji), SP6 (SYJ), SP9 (yin ling quan)	
Liver Qi Stagnation	Difficult urine following emotional stress, depression, distention of ABD and hypochondrium. P: wiry	Soothe Liver, regulate Qi, unblock urinary passage	LR3 (tai chong), BL39 (wei yang), REN3 (zhong ji), BL28 (pang guang shu), GB34 (yang ling quan)	
Blockage of Urinary Tract	Dribbling or weak, interrupted or total retention, distension. T: purple P: choppy	Transform stasis, dissipate accumulation, unblock the obstruction	REN3 (zhong ji), SP6 (SYJ), ST28 (shui dao), KI5 (shui quan), ST36 (zu san li)	
Spleen Qi Sinking	Distension and heaviness in lower ABD, scanty and hesitant output, weak SP Qi signs (fatigue, loss of appetite). T: pale P: weak	Raise clear Yang, descend turbid Yin, promote urination	BL20 (pi shu), ST36 (ZSL), SP9 (yin ling quan), REN3 (zhong ji), BL22 (san jiao shu)	
Kidney Yang Deficiency	Anuria or dribbling and weak stream, KD Yang Xu signs (cold intolerance, pale complexion, sore back/knees). T: pale P: deep, weak	Warm and supplement KD Yang, promote urination	BL23 (shen shu), REN4 (guan yuan), KD10 (yin gu), REN6 (qi hai), BL22 (san jiao shu)	

Jaundice (huang dan)

Definition:
Characterized by a yellowish discoloration of the sclera, skin and urine due to obstruction of bile and abnormal deposition of bile pigments into the body fluid and blood (stool will be grey/white re: no bile in stool). Liver and Gallbladder are unable to direct the free flow and distribution of Qi and drainage of bile is obstructed.
Characteristic signs: "3 yellow and 1 white" (yellow eyes, yellow skin, dark yellow urine + whie/pale stool) plus poor appetite, greasy food aversion, nausea, ABD distension.

Red flags:
Always refer for Western medical assessment and care. Jaundice accompanied by the following symptoms requires immediate Western medical care:
- Severe abdominal pain and tenderness
- Changes in mental function, such as drowsiness, agitation, or confusion
- Blood in stool or tarry black stool
- Blood in vomit
- Fever
- A tendency to bruise or to bleed easily, sometimes resulting in a reddish purple rash of tiny dots or larger splotches

Western Medicine Relevant Diseases:
Jaundice occurs when there is too much bilirubin (a yellow pigment) in the blood—a condition called hyperbilirubinemia. Bilirubin is formed when hemoglobin is broken down as part of the normal process of recycling old or damaged red blood cells. Bilirubin is carried in the bloodstream to the liver, where it binds with bile. Bilirubin is then moved through the bile ducts into the digestive tract, so that it can be eliminated from the body. Most bilirubin is eliminated in stool, but a small amount is eliminated in urine. If bilirubin cannot be moved through the liver and bile ducts quickly enough, it builds up in the blood and is deposited in the skin. The result is jaundice.

Many people with jaundice also have dark urine and light-colored stool. These changes occur when a blockage or other problem prevents bilirubin from being eliminated in stool, causing more bilirubin to be eliminated in urine.

If bilirubin levels are high, substances formed when bile is broken down may accumulate, causing itching all over the body. But jaundice itself causes few other symptoms in adults. Also, many disorders that cause jaundice can also cause other symptoms or serious problems. These may include nausea, vomiting and abdominal pain, and spider angiomas. Serious problems can include:
- Ascites: Accumulation of fluid within the abdomen
- Coagulopathy: A tendency to bleed or bruise
- Hepatic encephalopathy: Deterioration of brain function because the liver malfunctions, allowing toxic substances to build up in the blood, reach the brain, and cause changes in mental function (such as confusion and drowsiness)
- Portal hypertension: High blood pressure in the veins that bring blood to the liver, which can lead to bleeding in the esophagus and sometimes stomach

Jaundice has many causes. Most causes involve disorders and drugs that
- Damage the liver
- Interfere with the flow of bile
- Trigger hemolysis, thus producing more bilirubin than the liver can handle

The most common causes of jaundice are:

Etiology and Pathogenesis:
- Exterior pathogenic factors -- damp heat, damp cold (or any EPI) - block free flow of Qi in LR and GB
- Improper diet –generates damp heat internally by hindering SP/ST - damp heat disturbs LV/GB by obstructing free flow of Qi
- SP/ST yang xu – constitutional or prolonged illness – internal cold & damp – obstructs middle burner
- Blood stasis, stones, parasites – anything obstructing middle burner – abnormal secretion and drainage of bile resulting in jaundice

TCM Differentiation and Treatment:
In TCM, Jaundice is divided into Yin and Yang types. Clinically, Yang and Yin jaundice may transform creating complicated patterns involving both heat and cold, excess and deficiency.

Pattern	Signs and Symptoms	Treatment Principle	Acupuncture	Formula
Yin Type	-damp cold or Yang Qi weak -acute or chronic – but usually long course -dark yellow, smoked, pale yellow -often no fever -tired, weak, SOB, cold, edema -weak pulse -nausea, vomit -possible rib distension and pain T: pale and yellow tongue P: weak, tight	Strengthen SP, harmonize ST, warm and transform cold-damp, dispel jaundice	Principle Points: DU9 (zhi yang), SI4 (wan gu), BL18 (gan shu), BL19 (dan shu), GB34 (yang ling quan), SP 9 (yin ling quan), PC6 (nei guan) for nausea, REN 12 (zhong wan) for poor appetite, ST37 (shang ju xu) for diarrhea	
Yang Type	-mainly damp heat from exterior pathogens -bright yellow, vivid (like an orange peel) -often high fever, excess/severe heat -acute, fast developing -nausea, vomit T: red, yellow (greasy) coat P: rapid Further classified by: Acute Heat Toxin: sudden onset, golden yellow discoloration, rapid development, high fever, extreme thirst, costal pain, possible LOC, delirium, hemorrhaging, hematuria. Heat Predominant: bright yellow discoloration, fever, thirst, nausea, vomiting, chest oppression, distension of ABD, dark yellow scanty urine, constipation. Damp Predominant: yellow discoloration (but not as bright as with heat), heaviness, nausea, loss of appetite, vomiting, ABD distension, loose stools, dark scanty urine.	Drain damp, promote urination, clear heat (or toxic heat), cool blood, dispel jaundice	For yang type + LR2 (xing jian), GB43 (xia xi), ST44 (nei ting), LI4 (he gu), LI11 (qu chi), DU14 (da zhui) For yin type + REN6 (qi hai) REN8 (shen que), BL20 (pi shu), BL48 (yang gang)	

Lumbago (yao tong)

Definition:
Lumbago, or lower back pain is a subjective sensation of discomfort or pain that may be unilateral, bilateral or centered on the lumbar vertebrae. Lower back pain is strongly influenced by the KI.

Red Flags:
In people with low back pain, certain symptoms and characteristics are cause for concern. They include:
- A history of cancer
- Pain for more than 6 weeks
- Numbness, weakness in one or both legs, retention of urine, or incontinence (possible nerve damage)
- Fever
- Weight loss
- Severe pain at night
- Pain in people aged 55 or older without an obvious explanation (such as an injury)
- Use of drugs that suppress the immune system, HIV infection or AIDS, use of injected drugs, recent surgery, or a wound (increase the risk of infection)
- Difficulty breathing, paleness, light-headedness, sudden sweating, a racing heartbeat, or loss of consciousness (possible abdominal aortic aneurysm)
- Vomiting, severe abdominal pain, or stool that is black or bloody (possible digestive disorder)
- Difficulty urinating, blood in the urine, or severe pain radiating into the groin (possible urinary tract disorder)

Western Medicine Relevant Diseases:
Most back pain is caused by disorders of the spine and the muscles, ligaments, and nerve roots around it or the disks between vertebrae. Often, no single specific cause can be identified. Many factors such as fatigue, obesity, and lack of exercise can worsen back pain. Also, any painful disorder of the spine may cause spasm of muscles around the spine. Occasionally, back pain is due to disorders outside the spine, such as those of the kidneys and urinary tract, digestive tract, and blood vessels.

The most common cause of low back pain is muscle strains and ligament sprains, which may result from lifting, exercising, or moving in an unexpected way.

Other common causes of low back pain include:
- Osteoarthritis: causes the cartilage that covers and protects the vertebrae to deteriorate. This disorder is thought to be due, at least in part, to the wear and tear of years of use.
- Compression fractures: commonly develop when bone density decreases because of osteoporosis. Vertebrae are particularly susceptible to the effects of osteoporosis.
- A ruptured or herniated disk: If a disk is suddenly squeezed by the vertebrae above and below it, the interior of the disk can squeeze through the tear in the covering, so that part of the interior herniates. This bulge can compress, irritate, and even damage the spinal nerve root next to it, causing more pain.
- Lumbar spinal stenosis: is narrowing of the spinal canal in the lower back. It is caused by such disorders as osteoarthritis, spondylolisthesis, rheumatoid arthritis, ankylosing spondylitis, and Paget disease of bone.
- Spondylolisthesis is partial displacement of a vertebra in the lower back. It usually occurs in people who have a common bone birth defect (spondylolysis) that weakens part of the vertebrae.

Less common causes that are serious include:
- Spinal infections
- Spinal tumors
- An aortic aneurysm
- Certain digestive disorders, such as a perforated peptic ulcer, diverticulitis, and pancreatitis
- Certain urinary tract disorders, such as kidney infections, kidney stones, and prostate infections
- Certain disorders involving the pelvis, such as ectopic pregnancy, pelvic inflammatory disease, and cancer of the ovaries or other reproductive organs

Less common causes that are not as serious include shingles and several types of inflammatory arthritis.

Etiology and Pathogenesis:
- Exterior pathogens – especially damp (cold or heat) invading the channels and inhibiting circulation of Qi and Blood causing lumbago

- Qi stagnation and blood stasis – caused by traumatic injuries or prolonged and chronic illness – obstructs Qi flow and can lead to Blood stasis and lumbago
- Kidney deficiency/essence deficiency – aging, constitutional, illness, too much sex – deplete KD essence and fail to nourish lower back, sinews and bones

TCM Differentiation and Treatment:

Pattern	Signs and Symptoms	Treatment Principle	Acupuncture	Formula
	-acute or chronic flare -local pain, often red, hot, swollen, burning pain and heaviness -fever common T: red/yellow P: rapid	Clear heat, drain damp, open channel to stop pain	Local back points, e.g.: Ashi points, Jiaji (lumbar 2, 3, 4, 5), BL23 (shen shu), BL24 (qi hai shu), BL25 (da chang shu), Ba Liao points, GB30 (huan tiao), BL52 (zhi shi), DU3 (yao yang guan) Also distal: SI3 (hou xi), DU26 (shui gou), BL 40 (wei zhong), BL60 (kun lun), BL62 (shen mai) clear heat: + LI4 (he gu), LI11 (qu chi) drain damp + SP9 (yin ling quan), ST40 (feng long)	
	-slow onset, often chronic -cold weather worse, warm better -pain dull or sharp, often patient stiffness P: tight	Expel damp-cold, warm and open channel to stop pain	Local and distal points, as above. + GB20 (feng chi), SJ5 (wei guan) (EPI), ST36 (ZSL), ST40 (feng long)	
	-sharp, fixed low back pain -worse at night -limited ROM -possible history of injury T: dark purple P: choppy	Invigorate blood, transform stasis, alleviate pain	Local and distal points, as above. + SP10 (xue hai), BL17 (ge shu)	
	-chronic dull pain -back weak (or stiffness) -with Yang qi weak/cold invading – sharp pain: cold makes worse, exertion worse, pale, tired, weak -with BL stasis – sharp pain -with Yin Xu – whole body, night sweat, hot flash, red/yellow tongue, often senior	KD Yang Qi Xu: tonify yang Qi, strengthen marrow, stop pain KD Yin Xu: nourish yin, stop pain	BL23 (shen shu), DU4 (ming men), KI3 (tai xi)	

Lung Distention (fei zhang)

Definition:
Lung distension is a chronic, obstructive pulmonary disease (COPD). Various chronic pulmonary disorders are caused by smoking and aging. Symptoms include: chronic cough, dyspnea with phlegm, distended chest and chest fullness, restlessness and palpitations.

Western Medicine Relevant Diseases:
TCM Lung Distention patterns relate to the characteristics of the Western medical condition of COPD, and its complications. COPD is persistent obstruction of the airways occurring with emphysema, chronic obstructive bronchitis, or cor pulmonale.

COPD leads to a decrease in the rate of airflow from the lungs when the person exhales, which is called chronic airflow obstruction. COPD includes the diagnoses of chronic obstructive bronchitis and emphysema. Many people have both disorders.
- Chronic bronchitis is defined as cough that produces sputum repeatedly during two successive years. When chronic bronchitis involves airflow obstruction, it qualifies as chronic obstructive bronchitis.
- Emphysema is defined as widespread and irreversible destruction of the alveolar wall and enlargement of many of the alveoli.

Chronic asthmatic bronchitis is similar to chronic bronchitis. People have wheezing, a cough that produces sputum, and partially reversible airflow obstruction. It occurs predominantly in people who smoke and have asthma.

The bronchioles of the lungs contain smooth muscles and are normally held open by their attachments to alveolar walls. In emphysema, the destruction of alveolar wall attachments results in collapse of the bronchioles when a person exhales, causing airflow obstruction that is permanent and irreversible. In chronic bronchitis, the glands lining the larger airways (bronchi) of the lungs enlarge and increase their secretion of mucus. Inflammation of the bronchioles develops and causes smooth muscles in lung tissue to spasm, further obstructing airflow. Inflammation also causes swelling of the airway passages and secretions in them, further limiting airflow. Eventually, the small airways in the lung become narrowed and destroyed.

Airflow obstruction in COPD causes air to become trapped in the lungs after a full exhalation, increasing the effort required to breathe. Also in COPD, the number of capillaries in the walls of the alveoli decreases. These abnormalities impair the exchange of oxygen and carbon dioxide between the alveoli and the blood. In the earlier stages of COPD, oxygen levels in the blood may be decreased, but carbon dioxide levels remain normal. In the later stages, carbon dioxide levels increase and oxygen levels fall.

The most significant cause of COPD is
- Cigarette smoking

Working in an environment polluted by chemical fumes or dust or by heavy smoke from indoor cooking fires may increase the risk of COPD. Exposure to air pollution and to smoke from nearby cigarette smokers may cause flare-ups in people who have COPD, but probably does not cause COPD.

In people with COPD, a mild cough that produces clear sputum develops during their 40s or 50s. The cough and sputum production are usually worse when the person first gets out of bed in the morning. Cough and sputum production can persist throughout the day. Shortness of breath may occur during exertion. Sometimes, shortness of breath first occurs only when the person has a lung infection (usually bronchitis), during which time the person coughs more and has an increased amount of sputum. The color of the sputum changes from clear or white to yellow or green.

By the time people with COPD reach their middle to late 60s, especially if they continue smoking, shortness of breath during exertion becomes more troublesome.
Pneumonia and other lung infections occur more often. Infections may result in severe shortness of breath even when the person is at rest and may require hospitalization. Shortness of breath during activities of daily living may persist after the person has recovered from the lung infection. About one third of people with severe COPD experience severe weight loss. The cause of weight loss is not clear, and causes may differ among different people. Possible causes include shortness of breath that makes eating difficult and increased levels in the blood of a substance called tumor necrosis factor. Swelling of the legs develops in people who have cor pulmonale. People with COPD may intermittently cough up blood, which is usually due to inflammation of the bronchi, but which always raises the concern of lung cancer. Morning headaches may occur because breathing decreases during sleep, which causes increased retention of carbon dioxide and decreased levels of oxygen in the blood.

As COPD progresses, some people, especially those who have emphysema, develop unusual breathing patterns. Some people breathe out through pursed lips. Others find it more comfortable to stand over a table with their arms outstretched and their weight on their palms or elbows to improve the function of some of the respiratory muscles. Over time, many people develop a barrel chest as the size of the lungs increases because of trapped air. Low oxygen levels in the blood can result in cyanosis. Fragile areas in the lungs may rupture, causing pneumothorax.

A flare-up (or exacerbation) of COPD is a worsening of symptoms, usually cough, increased sputum, and shortness of breath. Sputum color often changes to yellow or green, and fever and body aches sometimes occur. Shortness of breath may be present when the person is at rest and may be severe enough to require hospitalization. Severe air pollution, common allergens, and viral or bacterial infections may cause flare-ups. During severe flare-ups, people may develop acute respiratory failure. Among the possible symptoms are severe shortness of breath (a feeling likened to being drowned), severe anxiety, sweating, cyanosis, and confusion.

If low oxygen levels are not treated with supplemental oxygen, complications can occur. Low oxygen levels in the blood, if not treated, stimulate the bone marrow to send more red blood cells into the bloodstream causing secondary polycythemia (increase RBCs in blood stream). The low oxygen levels in the blood also constrict the blood vessels leading from the right side of the heart to the lungs, thereby increasing the pressure in these vessels. As a result of the increased pressure, called pulmonary hypertension, cor pulmonale can occur. People with COPD also have an increased risk of developing arrhythmias and lung cancers.

Etiology and Pathogenesis:
- Aging, chronic disease – weaken Lung, Spleen, Kidney – lead to turbid phlegm build up – obstructs Lung Qi – leads to Lung Qi deficiency (and often Heart Qi or Yang deficiency)
  - Exogenous pathogens and weak Wei Qi further aggravate condition

TCM Differentiation and Treatment:

Pattern	Signs and Symptoms	Treatment Principle	Acupuncture	Formula
Exterior Wind Cold Triggering Latent Cold Congested Fluids	Productive cough with copious frothy white sputum, breathlessness, orthopnea, condition aggravated by cold weather, aversion to cold, fever, no sweating, body aches. T: white greasy coat P: wiry, tight	Disperse cold, release exterior, warm the Lung and transform congested fluids	For those with significant, productive cough with copious sputum, refer to cough for treatment. For those with significant breathlessness and rapid respirations, refer to wheezing.	
Exterior Wind Cold with Phlegm Heat in the Lungs	Productive cough, tachypnea, copious sputum that is yellow viscous or blood tinged and difficult to expectorate, aversion to cold, fever, body ache, thirst. T: yellow, greasy coat P: rapid floating or rapid slippery	Disperse Lung Qi, release pathogens, clear heat, transform phlegm		
Lung Deficiency	Weak cough with thin sputum, shallow and rapid respiration, SOB, spontaneous sweat, aversion to wind, easily catch cold, dry cough, thirst, dry throat, malar flush. T: dry red or pale P: thready weak, or rapid thready	Augment the Qi, nourish Yin, tonify the Lung		
Kidney Deficiency	Primary symptoms of dyspnea, inhalation more difficult than exhalation; if Yang deficiency, lassitude, fatigue, cold intolerance, dusky complexion, pale tongue, weak thready pulse; if Yin deficiency, irritable, red face, dry mouth, blood tinged sputum, dry red tongue, rapid thready pulse.	Tonify and assist Kidney in receiving Qi		
Spleen and Kidney Yang Deficiency	Stifling and suffocating sensation in the chest, tachypnea or breathlessness, palpitations, thirst with no desire to drink, general edema, flabby pale tongue and deep thready pulse.	Warm the Yang, tonify the Spleen and Kidney		

Malaria (nue ji)

Definition:
Malaria is an infectious disease characterized by cycles of recurring chills alternating with high fever. It is most prevalent during summer and autumn, but can occur in all seasons. The main cause is infection by malarial evils.

Red Flags:
Referral for Western medical treatment required.

Western Medicine Relevant Diseases:
Malaria is a protozoan infection that is spread by the bite of an infected female mosquito. Very rarely, the disease is transmitted from an infected mother to her fetus, through transfusion of contaminated blood, through transplantation of a contaminated organ, or through injection with a needle previously used by a person with malaria.

The initial symptoms of all forms of malaria are similar. As the infected red blood cells rupture and release parasites, a person typically develops a shaking chill followed by a fever that can exceed 104° F (40° C). Fatigue and vague discomfort (malaise), headache, body aches, and nausea are common. The fever typically falls after several hours, and heavy sweating and extreme fatigue follow. Fevers occur unpredictably at first, but with time, they may become periodic.

Etiology and Pathogenesis:
- Invasion of malarial evils with simultaneous invasion of other external evils (wind, cold, summer heat, damp)
- Injury to SP/ST resulting in depletion of Qi and blood, accumulation of phlegm – weakens body

TCM Differentiation and Treatment:

Pattern	Signs and Symptoms	Treatment Principle	Acupuncture	Formula
Typical Malaria	Cyclic bouts of chills and fever progressing into chills, then replaced by signs of internal and external heat: flushed face, red lips, dry mouth, extreme thirst, profuse sweating. Yawning, fatigue, lassitude. T: red, greasy coat P: wiry	Relieve Shao Yang symptoms, dispel evils, terminate malaria		

Mania (dian kuang)

Definition:
Manic-depressive psychosis is a bipolar affective disorder with severe alterations in mood that are usually episodic and recurrent. Mood fluctuates between depression and mania. In TCM, *dian* means depressive, non-violent behavior and *kuang* means hyperactive, manic, shouting, violent behavior.

Red Flags:
Primary care by Western medical specialist required. See red flags of depression.

Western Medicine Relevant Diseases:
TCM mania includes a wide variety of Western medical conditions, including:
- Schizophrenia and delusional disorder: Schizophrenia is a mental disorder characterized by loss of contact with reality (psychosis), hallucinations (usually, hearing voices), firmly held false beliefs (delusions), abnormal thinking and behavior, reduced expression of emotions, diminished motivation, a decline in mental function (cognition), and problems in daily functioning, including work, social relationships, and self-care.
- Mood disorders: Mood disorders are mental health disorders that involve emotional disturbances consisting of long periods of excessive sadness (depression), excessive joyousness or elation (mania), or both. Depression and mania represent the two extremes of mood disorders.
- Delirium and dementia are the most common causes of mental (cognitive) dysfunction. Although delirium and dementia may occur together, they are quite different: delirium begins suddenly, causes fluctuations in mental function, and is usually reversible and dementia begins gradually, is slowly progressive, and is usually irreversible. Both delirium and dementia may occur at any age but are much more common among older people.
- Alzheimer's disease: a type of dementia with a progressive loss of mental function, characterized by degeneration of brain tissue, including loss of nerve cells, the accumulation of an abnormal protein called beta-amyloid, and the development of neurofibrillary tangles.

Etiology and Pathogenesis:

TCM Differentiation and Treatment:

Pattern	Signs and Symptoms	Treatment Principle and Acupuncture	Formula
Dian Syndrome	Two types: a) Qi Stagnation and phlegm (cold) blocking heart orifices: -depressive, apathetic, incoherent speech, subdued, anxiety, mood swings T: pale P: slippery b) SP and HT Deficiency: -protracted disease, disturbed thoughts, incoherent speech, depression, crying, panic, palpitations, pale complexion, fatigue, loss of appetite T: pale P: weak	Treatment principle: a) Regulate Qi, drain phlegm, open orifices b) Strengthen SP, nourish HT, calm spirit Principle points: Local: DU26 (shui gou), DU24 (shen ting), DU20, (bai hui), Sishencong On channel: P6 (nei guan), HT6 (yin xi) or P7 (da ling), HT7 (shen men) Phlegm + ST36 (ZSL), ST40 (feng long), PC5 (jian shi) Qi +LI4, LV3 (4 gates) SP and HT deficiency + BL20 (pi shu), BL15 (xin shu), SP 10 (xue hai), SP3 (tai bai), SP6 (SYJ)	
Kuang Syndrome	Two types: a) Excess attack - phlegm and fire blocking Heart orifices: -acute onset, flushed face, red eyes, aggressive behavior, irritable, agitated, insomnia, headache T: red, greasy coat P: slippery and rapid b) Deficiency type - chronic heat, Yin and Qi weak: -protracted disease, emotional instability, anxiety, panic attacks, palpitations, five center heat, emaciation, often senior, tired, SOB, night sweat, hot flash T: red P: weak and rapid	Treatment principle: a) Clear fire, drain phlegm, open orifices to calm heart spirit b) Clear fire and phlegm, nourish Yin, calm heart Principle Points: Local: DU26 (shui gou), DU24 (shen ting), DU20, (bai hui), Sishencong Excess + PC8 (lao gong), HT6 (yin xi), HT7 (shen men), LR2 (xing jian), LI4 (he gu) Deficient + SP6 (SYJ), ST36 (ZSL), K3 (tai xi), KI6 (zhao hai), LV2-LI4 (xing jian + he gu), ST40 (feng long), BL15 (xin shu), BL23 (shen shu)	

Palpitations (xin ji)

Definition:
Patterns in which the patient experiences a subjective sensation of a rapid or irregular heart beat. May be accompanied by anxiety or panic. Palpitations include changes in heart rate or rhythm. They are often brought on by emotional stress or exhaustion, but may also be due to organic heart disorders.

Red Flags:
In people with palpitations, certain symptoms and characteristics are cause for concern and merit referral. They include:

Western Medicine Relevant Diseases:
In Western medicine, palpitations are defined as the perception of cardiac activity. They are often described as a fluttering, racing, or skipping sensation. They are common and some patients find them unpleasant and alarming.

The mechanisms responsible for the sensation of palpitations are unknown. Ordinarily, sinus rhythm at a normal rate is not perceived, and palpitations thus usually reflect changes in cardiac rate or rhythm.

Some patients simply have heightened awareness of normal cardiac activity, particularly when exercise, febrile illness, or anxiety increases heart rate. However, in most cases, palpitations result from arrhythmia. Arrhythmias range from benign to life threatening. The most common arrhythmias include:
- Premature atrial contractions (PACs)
- Premature ventricular contractions (PVCs)

Both of these arrhythmias usually are harmless. Some arrhythmias occur spontaneously in patients without serious underlying disorders, but others are often caused by a serious cardiac disorder.

Serious cardiac causes include myocardial ischemia or other myocardial disorders, congenital heart disease (e.g. Brugada syndrome, arrhythmogenic right ventricular cardiomyopathy, congenital long QT syndrome), valvular heart disease, and conduction system disturbances (e.g. disturbances that cause bradycardia or heart block). Patients with orthostatic hypotension commonly sense palpitations caused by sinus tachycardia upon standing.

Non-cardiac disorders that increase myocardial contractility (e.g. thyrotoxicosis, pheochromocytoma, anxiety) may cause palpitations.

Some drugs, including digitalis, caffeine, alcohol, nicotine, and sympathomimetics (e.g. albuterol, amphetamines, cocaine, dobutamine, epinephrine, ephedrine, isoproterenol, norepinephrine, and theophylline), frequently cause or exacerbate palpitations.

Metabolic disturbances, including anemia, hypoxia, hypovolemia, and electrolyte abnormalities (e.g. diuretic-induced hypokalemia), can trigger or exacerbate palpitations.

Etiology and Pathogenesis:
- Constitutional Heart and Gallbladder deficiency (lack of confidence, timidity) – heart malnourished and spirit easily disturbed

- Severe blood loss or injury to Spleen - Heart blood deficiency – malnourishment of heart
- Excessive sexual activity, aging – injures KI essence – KI water cannot nourish HT fire – HT fire overactive
- Chronic/severe illness – exhausts Heart Yang
- Cold congested fluids overflowing to the heart – KI Yang fails to warm and steam water, fluids become congested and spill into upper jiao – block circulation and result in heart dysfunction
- Blood stasis – from HT Yang xu, bi syndromes – blocks heart vessels and impairs circulation

TCM Differentiation and Treatment:

Pattern	Signs and Symptoms	Treatment Principle	Acupuncture	Formula
Heart and GB Qi Deficiency	Palpitations, easily frightened, fearful, insomnia, excessive dreaming. P: slightly rapid, weak	Supplement HT and GB Qi, quiet the spirit	BL15 (xin shu), REN14 (ju que), HT7 (shen men), PC6 (nei guan), PC7 (da ling), HT5 (tong li), GB40 (qiu xu)	
Heart Blood Deficiency	Palpitations, dizziness, vertigo, pale complexion, fatigue, insomnia, forgetfulness. T: pale P: weak, thready	Boost Qi, supplement blood, nourish HT, quiet spirit	BL15 (xin shu), REN14 (ju que), HT7 (shen men), PC6 (nei guan), BL20 (pi shu), ST36 (ZSL), BL17 (ge shu)	
Yin Deficiency with Empty Fire	Palpitations, irritability, insomnia, dizzy, vertigo, five center heat, low backache, tinnitus. T: red with no coat P: rapid, thready	Nourish yin, clear fire, tonify HT, calm spirit	BL15 (xin shu), REN14 (ju que), HT7 (shen men), PC6 (nei guan), BL14 (jue yin shu), BL23 (shen shu), KI3 (tai xi)	
Heart Yang Deficiency	Palpitations, chest pain or oppression, SOB, pale complexion, cold extremities. T: pale P: weak or deep and thready	Warm and supplement HT yang, quiet spirit	BL15 (xin shu), REN14 (ju que), HT7 (shen men), PC6 (nei guan), REN6 (qi hai), REN4 (guan yuan)	
Cold Congested Fluids Overflow to Heart	Palpitations, dizziness, vertigo, expectoration of phlegm and mucus, fullness of chest, cold extremities, nausea, vomit clear fluids. P: slippery, wiry	Warm and activate HT yang to transform congested fluids	BL15 (xin shu), REN14 (ju que), HT7 (shen men), PC6 (nei guan), REN9 (shui fen), SP9 (yin ling quan), REN4 (guan yuan)	
Heart Blood Stasis	Palpitations, chest oppression, pain, purple lips and nails. T: purple with petechiae P: choppy, knotted, intermittent	Invigorate Blood, transform stasis, unblock channels	BL15 (xin shu), REN14 (ju que), HT7 (shen men), PC6 (nei guan), SP10 (xue hai), REN6 (qi hai), SP6 (SYJ)	

Pulmonary Abscess (fei yong)

Pulmonary abscess

Definition:
Suppurated sores and boils in the lung characterized by chest pain, fever, and coughing up foul smelling opaque sputum. In severe stages, there may be blood and sputum.

Red Flags:
Referral required.

Western Medicine Relevant Diseases:
A lung abscess is a pus-filled cavity in the lung surrounded by inflamed tissue and caused by an infection. A lung abscess is usually caused by bacteria that live in the mouth or throat, and are aspirated into the lungs, resulting in an infection. Often, periodontal disease is the source of the bacteria that cause a lung abscess.

The body has many defenses (such as a cough) to help prevent bacteria from getting into the lungs. Infection occurs primarily when a person is unconscious or very drowsy because of sedation, anesthesia, alcohol or drug use, or a disease of the nervous system and is thus less able to cough to clear the aspirated bacteria. In people whose immune system functions poorly, a lung abscess may be caused by organisms that are not typically found in the mouth or throat, such as fungi or Mycobacterium tuberculosis (the organism that causes tuberculosis). Other bacteria that can cause lung abscesses are streptococci and staphylococci, including methicillin-resistant Staphylococcus aureus (MRSA), which is a serious infection.

Obstruction of the airways also can lead to abscess formation. If the branches of the bronchi are blocked by a tumor or a foreign object, an abscess can form because mucus can accumulate behind the obstruction. Bacteria sometimes enter these secretions. The obstruction prevents the bacteria-laden secretions from being coughed back up through the airway.

Less commonly, abscesses result when bacteria or infected blood clots travel through the bloodstream to the lung from another infected site in the body (septic pulmonary emboli).

Usually, people develop only one lung abscess as a result of aspiration or airway obstruction. If several abscesses develop, they are usually in the same lung. When an infection reaches the lungs through the bloodstream, however, many scattered abscesses may develop in both lungs.

Eventually, most abscesses rupture into an airway, producing a lot of sputum that gets coughed up. A ruptured abscess leaves a cavity in the lung that is filled with fluid and air. Sometimes an abscess ruptures into the space between the lungs and the chest wall pleural space, filling the space with pus. Very rarely, if an abscess destroys a blood vessel wall, it may lead to serious bleeding.

Symptoms most commonly start slowly. However, depending on the cause of the abscess, symptoms can occur suddenly. Early symptoms resemble those of pneumonia and include:
- Fatigue
- Loss of appetite
- Sweating during the night
- Fever
- A cough that brings up sputum

The sputum may be foul smelling (because bacteria from the mouth or throat tend to produce foul odors) or streaked with blood. People also may feel chest pain as they breathe, especially if the lining on the outside of the lungs and inside of the chest wall (pleura) is inflamed. Many people have these symptoms for weeks or months before seeking medical attention. These people have chronic abscesses and, in addition to the other symptoms, lose a substantial amount of weight and have daily fever and night sweats. In contrast, lung abscesses caused by Staphylococcus aureus or MRSA can be fatal within days or sometimes even hours.

Etiology and Pathogenesis:
- Wind-heat attacking Lung or Phlegm heat hidden in Lung – cause LU Qi dysfunction, heat toxicity accumulation, phlegm and stasis – lead to Lung abscess

TCM Differentiation and Treatment:

Pattern	Signs and Symptoms	Treatment Principle	Acupuncture	Formula
	Aversion to cold, fever, productive cough, sticky sputum, painful chest, dyspnea. T: thin white or yellow coat P: floating, rapid and slippery	Clear the LU and disperse pathogens, release exterior	DU14 (da zhui), LI11 (qu chi), SJ5 (wei guan), LI4 (he gu), LU7 (lie que), BL13 (fei shu)	
	High fever, sweating, irritability, cough, opaque or yellow-green sputum, stifling and painful chest, foul smell in throat, dry mouth and throat. T: yellow, greasy P: slippery, rapid	Clear heat and toxicity, transform stasis, reduce abscess	REN22 (tian tu), LU5 (chi zi), ST40 (feng long), LU7 (lie que), LI11 (qu chi), BL13 (fei shu), LU6 (kong zui)	
	Productive cough with copious purulent bloody sputum, which is foul smelling, painful chest, irritable, dyspnea, fever, red face, thirst. T: red, yellow greasy coat P: slippery and rapid	Promote purulent discharge and relieve toxicity	REN22 (tian tu), LU5 (chi zi), ST40 (feng long), LU7 (lie que), LI11 (qu chi), BL13 (fei shu), LU6 (kong zui)	
	Condition improving, reduced signs and symptoms. May be Yin deficiency signs. T: red P: thready and forceless	Nourish the Yin and tonify Lung	BL13 (fei shu), LU1 (zhong fu), LU7 (lie que), KD6 (zhao hai), LU9 (tai yuan), SP3 (tai bai)	

Pulmonary Tuberculosis (fei lao)

Definition:
This is a communicable chronic consumptive disease of the lung, with coughing, spitting blood, tidal fever, night sweating, and emaciation.

Red Flags:
Referral required.

Western Medicine Relevant Diseases:
Tuberculosis (TB) is a disease with many presentations and manifestations. It is the most common cause of infectious disease-related mortality worldwide. TB usually affects the lungs, but it can affect other organs as well.

TB is caused by bacteria called *Mycobacterium tuberculosis. Mycobacterium tuberculosis* lives only in people and are not normally transmitted by animals, insects, soil, or other nonliving objects. People are infected with tuberculosis almost exclusively by breathing air contaminated by a person who has active disease. Touching someone who has the disease does not spread TB because *Mycobacterium tuberculosis* bacteria are spread almost exclusively through the air.

Cough is the most common symptom of pulmonary tuberculosis. The cough may produce a small amount of green or yellow sputum, usually when people awaken in the morning. Eventually, the sputum may be streaked with blood, although large amounts of blood are rare. People may awaken in the night and be drenched with a cold sweat, with or without fever. People also feel generally unwell, with decreased energy and appetite. Weight loss often occurs after they have been ill for a while.

Rapidly developing shortness of breath plus chest pain may signal the presence of air (pneumothorax) or fluid (pleural effusion) in the space between the lungs and the chest wall. About one third of tuberculosis infections first show up as pleural effusion. Eventually, many people with untreated tuberculosis develop shortness of breath as the infection spreads in the lungs.

Etiology and Pathogenesis:
Involves both external and internal factors. Internal factors include a weakened constitution, Qi and Blood deficiency, and Yin and Essence deficiency. The external factor is invasion of a parasite. The primary site of illness is the Lung.
The basis of the pathogenesis is Yin depletion. Eventually, this leads to KI, HT, and LR involvement with systemic Yin deficiency fire. When damage to the LU also involves the SP, both Qi and Yin deficiency can result. In all cases, the advanced stages will have injury to the LU, SP, and KI, and weakening of both Yin and Yang.

TCM Differentiation and Treatment:

Pattern	Signs and Symptoms	Treatment Principle	Acupuncture	Formula
	Dry cough, scanty phlegm, possibly blood streaked phlegm, dull chest pain, afternoon tidal fever, flushed cheeks, night sweats, dry throat and mouth. T: dry P: rapid, thready	Nourish Yin, moisten LU, relieve coughing, expel pathogen	BL13 (fei shu), LU9 (tai yuan), BL43 (gao huang shu), LU5 (chi ze), LU7 (lie que) Blood expectoration + LU6 (kong zui), BL17 (ge shu) Night sweats + HT6 (yin xi), KD7 (fu liu)	
	Choking cough, rapid breathing, sticky scanty yellow phlegm, spitting red blood, steaming bone tidal fever, five center heat, flushed cheeks, night sweating, irritability, insomnia, emaciation. T: red, no coat P: rapid, thready	Moisten Yin, clear fire, relieve coughing, expel pathogen	BL13 (fei shu), BL23 (shen shu), BL43 (gao huang shu), KD3 (tai xi), LU10 (yu ji), LR2 (xing jian) Tidal fever + DU14 (da zhui)	
	Weak cough, SOB, weak voice, phlegm with light blood, mild tidal fever, night sweats, spontaneous sweats, pale complexion, tired, poor appetite. T: tender, tooth marks P: rapid, thready	Benefit Qi, nourish Yin, expel pathogen	BL13 (fei shu), BL20 (pi shu), BL43 (gao huang shu), ST36 (ZSL), SP6 (SYJ)	
	Choking cough, spitting blood, tidal fever, night sweats, loss of voice, frail, cold, spontaneous sweat, SOB, low food intake. T: red or pale P: faint, thready	Nourish Yin, warm Yang, supplement deficiency, expel pathogen	BL13 (fei shu), BL20 (pi shu), BL43 (gao huang shu), BL23 (shen shu), REN4, (guan yuan), ST36 (ZSL)	

Seminal Emission (yi jing)

Definition:
Seminal emission is the spontaneous discharge of semen not induced by sexual activity. This may occur at night or during the day while awake. Seminal emission is considered normal if it occurs less than twice a month without any other symptoms.

Red Flags:
If seminal emission disturbs daily activities, or is accompanied by dizziness, listlessness, insomnia, sore and weak lower back and knees, then medical evaluation and treatment may be necessary.

Western Medicine Relevant Diseases:
Spontaneous discharge of semen may be a symptom in certain biomedical disorders such as: prostatitis (prostate infection), prostatic hypertrophy (enlarged prostate gland), spermatocystitis (inflammation of seminal vesicles), and orchitis (inflammation of the testicles).

Etiology and Pathogenesis:

TCM Differentiation and Treatment:

Pattern	Signs and Symptoms	Treatment Principle	Acupuncture	Formula
Lack of Communication between Heart and Kidney	Nocturnal emissions with erotic dreams, insomnia, irritability, dizziness blurred vision, palpitations, dry mouth, and scanty urine. T: red P: thready, rapid	Clear heat, nourish yin, calm spirit	BL15 (xin shu), BL23 (shen shu), HT7 (shen men), KD3 (tai xi), PC6 (nei guan), SP6 (SYJ), REN4 (guan yuan)	
Damp Heat	Frequent seminal emission, dark turbid urine burning sensation when urinating, bitter taste, heavy body, foul stools, nausea. T: yellow, greasy P: rapid, slippery	Clear heat, drain damp	REN3 (zhong jj), BL34 (ba liao), SP9 (yin ling quan), SP6 (SYJ), LR3 (tai chong), PC6 (nei guan), LI11 (qu chi)	
Qi deficiency failing to hold the Essence	Seminal emissions when fatigued, sallow complexion, heavy and fatigued limbs, palpitations, insomnia, poor appetite, loose stool. T: pale P: weak	Harmonize and tonify HT and SP, support Qi, bind the Essence	BL20 (pi shu), BL23 (shen shu), REN6 (qi hai), ST36 (ZSL), SP6 (SYJ)	
Kidney Yang Deficiency	Frequent nocturnal emissions, cold extremities, impotence, premature ejaculation, pale complexion. T: pale P: deep, thready	Supplement KD Yang, secure Essence	BL23 (shen shu), REN4 (guan yuan), SP6 (SYJ), REN6 (qi hai), KD12 (da he), DU4 (ming men)	

Spontaneous Sweats, Night Sweats (zi han, dao han)

Definition:
Abnormal, or spontaneous sweats and night sweats, is pathological perspiration due to disharmony between Yin and Yang and an unconsolidated superficial layer between the skin and muscles.

Red Flags:
- Signs of dehydration

Western Medicine Relevant Diseases:
Sweat is made by sweat glands in the skin and carried to the skin's surface by ducts. Sweating helps keep the body cool. Sweat is composed mostly of water, but it also contains salt (mostly sodium chloride) and other chemicals. When a person sweats a lot, the lost salt and water must be replaced. In Western medicine, excessive sweating is called hyperhidrosis.

Excessive sweating may affect the entire surface of the skin but is often limited to certain parts of the body (called focal excessive sweating). The parts most often affected are the palms of the hands, soles of the feet, forehead, and armpits. Sweating in these areas is usually caused by anxiety, excitement, anger, or fear.

Certain disorders can increase such sweating, such as diabetes that affects the nerves, shingles affecting the face, brain disorders, certain disorders affecting the autonomic nervous system in the neck, and certain injuries affecting the nerves to the salivary gland in front of the ear (the parotid gland).

Excessive sweating that affects most of the body is called generalized excessive sweating. Usually, no specific cause is found. However, a number of disorders can cause generalized excessive sweating, for example: endocrine disorders (hyperthyroidism, hypoglycemia, pituitary gland disorders), certain drugs, nervous system disorders, lymphoma and leukemia, infections, pregnancy, and menopause.

Etiology and Pathogenesis:

TCM Differentiation and Treatment:

Pattern	Signs and Symptoms	Treatment Principle	Acupuncture	Formula
Lung Qi deficiency	Aversion to wind, sweating with mild exertion, susceptible to catching colds, fatigue, poor appetite. T: thin white coat P: weak	Tonify Qi, consolidate exterior	LU Qi xu + BL13 (fei shu), BL20 (pi shu), ST36 (ZSL), REN6 (qi hai) Harmonize Qi + SJ5 (wei guan), SP6 (SYJ), ST36 (ZSL) Yin xu + BL13 (fei shu), BL23 (shen shu), KD7 (fu liu), KD3 (tai xi), LV2 (xing jian) Excess heat + DU14 (da zhui) Damp heat + LI11 (qu chi), LI4 (he gu), KD7 (fu liu) Consider calming the shen for anxiety if applicable as well.	
Disharmony between protective and nutritive Qi	Persistent sweating, maybe localized, slight aversion to wind, low-grade fever, body ache, H/A. T: thin white coat P: floating	Harmonize Qi, reduce sweating		
Yin deficiency and empty fire	Night sweating, insomnia, five center heat, tidal fever, malar flush, emaciation. T: red, scanty coat P: thready, rapid	Nourish Yin, reduce empty fire, restrain sweating		
Excess heat flaring	Persistent, profuse sweating, irritable, restless, hot chest, thirst, scanty urine, constipation. T: red, yellow coat P: rapid	Clear heat, drain fire, stop sweating		
Damp heat accumulation	Sticky sweat that leaves yellow stains, irritable, bitter taste, fever, thirst with no desire to drink, scanty urine. T: red, greasy coat P: rapid, slippery	Clear heat, drain damp, stop sweating		

Stranguria (lin zheng)

Stranguria
(also called Painful Urinary Syndrome)

Definition:
This is a group of symptoms characterized by discomfort, oliguria, increased urgency, increased frequency, difficult, or painful urination.

Red Flags:
- Acute loin pain coming in waves, possible vomiting and collapse. This is characteristic of an obstructed kidney stone. The pain may radiate round to the suprapubic region particularly if the stone moves some way down the ureter.
- Blood in the urine (haematuria) or sperm (haemospermia)
- Recurrent or persistent urinary tract infections. Symptoms including some or all of: cloudy urine, burning on urination, abdominal discomfort, blood in urine and fever.
- Features of moderate prostatic obstruction. Enlargement of the prostate gland leads to symptoms such as increasing difficulty urinating, and nocturia. Benign prostatic enlargement is common and the symptoms can respond to acupuncture treatment. However, the same symptoms can be caused by a prostatic tumor.
- Features of acute pyelonephritis: Fever, malaise, loin pain and cloudy urine suggest an infection of the kidneys requiring antibiotic treatment.
- Features of a urinary tract infection in anyone in the following vulnerable groups:
    - Pre-existing disorder of the urinary system
    - diabetes
    - pregnancy

Western Medicine Relevant Diseases:
In Western medicine, painful urinary syndrome may correspond to conditions such as urinary tract infections, or urinary calculi.

Urinary tract infections (UTIs) can be divided into: upper tract infections, which involve the kidneys (pyelonephritis), and lower tract infections, which involve the bladder (cystitis), urethra (urethritis), and prostate (prostatitis). Although urethritis and prostatitis are infections that involve the urinary tract, the term UTI usually refers to pyelonephritis and cystitis.

Bacteria is the cause of most cases of cystitis and pyelonephritis. The most common nonbacterial pathogens are fungi (usually candida), and, less commonly, mycobacteria, viruses, and parasites. Nonbacterial pathogens usually affect patients who are: immune-compromised, have diabetes, obstruction, or structural urinary tract abnormalities, or have had recent urinary tract instrumentation.

Urinary calculi are hard masses that form in the urinary tract and may cause pain, bleeding, or an infection or block of the flow of urine. Tiny stones may cause no symptoms, but larger stones can cause excruciating pain between the ribs and hips in the back.

Stones may form because the urine becomes too saturated with salts that can form stones or because the urine lacks the normal inhibitors of stone formation.

Stones are more common among people: with certain disorders (e.g. hyperparathyroidism, dehydration), whose diet is very high in animal-source protein or vitamin C, or who do not consume enough water or calcium. People who have a family history of stone formation are more likely to have calcium stones. Surgery for weight loss (bariatric surgery) may also increase risk of stone formation.

Etiology and Pathogenesis:
- Diet – excess consumption of sweets, sugar, dairy, greasy foods – leads to formation of dampness – slows and Qi transformation and obstructs bladder; or excess consumption of spicy foods and alcohol may generate heat that combines with damp – causes damp heat in lower burner
- Aging, weak constitution overexertion, excessive sexual activity – lead to Spleen and Kidney deficiency - causes Qi sinking and failure to secure (and may also cause yin deficiency with empty fire)
- Emotional stress – leads to Qi stagnation – can transform into Liver fire – may be transmitted to Bladder

TCM Differentiation and Treatment:

Pattern	Signs and Symptoms	Treatment Principle	Acupuncture	Formula
	Frequent, scanty, difficult urination, burning pain on urination, dark urine with strong smell, hypogastric pain, bitter taste, nausea, constipation, thirst. T: red, yellow greasy coat P: rapid, slippery (in addition, may be caused by LR Fire or HT fire, with related signs and symptoms of these patterns)	Clear heat, drain damp, open water passages	REN3 (zhong ji), BL28 (pan guang shu), BL22 (san jiao shu), SP9 (yin ling quan), BL63 (jin men), BL66 (tong gu), LI11 (qu chi)	
	Stones or sand in urine, difficult urination that may stop suddenly, spasmodic pain in urethra while urinating, hypogastric pain, blood in urine. T: red, yellow coat P: wiry, rapid	Clear heat, drain damp, open water passages, expel stones	BL22 (san jiao shu), ST28 (shui dao), SP9 (yin ling quan), REN3 (zhong ji), BL28 (pang guang shu), BL63 (jin men), BL39 (wei yang)	
	Excess type: difficult, painful urination, distension of lower ABD, fullness and discomfort of chest/hypochondriac regions, irritability, wiry and deep pulse. Deficient type: Difficult urination, weak stream, tiredness, heavy sensation in lower ABD, pale tongue, weak pulse.	Excess type: more Qi, eliminate stagnation open water passages Deficient type: tonify and raise Qi, open water passages	REN3 (zhong ji), REN5 (shi men), BL28 (pang guang sue), LR3 (tai chong), LR5 (li gou), LR8 (qiu quan), BL64 (jing gu) Deficient type: KD1 (yong quan), GB34 (yang ling quan), REN5 (shi men), DU20 (bai hui) For females: LU7 (lie que) & KD6 (zhao hai) (ren mai) For males: SI3 (hou xi) & UB62 (shen mai (du mai)	
	Excess type: Difficult urination, burning pain on urination, blood in urine, fullness and pain in hypogastrium, mental restlessness, red tongue, rapid pulse. Deficient type: Pale blood in urine, slight discomfort on urination, not much pain, sore back, depression, feel heat in evening, red and peeled tongue, rapid and floating-empty pulse.	Excess type: clear heat, cool blood, stop bleeding, open water passages Deficient type: clear empty heat, cool blood, nourish yin, stop bleeding, open water passages	LR3 (tai chong), KD2 (ran gu), REN3 (zhong ji), BL28 (pang guang shu), BL63 (jin men), SP10 (xue hai), BL17 (ge shu), SP6 (SYJ) Deficient + REN4 (guan yuan), KD6 (zhao hai)	

© 2017 LIFT Education Academy www.lifteducation.academy

	Excess: Turbid, milky, or cloudy urine, possible blood, difficult urination with burning pain, ABD distension, red tongue with sticky coat, slippery rapid pulse. Deficient: Chronic lin syndrome with turbid urine and mild pain, emaciation, weak low back/knees, dizziness, fatigue, pale tongue, weak pulse.	Excess: drain damp, clear heat, separate clear and turbid, open water passages Deficient: tonify Qi, strengthen KD, separate clear and turbid, open water passages	REN3 (zhong ji), BL28 (pang guang shu), BL22 (san jiao shu), REN6 (qi hai), REN9 (shui fen), ST28 (shui dao), SP6 (SYJ), SP9 (yin ling quan) Deficient + BL23 (shen shu), KD7 (fu liu)	
	Difficult urination with dribbling that occurs with exertion, fatigue, lassitude, sore back/knees, pale tongue, weak pulse.	Tonify and raise Qi, strengthen KD, open water passages.	BL23 (shen shu), REN4 (guan yuan), BL28 (pang guang shu), DU20 (bai hui), ST36 (ZSL), SP6 (SYJ), SP9 (yin ling quan), KD3 (tai xi), DU4 (ming men)	

Tinnitus and Deafness (er ming er long)

Definition:
Tinnitus and deafness are both hearing disorders. Tinnitus refers to the subjective sensation of ringing in the ears, and deafness is a decrease or loss in hearing. These may be symptoms of other diseases or may occur in isolation.

Red Flags:
Certain symptoms and characteristics merit referral. They include:

Western Medicine Relevant Diseases:
In Western medicine, tinnitus is defined as noise in the ears that may be experienced as buzzing, ringing, roaring, whistling, or hissing sound and is often associated with hearing loss. Subjective tinnitus is perception of sound in the absence of an acoustic stimulus and is heard only by the patient. Objective tinnitus is uncommon and results from noise generated by structures near the ear.

Subjective tinnitus is by far the most common type. It is caused by abnormal activity in the auditory cortex. It is not fully understood how this abnormal activity develops. Objective tinnitus is much less common. It represents actual noise created by structures near the ear. Other people can sometimes hear the sounds of objective tinnitus if they listen closely.

The most common causes of subjective tinnitus include:
- Exposure to loud noises or explosions
- Aging
- Certain drugs that damage the ear
- Meniere disease

Other causes include middle ear infections, disorders that block the ear canal (such as an external otitis, excessive ear wax, or foreign bodies), problems with the eustachian tube due to allergies or other causes of obstruction, and otosclerosis (a disorder of excess bone growth in the middle ear). An uncommon but serious cause is an acoustic neuroma, a noncancerous (benign) tumor of part of the nerve leading from the inner ear.

Objective tinnitus usually involves noise from blood vessels near the ear. In such cases, the sound comes with each beat of the pulse. Causes include:
- Turbulent flow through the carotid artery or jugular vein
- Certain middle ear tumors that are rich in blood vessels
- Malformed blood vessels of the membrane covering the brain

Deafness, or hearing loss, has many causes in Western medicine. Different parts of the hearing pathway can be affected, and loss is classified as conductive, sensorineural, or mixed, depending on the part of the pathway that is affected.

Conductive hearing loss occurs when something blocks sound from reaching the sensory structures in the inner ear. The problem may involve the external ear canal, the eardrum (tympanic membrane—TM), or the middle ear.

Sensorineural hearing loss occurs when sound reaches the inner ear, but either sound cannot be translated into nerve impulses (sensory loss) or nerve impulses are not carried to the brain (neural loss). The distinction between sensory and neural loss is important because sensory hearing loss is sometimes reversible and is seldom life threatening. A neural hearing loss rarely goes away and may be due to a potentially life-threatening brain tumor—commonly a cerebellopontine angle tumor.

Mixed loss involves both conductive and sensorineural loss. It may be caused by severe head injury, chronic infection, or one of many rare genetic disorders.

The most common causes are:
- Earwax accumulation
- Noise (can cause sudden or gradual hearing loss)
- Aging
- Ear infections are a common cause of temporary mild to moderate hearing loss

Less common causes include autoimmune disorders, congenital disorders, drugs that damage the ear, injuries, or tumors.

Etiology and Pathogenesis:
Excess patterns may result from:
- Emotional stress stirring Liver and Gallbladder fire which rises to disturb the ears
- Invasion of the ear by wind heat – EPI blocks orifices
- Excessive consumption of alcohol and rich foods leading to stagnation of phlegm fire

Deficiency patterns may result from:
- Constitutional issues or extended illness leading to weak Kidney essence
- Poor diet and excessive work causing inability of Spleen and Stomach Qi to rise and nourish the ears

TCM Differentiation and Treatment:

Pattern	Signs and Symptoms	Treatment Principle	Acupuncture	Formula
Wind Heat Attack	Initial symptoms of common cold, sudden onset decrease in hearing, ear slightly red. P: floating rapid	Expel wind heat	Local: GB2 (ting hui), SI19 (ting gong), SJ21 (er men) Wind heat + LI4 (he gu), SJ5 (wei guan), GB20 (feng chi), LI6 (kong zui)	
Liver Fire Rising	Sudden onset, worse with emotion, tinnitus usually high pitch or can like ocean waves or thunder (whatever it is, it is LOUD), ear distension and pain, H/A, dizziness, red eyes/face, bitter taste, dry throat, heat signs. P: wiry, rapid	Clear Liver Fire	Local: GB2 (ting hui), SI19 (ting gong), SJ21 (er men) + LR2 (xing jian), LR3 (tai chong), GB43 (xia xi), GB34 (yang ling quan)	
Phlegm Fire	Tinnitus, ear blocked and decreased hearing, dizzy spells, foggy/heavy sensations in head, chest oppression, cough with phlegm, incomplete bowel movements. T: red, greasy coat P: wiry, slippery, rapid	Clear fire, drain phlegm	Local: GB2 (ting hui), SI19 (ting gong), SJ21 (er men) +ST40 (feng long), PC8 (lao gong), LI4 (he gu)	
Kidney Essence Depletion	Chronic tinnitus like cicadas, intermittent, worse at night, gradual hearing loss, dizziness, vertigo, insomnia, sore back/knees. T: red, little coat P: thready	Tonify KD, secure essence	Local: GB2 (ting hui), SI19 (ting gong), SJ21 (er men) +UB23 (shen shu), REN4 (guan yuan), KD3 (tai xi), SP6 (SYJ), ST36 (ZSL), GB39 (xuan zhong)	
Spleen and Stomach Qi Deficiency	Tinnitus and deafness worse with overwork, tiredness, poor appetite, loose stools, epigastric distension, sallow complexion. T: pale P: weak	Strengthen ST and SP, boost Qi	Local: GB2 (ting hui), SI19 (ting gong), SJ21 (er men) + BL20 (pi shu), BL21 (wei shu), SP6 (SYJ), ST36 (ZSL), REN6 (qi hai)	

Vertigo (xuan yun)

Vertigo

Definition:
Refers to subjective symptoms of blurred vision and a sensation of turning in space or having objects moving around. May range from mild lightheadedness, to severe vertigo with loss of balance.

Red Flags:
In people with dizziness or vertigo, certain symptoms and characteristics may require referral:
- Headache
- Neck pain
- Difficulty walking
- Loss of consciousness
- Other neurologic symptoms (such as trouble hearing, seeing, speaking, or swallowing or difficulty moving an arm or leg)

Western Medicine Relevant Diseases:
Dizziness and vertigo are usually caused by disorders of the parts of the ear and brain that are involved in maintaining balance:
- Inner ear
- Brain stem and cerebellum
- Nerve tracts connecting the brain stem and cerebellum or within the brain stem

The inner ear contains structures (semicircular canals, saccule, and utricle) that enable the body to sense position and motion. Information from these structures is sent to the brain through the vestibulocochlear nerve (8th cranial nerve, which is also involved in hearing). This information is processed in the brain stem, which adjusts posture, and the cerebellum, which coordinates movements, to provide a sense of balance. A disorder in any of these structures can cause dizziness, vertigo, or both. Disorders of the inner ear sometimes also cause decreased hearing and/or tinnitus.

Also, any disorder that affects brain function in general (for example, low blood sugar, low blood pressure, severe anemia, or certain drugs) can make people feel dizzy. Although symptoms may be disturbing and even incapacitating, very few cases result from a serious disorder.

The most common causes of dizziness and vertigo include:

Very often, no particular cause is found, and symptoms go away without treatment.

Less common causes include a tumor of the vestibulocochlear nerve (acoustic neuroma); a tumor, stroke, or transient ischemic attack (TIA) affecting the brain stem; an injury to the eardrum, inner ear, or base of the skull; multiple sclerosis; low blood sugar; and pregnancy.

Etiology and Pathogenesis:
- Constitutional Yang excess, or Liver Yin deficiency and Kidney Yin deficiency – fail to nourish Liver - Yang rising disturbs orifices
- Chronic illness, excessive bleeding, or Spleen Qi deficiency – lead to Qi and Blood deficiency – induces dizziness

- Congenital deficiency or overwork or aging – leads to Kidney Essence deficiency – lack of generation of marrow – malnourishment of orifices
- Improper diet, or SP and ST deficiency – leads to phlegm dampness accumulation – prevents clear Yang from rising

TCM Differentiation and Treatment:

Pattern	Signs and Symptoms	Treatment Principle	Acupuncture	Formula
Liver Yang Rising	Dizziness, distending H/A, worse with emotion, tinnitus, flushed face, irritable, bitter taste. T: red P: rapid, wiry	Pacify Liver, subdue Yang and nourish Liver and Kidney	GB20 (feng chi), BL18 (gan shu), BL23 (shen shu), KD3 (tai xi), LR2 (xing jian), GB41 (zu lin qi)	
Phlegm Damp Obstruction	Dizziness with heavy or muzzy sensation in head, difficulty concentrating, obesity, stuffy chest, nausea, poor appetite. T: greasy coat P: slippery	Dry damp, resolve phlegm, tonify SP and ST	ST8 (tou wei), BL20 (pi shu), REN12 (zhong wan), PC6 (nei guan), ST40 (feng long)	
Qi and Blood Deficiency	Dizziness worse with exertion, pale complexion, dull pale lips and nails, SOB, insomnia, poor memory, fatigue, poor appetite. T: pale P: thready, weak	Tonify Qi and nourish blood	DU20 (bai hui), BL20 (pi shu), REN4 (guan yuan), ST36 (ZSL), SP6 (SYJ), BL17 (ge shu),	
Kidney Essence Deficiency	Chronic dizziness, empty head, fatigue, tinnitus, insomnia, poor memory, sore back/knees, may be Yin deficient signs or Yang deficient signs.	Tonify Kidney, nourish Yin or assist Yang	DU20 (bai hui), BL23 (shen shu), REN4, (guan yuan), KD6 (zhao hai)	

Vomiting (ou tu)

Definition:
Vomiting is a common condition presented in a wide range of illnesses. In TCM, it is the ejection of the stomach contents due to a disharmony of the Stomach and rebellion of Stomach Qi.

Red Flags:
- Signs of dehydration (such as thirst, dry mouth, little or no urine output, and feeling weak and tired)
- Headache, stiff neck, confusion, or decreased alertness
- Constant abdominal pain
- Tenderness when the abdomen is touched, or distended (swollen) abdomen
- Recent head injury

Western Medicine Relevant Diseases:
In Western medicine, vomiting is a forceful contraction of the stomach that propels its contents up the esophagus and out the mouth.

In addition to being uncomfortable, vomiting can cause complications:
- Inhaled vomitus (aspiration)
- Torn esophagus (Mallory-Weiss tear from vomiting – causes bleeding)
- Dehydration and electrolyte abnormalities
- Under-nutrition and weight loss

The most common causes of nausea and vomiting are:
- Gastroenteritis (infection of the digestive tract)
- Drugs
- Toxins

Nausea and vomiting commonly occur with any dysfunction of the digestive tract but are particularly common with gastroenteritis. A less common digestive tract disorder is obstruction of the intestine, which causes vomiting because food and fluids back up into the stomach due to the obstruction. Many other abdominal disorders that cause vomiting also cause significant abdominal pain, for example, appendicitis or pancreatitis.

Many drugs, including alcohol, opioid analgesics, and chemotherapy drugs, can cause nausea and vomiting. Toxins, such as lead or those found in some foods and plants, can cause severe nausea and vomiting.

Less common causes of nausea and vomiting include
- Brain or central nervous system disorders
- Motion sickness
- Metabolic changes or systemic illness
- Psychological disorders
- Cyclic vomiting syndrome

The vomiting center in the brain can also be activated by certain brain or central nervous system disorders, including infections (such as meningitis and encephalitis), migraines, and disorders that increase pressure inside the skull (intracranial pressure). Disorders that increase intracranial pressure include brain tumors, brain hemorrhage, and severe head injuries.

Nausea and vomiting may also occur when there are metabolic changes in the body, such as during early pregnancy, or when people have unmanaged diabetes or severe liver failure or kidney failure.

Psychological problems also can cause nausea and vomiting. This is known as functional or psychogenic vomiting. Such vomiting may be intentional. For instance, people who have bulimia make themselves vomit to lose weight.

Etiology and Pathogenesis:
- Exterior pathogens
- Improper diet
- Emotional stress
- Spleen and Stomach deficiency

TCM Differentiation and Treatment:

Pattern	Signs and Symptoms	Treatment Principle	Acupuncture	Formula
	Sudden onset vomiting with aversion to cold, fever, H/A, general aches, chest oppression, epigastric fullness. P: floating	Dispel EPI, release exterior, relieve vomiting	LI4 (he gu), DU14 (da zhui), REN12 (zhong wan), PC6 (nei guan), ST36 (ZSL), DU20 (bai hui)	
	Vomiting of acid, fluid or undigested contents of the stomach, distention and fullness of ABD, loss of appetite, foul stools. T: greasy P: slippery	Disperse food, harmonize ST, descend rebellious Qi	REN12 (zhong wan), ST36 (ZSL), PC6 (nei guan), REN11 (jian li), REN21 (xuan ji), SP14 (fu jie)	
	Vomiting of clear liquid and mucus, epigastric fullness, loss of appetite, dizziness. T: greasy P: slippery	Warm and transform congested fluids, harmonize ST, descend rebellious Qi	SP9 (yin ling quan), SP4 (gong sun), ST40 (feng long), REN12 (zhong wan), ST36 (ZSL), PC6 (nei guan)	
	Vomiting, acid regurgitation, chest oppression, hypochondriac pain. P: wiry	Soothe Liver, harmonize ST, descend rebellious Qi	REN12 (zhong wan), GB34 (yang ling quan), LR3 (tai chong), ST36 (ZSL), PC6 (nei guan)	
	Vomiting induced by improper diet or fatigue, sallow complexion, fatigue, weakness, cold extremities, loose stools. T: pale P: weak	Warm the middle burner, tonify SP & ST, descend rebellious Qi	BL20 (pi shu), BL21 (wei shu), REN12 (zhong wan), ST36 (ZSL), PC6 (nei guan), SP4 (gong sun)	
	Recurrent vomiting or dry heaves, hunger with no desire to eat, dry throat. T: red, scanty coat P: rapid, thready	Nourish ST Yin, descend rebellious ST Qi	REN12 (zhong wan), ST36 (ZSL), PC6 (nei guan), SP4 (gong sun), SP6 (SYJ), KD3 (tai xi)	

Watery Phlegm/sputum (tan yin)

Definition:
Watery phlegm refers to the retention of un-metabolized water in specific regions of the body. Dysfunction of one (or more) of the three main water-metabolizing organs (LU, SP, KI) often plays an important role. The fluids are watery, dilute and frothy. Congested fluids are classified into different categories in TCM, depending on the location of fluid accumulation. Tai Yin is accumulation in the Stomach and Intestines. A splashing sound may be heard in the abdomen.

(As defined by Shi and Zeng, *Essentials of Chinese Medicine: Internal Medicine*, 2nd Edition)

Red Flags:
Worsening of condition with extreme exhaustion, difficult breathing, fever, or signs of organ failure.

Western Medicine Relevant Diseases:
Watery phlegm, or congested fluids in general, is a symptom found in many chronic conditions described elsewhere in this document, including: chronic bronchitis, pleurisy, or cor pulmonale (right ventricular enlargement secondary to a lung disorder that causes pulmonary artery hypertension. Right ventricular failure follows.). Any long-term illnesses that affect the lungs, heart, or kidneys could create congested fluids in the body.

More specifically, Tan Yin, or accumulation in the Stomach and Intestines, may result from gastrointestinal dysfunction or bowel obstruction.

Etiology and Pathogenesis:
- Exterior cold-damp – damages protective Yang and Lung Qi – lodges in muscular layer – LU and SP cannot metabolize water
- Improper diet, especially cold and raw foods – injures Spleen – disrupts SP T&T – fluids congest
- Exhaustion, fatigue, chronic illness – damage KI and SP Yang – cause dysfunction of water metabolism
- Obstruction of San Jiao – interrupts flow of water – congested fluids develop

TCM Differentiation and Treatment:
Note: important to differentiate with edema.

Pattern	Signs and Symptoms	Treatment Principle	Acupuncture	Formula
Spleen Yang Deficiency	Fullness in costal and hypochondriac regions, epigastric distention, splashing fluid sounds in the stomach, discomfort better with warmth, nausea, vomiting of clear watery emesis, cold sensations. T: swollen P: thready, slippery	Warm the Spleen, transform congested fluids		
Fluid Retention in Stomach and Intestines	Stiffness, fullness and pain in epigastrium and ABD, splashing fluid sounds in ABD, ABD distension, constipation, dry mouth and throat. T: greasy coat P: deep and wiry	Drain and force out congested fluids		

Wheezing Syndrome (xiao zheng)

Definition:
Wheezing is a paroxysmal episode of difficult breathing that produces whistling sounds. This is a recurrent condition that may last minutes to days. Accompanying symptoms include: rattling sound of sputum in the throat, rapid and shallow breathing, tachypnea, dyspnea, and the need to sit upright to breathe.

Red Flags:
In people with wheezing, the following symptoms are of particular concern and should be referred to emergency care:

Western Medicine Relevant Diseases:
In Western medicine, wheezing results from a narrowing or partial blockage somewhere in the airways. The narrowing may be widespread (as occurs in asthma, chronic obstructive pulmonary disease [COPD], and some severe allergic reactions), or only in one area (as may result from a tumor or a foreign object lodged in an airway).

Overall, the most common causes are asthma and COPD. Wheezing may occur in other disorders that affect the small airways, including heart failure (cardiac asthma), a severe allergic reaction (anaphylaxis), and inhalation of a toxic substance, or acute bronchitis.

COPD is described in the sections on dyspnea and lung distension.

Asthma is a condition in which the airways narrow—usually reversibly—in response to certain stimuli. Coughing, wheezing, and shortness of breath that occur in response to specific triggers are the most common symptoms.

The most important characteristic of asthma is narrowing of the airways that can be reversed. Cells lining the bronchi, called receptors, sense substances and stimulate the underlying muscles to contract or relax, thus altering the flow of air. The two main types of receptors are important in asthma:
- Beta-adrenergic receptors respond to chemicals such as epinephrine and make the muscles relax, dilating the airways and increasing airflow.
- Cholinergic receptors respond to a chemical called acetylcholine and make the muscles contract, decreasing airflow.

Narrowing of the airways is often caused by abnormal sensitivity of cholinergic receptors, which cause the muscles of the airways to contract when they should not. Certain cells in the airways, particularly mast cells, are thought to be responsible for initiating the response. Mast cells throughout the bronchi release substances such as histamine and leukotrienes, which cause smooth muscle to contract, mucus secretion to increase, and certain white blood cells to move to the area. Eosinophils, a type of white blood cell found in the airways of people with asthma, release additional substances, contributing to airway narrowing.

In an asthma attack, the smooth muscles of the bronchi contract, causing broncho-constriction. The tissues lining the airways swell due to inflammation and mucus secretion into the airways. The top layer of the airway lining can become damaged and shed cells, further narrowing the airway. A narrower airway requires the person to exert more effort to breathe.

Asthma triggers include:
- Allergens
- Infections
- Irritants
- Exercise
- Stress and anxiety

Etiology and Pathogenesis:
The main pathological factor in wheezing is latent phlegm that hides in the lung. The upward movement of phlegm propelled by

rebellious Qi narrows airways and causes wheezing. Factors that trigger wheezing include:
- EPI attacking the Lung – if not properly treated, this can lodge in Lung, produce phlegm and obstruct LU dispersing and descending
- Improper diet – especially too much cold/raw food, or greasy food – interrupts SP transformation and transportation generating phlegm that is stored in the Lung
- Deficiency post illness, or constitutional weakness – disrupt Lung or Kidney function – water metabolism is impaired – phlegm is generated

TCM Differentiation and Treatment:

Pattern	Signs and Symptoms	Treatment Principle	Acupuncture	Formula
Acute Phase Cold Pattern	Rapid breathing, wheezing, chest fullness/oppression, cough, scanty phlegm, bluish-white complexion, no thirst, feel cold, worse in cold weather. T: swollen, sticky white coat P: tight, slippery	Warm Lungs, disperse cold, resolve phlegm, and relieve wheezing.	LU7 (lie que), BL13 (fei shu), LU1 (zhong fu), LU6 (zong kui), REN22 (tian tu), REN17 (shan zhong), ST40 (feng long), PC6 (nei guan)	
Acute Phase Heat Pattern	Wheezing and heavy breathing, choking cough, thick sticky yellow phlegm, irritable, red face, bitter taste, thirst, feeling of heat. T: red, greasy coat P: slippery rapid	Clear heat, disperse LU Qi, transform phlegm, stop wheezing	LU5 (chi ze), LU10 (yu ji), LU6 (knog zui), LU1 (zhong fu), BL13 (fei shu), LI11 (qu chi), ST40 (feng long), REN22 (tian tu)	
Chronic Phase Lung deficiency	Sweating, aversion to wind, easily catch colds, slight wheezing sound in throat, SOB, slight cough, low voice, pale complexion, clear white sputum. T: pale P: weak, thready	Tonify LU, consolidate protective Qi	LU9 (tai yuan), BL13 (fei shu), DU12 (shen zhu), ST36 (ZSL), REN6 (qi hai), LU7 (lie que)	
Chronic Phase Spleen deficiency	Slight wheezing (may be brought on by cold, sweet, greasy foods), poor appetite, ABD distension, loose stool, tiredness, SOB. T: pale Pulse: weak	Tonify SP, resolve phlegm	ST36 (ZSL), SP3 (tai bai), BL20 (pi shu), BL21 (wei shu), REN12 (zhong wan), ST40, (feng long) LU7 (lie que), LU9 (tai yuan), BL13 (fei shu), REN6 (qi hai)	
Chronic Phase Kidney deficiency	SOB, slight wheezing, rapid breathing, worse with exertion, difficult inhalation, poor memory, tinnitus, weak/sore back, plus either KI Yang or KI Yin deficiency signs.	Tonify KD, strengthen KD grasping Qi	KI3 (tai xi), SP6 (SYJ), REN4 (guan yuan), BL23 (shen shu), BL13 (fei shu), DU12 (shen zhu), KI25 (shen cang)	

Wind Stroke (zhong feng)

Definition:
This is a disorder characterized by sudden loss of consciousness with unilateral weakness, numbness, paralysis, and dysphasia, or unilateral paralysis and facial paralysis without loss of consciousness. Wind stroke is sudden, acute, and has many symptoms and rapidly changing manifestations.

Red Flags:
People who have any of the following symptoms should see a doctor immediately, even if the symptom goes away quickly:
- Sudden weakness or paralysis on one side of the body
- Sudden loss of sensation or abnormal sensations on one side of the body
- Sudden difficulty speaking, including difficulty coming up with words and sometimes slurred speech
- Sudden confusion, with difficulty understanding speech
- Sudden dimness, blurring, or loss of vision, particularly in one eye
- Sudden dizziness or loss of balance and coordination, leading to falls

One or more of these symptoms are typically present in both hemorrhagic and ischemic strokes. Symptoms of a transient ischemic attack are the same, but they usually disappear within minutes and rarely last more than 1 hour.

Symptoms of a hemorrhagic stroke may also include:
- Sudden severe headache
- Nausea and vomiting
- Temporary or persistent loss of consciousness
- Very high blood pressure

Western Medicine Relevant Diseases:
The term wind-stroke in TCM corresponds to a cerebrovascular disorder in Western medicine, commonly known as a stroke.

Stroke occurs when an artery to the brain becomes blocked or ruptures, resulting in death of an area of brain tissue due to loss of its blood supply (cerebral infarction) and causing sudden symptoms such as: muscle weakness, paralysis, abnormal or lost sensation on one side of the body, difficulty speaking, confusion, problems with vision, dizziness, and loss of balance and coordination.

There are two types of strokes:
- Ischemic
- Hemorrhagic

Most strokes are ischemic, usually due to a blocked artery, often blocked by a blood clot. Brain cells, thus deprived of their blood supply, do not receive enough oxygen and glucose, which are carried by blood. The damage that results depends on how long brain cells are deprived of blood. If they are deprived for only a brief time, brain cells are stressed, but they may recover. If brain cells are deprived longer, brain cells die, and some functions may be lost, sometimes permanently. How soon brain cells die after being deprived of blood varies. They die after only a few minutes in some areas of the brain but not until after 30 minutes or more in other areas. In some cases, after brain cells die, a different area of the brain can learn how to do the functions previously done by the damaged area.

Transient ischemic attacks (TIAs) are often an early warning sign of an impending ischemic stroke. They are caused by a brief interruption of the blood supply to part of the brain. Because the blood supply is restored quickly, brain tissue does not die, as it does in a stroke, and brain function quickly returns.

Hemorrhagic strokes are due to bleeding in or around the brain. In this type of stroke, a blood vessel ruptures, interfering with normal blood flow and allowing blood to leak into brain tissue or around the brain. Blood that comes into direct contact with brain tissue irritates the tissue and, over time, can cause scar tissue to form in the brain, sometimes leading to seizures.

Etiology and Pathogenesis:
The etiology of wind-stroke is complex and this condition usually develops over many years. Some of the main factors include:
- Exterior pathogenic invasion – unconsolidated protective qi – body unable to defend – leads to wind stroke
- Improper diet or aging – impairs Spleen transformation and transportation – phlegm develops – phlegm covers the heart's orifices and obstructs flow in the channels – wind stroke
- Emotional stress – affect both the Heart and the Liver – Heart fire will flare up and Liver Yang will rise generating Liver wind – wind stroke

- Aging, chronic illness, weak constitution – cause Liver and Kidney Yin deficiency – leads to Liver Yang rising and Liver wind rebelling upward

Note: Maciocia suggests (in *The Practice of Chinese Medicine*) that the four main pathogenic factors involved in the pathogenesis of wind stroke are: wind, phlegm, fire, and stasis, and that at least three need to be present. He also notes that, besides these, there will be some deficiency of Qi, Blood, or Yin.

TCM Differentiation and Treatment:
When treating wind-stroke, it is important to differentiate between channel involvement and organ involvement.

Channel involvement means that only the meridians and collaterals are affected. Effects are limited, and it is relatively milder in severity. There is no loss of consciousness, but mainly numbness, weakness, facial paralysis, or alterations in speech.

Organ involvement means that there is loss of consciousness, and changes in cognition. This is a more severe condition that may include aphasia, difficulty swallowing, and hemiplegia.

The more severe type with organ involvement is further divided into closed, and abandoned/open disorders (also known as tense and flaccid). In a closed disorder, the person will have locked jaws, clenched fists, rigid limbs, fecal and urinary retention, and a forceful pulse. Fire and phlegm are the main pathogens locked inside. In an open disorder, there is flaccidity of the muscles, fecal and urinary incontinence, profuse sweating, and minute weak pulse due to a collapse of yang Qi.

Pattern	Signs and Symptoms	Treatment Principle	Acupuncture	Formula
Channel Involvement:				
Exterior Wind Invading	Sudden numbness of extremities, abrupt onset of facial paralysis, slurred speech, drooling from corner of mouth on affected side, aversion to cold, fever, muscle spasm, sore aching joints. T: thin white coat P: floating	Dispel wind, nourish blood, clear channels	DU20 (bai hui), GB20 (feng chi), DU14 (bai hui), LI4 (he gu) + local points	
Liver and Kidney Deficiency with Yang Rising	Sudden occurrence of facial paralysis, slurred speech or aphasia, numbness and heavy sensation of extremities, hemiplegia in severe cases, dizziness, H/A, vertigo, tinnitus, dry throat, constipation. T: red, scanty coat P: thready, rapid	Nourish Liver and Kidney, subdue Yang, extinguish wind, unblock channels	BL18 (gan shu), BL23 (shen shu), KD3 (tai xi), GB20 (feng chi), LR3 (tai chong), LI4 (he gu)	
Local points to open channel and recover function: -upper limbs: -hand: SI 4.5, LI 4.5, SJ4.5 -elbow: LI11 (qu chi) LI10 (shou san li), LU5 (chi ze) -shoulder: LI14 (bi nao), LI15 (jian yu), SJ14 (jian liao), SI9 (jian zhen) or SI10 (nao shu) -lower limbs: -feet: K1 (yong quan), ST41 (jie xi), BL60 (kun lun), KI3 (tai xi) -knee: ST36 (ZSL), ST34 (liang qiu), GB34 (yang ling quan) -whole limbs: GB30 (huan tiao), BL54 (zhi bian) -speaking disorder: DU15 (ya men), LI4 (he gu) -facial paralysis: SJ17 (yi feng), ST4 (di cang), ST6 (jia che), LI4 (he gu) -deafness: SJ17 (yi feng), GB2 (ting hui), LI4 (he gu) -dizziness: GB20 (feng chi)			

Organ Involvement:				
	Sudden loss of consciousness, locked jaws, clenched fists, rigid limbs, urinary retention, red face, fever, rattling sound in throat,	Clear heat, extinguish wind and open orifices	DU26 (shui gou), ST40 (feng long), KI3 (tai xi), LR3 (tai chong)	

	agitation. T: red, yellow greasy coat P: wiry, slippery, forceful		+ for heat, bleed hand jing well points	
	Sudden loss of consciousness, locked jaws, clenched fists, rigid limbs, urinary retention, pale complexion, dark lips, quiet and still, cold extremities, excessive sputum. T: white greasy coat P: deep, slippery	Resolve phlegm, extinguish wind, open orifices	+ for cold, DU20 (bai hui) jaw spasm + ST6 (jia che), ST7 (xia guan), LI4 (he gu) rigid tongue + HT5 (tong li)	
	Sudden loss of consciousness, flaccid extremities, closed eyes, open mouth, urinary and fecal incontinence, shallow breathing, profuse sweating and clammy skin. T: flaccid P: thready, weak	Supplement Qi, revive Yang, revive collapse	REN6 (qi hai), REN4 (guan yuan), REN8 (shen que), DU20 (bai hui)	
Sequelae Stage:				
Wind phlegm	Stiffness of tongue, difficulty speaking, numbness of limbs. T: white greasy coat P: slippery, wiry	Dispel wind, expel phlegm, clear orifices	GB20 (feng chi), ST40 (feng long), REN23 lian quan), HT5 (tong li), DU15 (ya men), scalp points	
Deficiency and Stagnation of Qi and Blood	Unilateral weakness, loss of sensory and motor coordination, fatigue, lassitude, numbness of extremities, facial paralysis, sallow complexion, poor appetite. T: purple, petechiae P: choppy, weak	Boost Qi, invigorate blood, unblock channels	DU20 (bai hui), REN6 (qi hai), SP10 (xue hai), SP6 (SYJ), LI15 (jian yu), LI11 (qu chi), SJ5 (wei guan), LI4 (he gu), GB34 (yang ling quan), ST36 (ZSL), BL60 (kun lun), scapl points	
Depletion of Kidney Essence	Slurred speech or aphasia, sore and weak low back/knees, palpitations, dizziness, blurred vision, SOB. T: scanty coat P: thready, weak	Supplement KD Essence, nourish Yin, open orifices	BL23 (shen shu), KI3 (tai xi), REN23 (lian quan), HT5 (tong li), DU15 (ya men), scalp points	

External Medicine

Acne (fen ci)

Definition:
In TCM, acne is considered a condition caused by accumulation of heat in the Lung, Spleen, and Stomach. Acne may appear as a black head with red skin around it, or a pustule with yellow or white build up inside. It may be itchy and/or painful. It often disappears on its own, but may leave scaring or "orange peel" type skin. It is more common in young people and is mostly found on the face, chest and upper back.

Western Medicine Relevant Diseases:
In Western medicine, acne vulgaris is a common chronic skin disease involving blockage and/or inflammation of pilosebaceous units (hair follicles and their accompanying sebaceous gland). Acne can present as non-inflammatory, open or closed comedones and by inflammatory papules, pustules, and nodules, or a mixture of both, affecting mostly the face but also the back and chest.

Acne develops as a result of the following factors: (1) follicular epidermal hyper-proliferation with plugging of the follicle, (2) excess sebum production, (3) the presence and activity of bacteria, and (4) inflammation.

Severe acne, characterized by multiple comedones, without the presence of systemic symptoms, is known as acne conglobata. This severe form of acne frequently heals with disfiguring scars. Acne vulgaris may have a psychological impact on any patient, regardless of the severity or the grade of the disease.

Etiology and Pathogenesis:
Acne may be caused by:

TCM Differentiation and Treatment:

Pattern	Signs and Symptoms	Treatment Principle	Acupuncture	Formula
Wind Heat in the Lung Meridian	Superficial acne that is red and painful or itchy, may have pustule, forehead and nose are particularly affected. May also have dry mouth and nose, dry stool/constipation. T: red, thin-yellow tongue coat, P: floating, and rapid/forceful	Open Lung, clear heat	LI4 (he gu), LI11 (qu chi), GB20 (feng chi), BL12 feng men), BL40 (wei zhong), LU5 (chi ze), BL13 (fei shu)	
Damp Heat in Yangming	Acne is swollen (and painful) with excretions, may have constipation, low appetite, bloating, distension T: red and swollen tongue, yellow greasy coat P: slippery/rapid.	Clear heat, resolve damp, unblock Fu organs	LI4 (he gu), LI11 (qu chi), ST40 (feng long), SP9 (yin ling quan), SP10 (xue hai), ST44 (nei ting)	
Spleen Deficiency	Acne is not fresh red, acne comes and goes, some turn to cysts, does not often turn to pustules, poor appetite, may feel heavy and tired. T: tongue coating can be thin and white, moist, tongue body pale P: weak, soggy, thin.	Tonify the Spleen, transform damp	ST36 (ZSL), SP9 (yin ling quan), LU9 (tai yuan), REN6 (qi hai), ST40 (feng long), BL20 (pi shu), LI4 (he gu), SP6 (SYJ)	

Acute Mastitis (ru yong)

Definition:
An acute, purulent infection of the breast. Breast may be red, hot, swollen, and tender or painful. Acute mastitis is common during the early stages of breast-feeding, particularly for first-time mothers.

Red Flags:
- refer if high fever, development of abscess, extreme lethargy or other signs of disease not responding to treatment (extreme lethargy)
- incision and drainage by a physician may be required in some circumstances

Western Medicine Relevant Diseases:
Mastitis is painful inflammation of the breast, usually accompanied by infection. Staphylococcal species are the most common causes. Mastitis symptoms may include high fever and breast symptoms: erythema, induration, tenderness, pain, swelling, and warmth to the touch.

Etiology and Pathogenesis:
- stagnation of Liver Qi from emotional stress causes damp heat, obstruction of qi and blood and hindrance of milk flow
- binding heat in the Stomach channel from rich food causes eruption in the channel
- nipple break and toxin attack, or nipple deformation, causes stagnation and hindrance of milk flow

Differentiation of stages:

TCM Differentiation and Treatment:

Pattern	Signs and Symptoms	Treatment Principle	Acupuncture	Formula
Mastitis due to Stomach Heat Accumulation	Red, swollen, painful breast, extreme thirst, bad breath, constipation, nausea T: red P: forceful	Resolve Stomach Heat	ST16 (ying chuang), ST39 (xia ju xu), ST40 (feng long), LI7 (wen liu), REN17 (shan zhong), SI1 (shao ze), LI4 (he gu)	
Liver Qi Stagnation	Red, swollen, painful breast, chest/hypochondriac pain, poor appetite, no desire to eat, bloating and other digestive upsets P: wiry pulse (or wiry rapid) T: normal (coating might be slightly yellow)	Sooth Liver	LR14 (qi men), PC1 (tian chi), GB21 (jian jing), LR2 (xing jian), PC6 (nei guan)	

Alopecia Areata (you feng)

Definition:
In TCM, *you feng* or "wind gloss scalp" refers to the loss of hair characterized by smooth and shiny scalp patches. These are typically round or oval shape, and the underlying skin is shiny, but otherwise normal (no scars or rashes). When severe, this may involve the entire scalp and even the eyebrows. This hair loss usually happens suddenly, and is unrelated to age. It is often caused by stress, anxiety, or insomnia.

Western Medicine Relevant Diseases:
In Western medicine, alopecia areata is described as the sudden loss of patches of hair when there is no obvious cause, such as a skin disorder. Alopecia areata is common, occurs in both sexes, and at all ages.
It is thought to be caused by an autoimmune reaction in which the body's immune defenses mistakenly attack the hair follicles. Alopecia areata is not the result of another disorder, but some people may also have an associated thyroid disorder or vitiligo (a skin pigment disorder).

Round, irregular patches of hair are suddenly lost. Around the edges of the patches are characteristic short, broken hairs, which resemble exclamation points. The site of hair loss is usually the scalp or beard. Sometimes all the scalp hair is lost (alopecia totalis), or hair is lost from around the side and back edges of the scalp (ophiasis). Rarely, all body hair is lost (a condition called alopecia universalis). The nails may become pitted or rough. The hair usually grows back in several months. In people with widespread hair loss, re-growth is less likely.

Etiology and Pathogenesis:
- Liver-Kidney Deficiency/Blood Deficiency (two explanations):
    - blood cannot nourish skin, skin cannot protect itself, wind enters the body + dryness and lack of nourishment causing loss of hair; or,
    - because hair is the surplus of blood, blood deficiency causes hair loss
- Liver Qi Stagnation from emotional stress – hinders Qi flow – Qi stagnation and Blood stasis develop and inhibit distribution of nutrients to hair

TCM Differentiation and Treatment:

Pattern	Signs and Symptoms	Treatment Principle	Acupuncture	Formula
	Sudden hair loss in patches of round or irregular shape, may also have dizziness, insomnia, and pale signs on body – eyelids, lips, tongue, fingernails, may have other areas of dryness, itchiness T: pale P: weak	Nourish Blood, Resolve Wind	BL17 (ge shu), SP6 (SYJ), ST36 (ZSL), BL43 (gau huang shu), KD6 (zhao hai), BL20 (pi shu), HT7 (shen men) (with Liver and Kidney deficiency + BL18 (gan shu), BL23 (shen shu)) + local ashi points and plum needles to tap over affected area	
	High stress leads to sudden hair loss, dull complexion, possible H/A, distension and pain of the chest and costal region. T: may be purple and may have enlarged veins or purple dots in certain areas P: choppy or thin	Move Blood, Move Qi, Soothe Liver and Resolve Stasis	SP10 (xue hai), SP6 (SYJ), BL17 (ge shu), REN17 (shan zhong), GB20 (feng chi), LI4 (he gu), LR3 (tai chong) + local ashi points and plum blossom needles over affected areas	

Anal Fissure (gang lie)

Definition:
Tear in lining of the anus, resulting in itching, discomfort, and stinging or burning pain during bowel movements. Often caused by passing hard or large stools, repeat diarrhea, or childbirth. Fissures cause the anal sphincter to go into spasm, which worsens pain and prevents healing.

Western Medicine Relevant Diseases:
In Western medicine, the exact etiology of anal fissures is unknown, but the initiating factor is thought to be trauma from the passage of a particularly hard or painful bowel movement. Low-fiber diets are associated with the development of anal fissures. Prior anal surgery is a predisposing factor.

Initial minor tears in the anal mucosa due to a hard bowel movement probably occur often. In most people, these heal rapidly without long-term sequelae. In patients with underlying abnormalities of the internal sphincter, however, these injuries progress to acute and chronic anal fissures. The most commonly observed abnormalities are hypertonicity and hypertrophy of the internal anal sphincter, leading to elevated anal canal and sphincter resting pressures.

The anus is the most poorly perfused part of the anal canal. In patients with hypertrophied internal anal sphincters, this delicate blood supply is further compromised, thus rendering the posterior midline of the anal canal relatively ischemic. This is thought to account for why many fissures do not heal spontaneously and may last for several months. Pain accompanies each bowel movement as this raw area is stretched and damaged by the stool. The internal sphincter also begins to spasm when a bowel movement is passed. This spasm has two effects: First, it is painful in itself, and second, it further reduces the blood flow to the posterior midline and the anal fissure, contributing to the poor healing rate.

Etiology and Pathogenesis:

TCM Differentiation and Treatment:

Pattern	Signs and Symptoms	Treatment Principle	Acupuncture	Formula
Blood Heat and Dryness	Constipation with dry, hard stools, pain during defecation, dripping fresh blood with stool, agitation, dry throat. T: dry, yellow coat P: rapid	Clear heat, moisten dryness	DU1 (chang qiang), BL57 (cheng shan), ST25 (tian shu), ST37 (shang ju xu), KD6 (zhao hai)	
Blood Deficiency and Intestinal Dryness	Painful anus, bleeding during bowel movement, dry stools that are difficult to pass, dry mouth. T: scanty coat P: fine	Nourish blood, moisten dryness	DU1 (chang qiang), BL57 (cheng shan), SP10 (xue hai), SP6 (SYJ)	

Bedsore (re chuang)

Definition:
Bedsores are ulcers on the skin that can range from mild to severe craters, extending into the muscles and bones.

Red Flags:
- For severe sores with signs of infection, Western medical support is required. If bedsores (called pressure sores in Western medicine) become infected, they may have an unpleasant odor. Pus may be visible in or around the sore. Some people may have a fever. The area around the pressure sore may become red or feel warm, and pain may worsen if the infection spreads to the surrounding skin (causing cellulitis). Infection delays healing of shallow sores and can be life threatening in deeper sores. Infection can even penetrate the bone and spread into the bloodstream (sepsis), causing fever or shaking chills. Pressure sores that do not heal may also cause sinus tracts to form. Sinus tracts are passages that connect the infected area of the skin surface or the sore to other structures, such as those deep in the body. For example, a sinus tract from a pressure sore near the pelvis can connect to the bowel.

Western Medicine Relevant Diseases:
Pressure sores can occur in people of any age who are bed-ridden, chair-bound, or unable to reposition themselves. They occur where there is pressure on the skin from a bed, wheelchair, cast, splint, poorly fitting prosthetic device, or other hard object. They tend to occur over or between bony areas where pressure on skin can be concentrated, such as over the hipbones, tailbone, heels, ankles, and elbows, but they can occur anywhere.

Pressure sores often develop in people after they have been hospitalized for a different problem. Pressure sores lengthen the time spent in hospitals or nursing homes. Pressure sores can be life threatening if they are untreated or if underlying health conditions prevent them from healing. Pressure sores are more common among older people.

Causes that contribute to the development of pressure sores include: pressure, traction, friction, moisture, and inadequate nutrition.

Etiology and Pathogenesis:
- Inability to move ones body causes stagnation of Qi and Blood – skin and muscles lose nourishment – pressure from external sources causes increased aggravation

TCM Differentiation and Treatment:

Pattern	Signs and Symptoms	Treatment Principle	Acupuncture	Formula
Qi and Blood Stagnation	Redness, chafing, and possible ulceration of skin. Fatigue, SOB, dryness and shedding of skin of effected limb. T: pale P: deep, thready, forceless	Move Qi and Blood	REN4 (guan yuan) or REN6 (qi hai), BL17 (ge shu), SP10 (xue hai), LI4 (he gu), surround the dragon (only on undisturbed skin) If accompanied by signs of Qi and Blood deficiency, add: BL20 (pi shu), ST36 (ZSL), SP6 (SYJ)	

Boil (ding chuang)

Definition:
This is an acute, local, suppurative inflammation appearing mainly on the skin of the face, hands, or feet (but can be found anywhere on the body). Small on the surface, but deep rooted and hard at the base.

Red Flags:
- If the person has a weakened immune system, the infection has spread into nearby skin (cellulitis), the person has many abscesses, or the abscess is on the middle or upper part of the face, antibiotics are required.

Western Medicine Relevant Diseases:
In Western medicine, relevant conditions are skin abscesses, which are pus-filled pockets in the skin resulting from bacterial infection. They may be superficial or deep, affecting just hair follicles or deeper structures within the skin. Most abscesses are caused by *Staphylococcus aureus* bacteria and appear to be pus-filled pockets on the skin surface. Bacteria enter the skin through a hair follicle, small scrape, or puncture, although often there is no obvious point of entry. People who live in crowded conditions, have poor hygiene or chronic skin diseases, or whose nasal passages contain *Staphylococcus* are more likely to have episodes of skin abscesses. A weakened immune system, obesity, old age, and possibly diabetes are also common risk factors. Some people may have recurring episodes of infection for unknown reasons.

Abscesses may be one to several inches in diameter. Furuncles (boils) are tender, smaller, more superficial abscesses that involve a hair follicle and the surrounding tissue. Furuncles are common on the neck, breasts, face, and buttocks. They are uncomfortable and may be painful when closely attached to underlying structures. Carbuncles are multiple furuncles that are connected to one another below the skin surface. If not treated, abscesses often come to a head and rupture, discharging a creamy white or pink fluid. Bacteria may spread from the abscess to infect the surrounding tissue and lymph nodes. The person may have a fever and feel generally sick.

Both furuncles and carbuncles may affect healthy young people but are more common among the obese, the immune compromised (including those with neutrophil defects), the elderly, and possibly those with diabetes. Clustered cases may occur among those living in crowded quarters with relatively poor hygiene or among contacts of patients infected with virulent strains. Predisposing factors include bacterial colonization of skin or nares, hot and humid climates, and occlusion or abnormal follicular anatomy (e.g., comedones in acne).

Etiology and Pathogenesis:
- Toxins (external fire toxins, insect bites) enter pores of skin – obstruct Qi and Blood
- Indulgence in spicy, rich foods, or alcohol – produces heat in viscera and bowels – leads to production of internal toxins

Stages of Boils:
- Early Stage: tiny dot, seed like, hard and deep-rooted; local numbness, itching, mild pain (*do not break in this stage)
- Middle Stage: after about 5-7 days, turns red, swollen, more painful, grows bigger (about 3-6cm in size) with very deep root; millet part may break and pus moves out; if zheng qi strong enough, pus will drain out, and fever etc improves; patient may have fever, thirst, constipation, thin/yellow/greasy tongue, rapid/slippery pulse
- Late Stage: favorable case about 7-10 days, swelling decreases, boil shrinks, pain disappears, general symptoms improve; if do not treat correctly, can result in serious infection

T

CM Differentiation and Treatment:

Pattern	Signs and Symptoms	Treatment Principle	Acupuncture	Formula
Exuberant Fire Toxin	Small, seed like lesion, yellow or purple in color, hard at root, sometimes presenting with pustules; possible local numbness, itching, or pain. With continued development, sores become red, hot, swollen, and increasingly painful. Possible fever, thirst, dry stools, dark urine. T: yellow coat (possibly greasy) P: rapid, wiry, slippery	Clear heat, resolve toxin, relieve pain		

Breast Cancer (ru yan)

Definition:
In classical TCM literature, breast cancer is called "Ru Yan," or "breast stone."

Red Flags:
Western medical primary care required. Supportive acupuncture treatment should only be provided by those with advanced training in this area, under medical supervision.

Western Medicine Relevant Diseases:
Breast cancer most often involves glandular breast cells in the ducts or lobules. Most patients present with an asymptomatic mass discovered during examination or screening mammography. Diagnosis is confirmed by biopsy.

Most breast cancers are epithelial tumors that develop from cells lining ducts or lobules; less common are non-epithelial cancers (e.g., angiosarcoma, primary stromal sarcomas, phyllodes tumor). Cancers are divided into carcinoma in situ and invasive cancer.

Carcinoma in situ: proliferation of cancer cells within ducts or lobules and without invasion of stromal tissue. There are 2 types:

Invasive carcinoma is primarily adenocarcinoma. About 80% is the infiltrating ductal type; most of the remaining cases are infiltrating lobular. Rare types include medullary, mucinous, metaplastic, and tubular carcinomas. Mucinous carcinoma tends to develop in older women and to be slow growing.

Inflammatory breast cancer is a fast-growing, often fatal cancer. Cancer cells block the lymphatic vessels in breast skin; as a result, the breast appears inflamed, and the skin appears thickened, resembling orange peel. Usually, inflammatory breast cancer spreads to the lymph nodes in the armpit. The lymph nodes feel like hard lumps. However, often no mass is felt in the breast itself because this cancer is dispersed throughout the breast.

Paget's disease of the nipple is a form of ductal carcinoma in situ that extends into the skin over the nipple and areola, manifesting with a skin lesion. Characteristic malignant cells called Paget cells are present in the epidermis. Women with Paget disease of the nipple often have underlying invasive or in situ cancer.

Etiology and Pathogenesis:
In TCM, the fundamental cause of breast cancer is emotional disturbances such as excessive thinking or anger, which lead to functional disorders of the Liver and Spleen. A common causative pattern is that excessive Heat from a deficient Liver, combined with Phlegm Dampness due to Spleen dysfunction, results in the blockage of Qi and Blood, which then "condenses" into breast cancer.
Another common causative pattern is when Liver Deficiency and Kidney Deficiency lead to Qi and Blood Deficiency. Chronic Qi and Blood deficiency then leads to Qi Stagnation and Blood Stasis, which causes the formation of lumps in the breast.
A third pattern is when Qi Stagnation and Phlegm accumulation lead to excessive Heat toxins, which then turn to hard breast lump masses.

TCM Differentiation and Treatment:

Pattern	Signs and Symptoms	Treatment Principle	Acupuncture	Formula
Liver Qi Stagnation	Hard masses without pain and redness	Soothe Liver and resolve masses	Points common to all cancer (tonify immunity: DU14 (da zhui), LI11 (qu chi), SP6 (SYJ), SP10, (xue hai) LR3 (tai chong) + LI4 (he gu) – 4 gates, PC6 (nei guan), GB41 (zu lin qi), BL18 (gan shu)	
Phlegm Heat Obstruction	Hard masses with sharp pain and swelling	Clear heat, drain phlegm and remove obstruction	ST40 (feng long), LI11 (qu chi), DU14 (da zhui), SP3 (tai bai)	
Liver Kidney Deficiency	Hard lumps with swelling and a dimpled appearance of the breast skin, discharges and indentation of the nipple	Tonify Liver and Kidney	REN4 (guan yuan), SP6 (SYJ), KI6 (zhao hai), LR3 (tai chong), LR8 (qu quan)	
Qi and Blood Deficiency	Hard lumps with swelling, ruptured abscesses, spreading to the surrounding areas.	Tonify Qi and Blood	ST36 (ZSL), BL17 (ge shu), SP6 (SYJ), BL20 (pi shu), DU20 (bai hui), REN4 (guan yuan)	

*For the purposes of your exam, please just treat the SIDE effects of breast cancer and never go in to the cancer site. Acu/herbs for cancer requires specialized training.

Breast Lump (ru pi)

Definition:
Solid breast lumps or masses of varying sizes and shapes. Most commonly found on upper outer quadrant of the breast.

Red Flags:
The following symptoms and characteristics merit referral:

Western Medicine Relevant Diseases:
A breast lump is a thickening or bump that feels different from surrounding breast tissue.
Lumps in the breasts are relatively common and usually not cancerous.

Lumps may be painless or painful. They are sometimes accompanied by discharge or changes in the skin, such as irregularities, redness, a dimpled texture, or tightened skin.

Breast lumps may be fluid-filled sacs or solid masses, which are usually fibroadenomas. Fibroadenomas are not cancerous, and cysts usually are not cancerous.

The most common causes include:
- Fibroadenomas: typically smooth, rounded, movable, painless lumps. They usually develop in women of childbearing age. Fibroadenomas may be mistaken for breast cancer, but they are not. Some types of fibroadenoma do not appear to increase the risk of breast cancer. Others may increase the risk slightly.
- Fibrocystic changes: includes pain, cysts, and general lumpiness in the breast. Women may have one or more of these symptoms. Breasts feel lumpy and dense and are often tender when touched. In most women, fibrocystic changes are related to the monthly fluctuations in levels of the female hormones estrogen and progesterone. These hormones stimulate breast tissue. Fibrocystic changes do not increase the risk of breast cancer.

Less commonly, lumps may sometimes result from:
- Breast infections, including collections of pus (abscesses), which are very rare except during the few weeks after childbirth
- A clogged milk gland (galactocele), which usually occurs up to 6 to 10 months after breastfeeding stops
- Injuries, which can result in the formation of scar tissue
- Breast cancer

Etiology and Pathogenesis:
- emotional stress – causes Liver Qi stagnation – Qi stagnation combines with phlegm – masses form
- Liver and Kidney deficiency – dysfunction of the Chong and Ren – allows accumulation of phlegm giving rise to masses

TCM Differentiation and Treatment:

Pattern	Signs and Symptoms	Treatment Principle	Acupuncture	Formula
Stagnation of Liver Qi and Accumulation of Phlegm	Lumps or masses in the breasts, irritability, impatience, dizziness, vertigo, chest oppression, insomnia, dream disturbed sleep, distention and pain of breasts, possible difficult menstruation. T: thin and greasy coat P: wiry, slippery	Soothe the Liver, resolve stagnation, transform phlegm, dissipate nodules	PC6 (nei guan), REN17 (shan zhong), ST40 (feng long), ST36 (ZSL), LR3 (tai chong), GB21 (jian jing)	
Liver and Kidney Deficiency with Accumulation of Phlegm	Lumps or masses in the breast, irregular menstruation, weak low back/knees, scanty pale menstrual discharge, possible amenorrhea. T: pale P: wiry, thready or deep, thready	Tonify Liver and Kidney, regulate the Chong Ren, transform phlegm, dissipate nodules	PC6 (nei guan), ST36 (ZSL), SP6 (SYJ), BL23 (shen shu), REN4 (guan yuan), BL18 (gan shu)	

Carbuncle (yong)

Definition:
Refers to an acute suppurative disease between the muscle and skin. Its clinical feature is that there is a millet grain-like pus dot on the swelling in the initial stage, with local burning sensation, redness and pain. The swelling spreads, with increasing pus dots. Once the ulceration ruptures, it looks like a lotus seedpod or honeycomb.

Western Medicine Relevant Diseases:
See description under boil.

Etiology and Pathogenesis:
This disease is mostly caused by internal accumulation of toxins in zang-fu organs and secondary invasion of exogenous wind-heat, damp-heat and fire, which gather in the superficial muscle to cause obstruction in the meridians and collaterals, disharmony of Nutritive Qi and Defensive Qi, and stagnation of qi and blood.

TCM Differentiation and Treatment:

Pattern	Signs and Symptoms	Treatment Principle	Acupuncture	Formula
Damp Heat Accumulation	Red swelling and burning pain in the infected area, numerous pus dots, yellowish purulent fluid, high fever in the evening, stuffy chest, abdominal fullness, poor appetite, dark urine. T: red, yellowish and greasy coating P: slippery and rapid	Clear away heat, dissipate dampness, dissolve toxin and diminish swelling		
Fire-Toxin Accumulation	Protruded red swelling in the local area, burning pain, suppuration, yellow pus, accompanied by fever, thirst, dark urine, constipation. T: red tongue, yellowish tongue coating P: rapid and forceful	Clear heat, expel fire, dissolve toxin and diminish swelling		
Yin-Deficiency and Fire-Hyperactivity	Flat swelling with diffuse base, purple color in the wound, serious pain, swelling difficult to ulcerate, or scanty purulent fluid with little blood after rupture, accompanied by fever worse in evening, dry mouth and throat, thirst, constipated stool. T: red, dry and yellowish tongue coating, P: thready, wiry and rapid pulse.	Nourish yin, heat, promote detoxification and diminish swelling		
Qi-Deficiency and Toxin-Accumulation	Flat swelling with diffuse base, dim and lusterless wound, stuffy and distending and painful sensation, difficult dissolution of purulent decay, or thin purulent fluid in gray dark color after ulceration, empty shell underneath the skin, accompanied by fever, thirst, low spirit, lusterless complexion, slightly red tongue, thin and whitish coating, thready and feeble pulse.	Benefit qi, heal the wound, promote pus discharge and diminish swelling		

Contact Dermatitis (jie chu xing pi yan)

Definition:
Acute inflammatory condition of the skin or mucosa that results from contact with certain irritant substances or stimulants. The condition occurs in all ages and both sexes, but there is a higher incidence in children than the elderly and women are more commonly affected than men. A characteristic of the disease is a history of exposure to allergenic substances prior to the inflammatory episode. Such substances or stimulants can include medicated plasters, ointment, lacquer, plants, certain materials used in clothing and contact with animals. The distribution of the lesions on the skin corresponds to the points of contact with the irritant and is largely limited to those areas.

The disease has an acute onset. Typical symptoms include itchiness, a burning sensation, and swelling and tenderness of the lesions. Systemic involvement can occur in severe cases. Once irritants are removed and proper treatment given, the condition will usually resolve within one to two weeks. However, further exposure to the causative agent will cause a re-occurrence.

Western Medicine Relevant Diseases:
Contact dermatitis is skin inflammation caused by direct contact with a particular substance. The rash is very itchy, is confined to a specific area, and often has clearly defined boundaries. There are two types: irritant contact and allergic contact.

Irritant contact dermatitis occurs when a chemical substance causes direct damage to the skin. Irritant contact dermatitis is more painful than itchy. Typical irritating substances are acids, alkalis (such as drain cleaners), solvents (such as acetone in nail polish remover), strong soaps, and plants (such as poinsettias and peppers). Skin can also be irritated by body fluids (such as urine and saliva).

Allergic contact dermatitis is a reaction by the body's immune system to a substance contacting the skin. When the skin first comes into contact with the substance, the skin becomes sensitized to that substance. Sometimes a person can be sensitized by only one exposure, and other times sensitization occurs only after many exposures to a substance. After a person is sensitized, the next exposure causes intense itching and dermatitis within 4 to 24 hours, although some people, particularly older people, do not develop a reaction for 3 to 4 days.

Thousands of substances can result in allergic contact dermatitis. The most common include substances found in
- Plants (such as poison ivy)
- Rubber (including latex)
- Antibiotics
- Fragrances
- Preservatives
- Some metals (such as nickel and cobalt)

Etiology and Pathogenesis:
Contact dermatitis can be caused by both endogenous and exogenous factors:
- Constitution or inborn susceptibility (endogenous causes): The incidence of contact dermatitis is influenced by body constitution and is more likely to occur in individuals with a congenital/inherited predisposition to the disorder. In cases of congenital deficiency, the skin and tissues beneath are loosely bonded. This means that the protective qi is weak and that the body is more prone to a flare-up of fire evil or to the development of internal wind evil. Contact with certain substances, such as lacquer, drugs, plastic, rubber products, dyes or plants, facilitates transformation of heat evil internally in the body. The conflict between blood and qi against the heat evil triggers the skin disease.
- Environmental pathogen invasion (exogenous causes) In situations where external pathogens are allowed to invade the body directly, excessive fire evil will develop and accumulate. Circulation of blood and qi in the surface areas of the body becomes disturbed and does not flow smoothly. This in turn damages the integrity and function of the skin causing dermatitis.

TCM Differentiation and Treatment:

Pattern	Signs and Symptoms	Treatment Principle	Acupuncture	Formula
Acute Stage	-initial contact, reaction may be minimal (or latent reaction that happens days after contact) -after second contact, reaction will be much stronger and more immediate -dermatitis will be located only in exposed area -clear, localized border -different manifestations: e.g. erythema, swollen, rashes, blisters, blebs, erosion -if there is a strong reaction, may have general symptoms, fever, chills, etc			
Chronic Stage	-long term recurring reactions -frequent contact with allergen and flare ups -roughness, thickness, lichenification of skin -difficult to differentiate with chronic eczema			

Digital Gangrene (tuo ju)

Definition:
Death of body tissue due to lack of blood flow or infection.

Red Flags:
If infection from gangrene gets into the blood, sepsis and septic shock may develop. This can be life threatening if not treated immediately. Symptoms of sepsis may include: low blood pressure, rapid heartbeat, shortness of breath change in body temperature, light-headedness, body pain and rash confusion, cold, clammy, and pale skin.

Western Medicine Relevant Diseases:
Gangrene is a condition that occurs when body tissue dies. It is caused by a loss of blood supply due to an underlying illness, injury, and/or infection. Fingers, toes, and limbs are most often affected, but gangrene can also occur inside the body, damaging organs and muscles. There are different types of gangrene and all require immediate medical attention.

There are two main types of gangrene:
Dry gangrene: More common in people with blood vessel disease, diabetes, and autoimmune diseases, dry gangrene usually affects the hands and feet. It develops when blood flow to the affected area is impaired, usually as a result of poor circulation. In this type, the tissue dries up and may be brown to purplish-blue to black in color and often falls off. Unlike other types of gangrene, infection is typically not present in dry gangrene. However, dry gangrene can lead to wet gangrene if it becomes infected.
Wet gangrene: Unlike dry gangrene, wet gangrene almost always involves an infection. Injury from burns or trauma where a body part is crushed or squeezed can rapidly cut off blood supply to the affected area, causing tissue death and increased risk of infection. The tissue swells and blisters and is called "wet" because of pus. Infection from wet gangrene can spread quickly throughout the body, making wet gangrene a very serious and potentially life-threatening condition if not treated quickly.

Etiology and Pathogenesis:
- Emotions, poor diet, or cold-damp attack turning to damp heat – leads to Qi stagnation and blood stasis (early stage)
- Liver and Kidney Yin Deficiency – leads to Qi and Yin Deficiency - stagnation and stasis (late stage)

TCM Differentiation and Treatment:

Pattern	Signs and Symptoms	Treatment Principle	Acupuncture	Formula
	Pale (dull, lusterless complexion), cold/chills, heaviness, aching, numbness, pain in extremities and extremities feel cold, intermittent limping (or pain and cramps), pulse on extremities may weaken, skin over affected area becomes pale, dry, cool.	Move blood, resolve stasis, unblock collaterals	BL17 (ge shu), BL26 (guan yuan shu), REN6 (qi hai), ST36 (ZSL), SP6 (SYJ), KD6 (zhao hai), GB40 (qiu xu) + local points to soothe and release stagnation -in hands, use baxie -in feet, use bafeng	
	Cold, sharp pain, muscle atrophy, limited movement, skin color changes to purplish discoloration, consistent pain, body hair drops, fingernails and toenails grow thick, pulse on feet may be weaker and may disappear, dizziness, back pain. P: deep, thin, choppy	Move blood, resolve stasis, unblock collaterals		
	Skin darker, more dull, more atrophy, skin may break or drop off, sharp pain consistently, fever, thirst, constipation, sallow complexion, fatigue. T: red P: disappears or thin and rapid, weak	Tonify Qi and nourish Yin	+ late stage: REN4 (guan yuan), KD3 (tai xi), HT8 (shao fu), SP10 (xue hai), DU12 (shen zhu), LU9 (tai yuan)	

Drug Rash (yao wu xing pi yan)

Definition:
Drug rash is an allergic reaction of the skin and membrane caused by injection, oral administration and inhalation of the drugs (including herbs). Can be the first sign of general hypersensitivity or toxic reaction involving other organs.

Red Flags:
- Acute allergic reaction (respiratory distress, swelling of the face and neck) requires emergency medical care.

Western Medicine Relevant Diseases:
Most drug rashes result from an allergic reaction to the drug. Usually the reaction is to a drug taken by mouth or injected. When the immune system comes into contact with a drug, it can become sensitive to that drug. Sometimes a person becomes sensitized to a drug after only one exposure, and other times sensitization occurs only after many exposures. Once a person is sensitized to a drug, later exposure to that drug triggers an allergic reaction, such as a rash.

Drug rashes vary in severity from mild redness with tiny bumps over a small area to peeling of the entire skin. Rashes may appear suddenly within minutes after a person takes a drug, or they may be delayed. Rashes may cause red, purple, blue, or gray discoloration. Some rashes are painful and may cause sores to form in the mouth. People with an allergic rash can have hives and/or other allergic symptoms, such as runny nose and watery eyes. They also may develop more significant symptoms such as wheezing or low blood pressure.

Etiology and Pathogenesis:
Drug rash belongs to the category of "Drug Poison" in TCM. It is mostly related to constitutional intolerance and occurs when drug poison enters the Ying-Nutrient System and Xue-Blood System, attacks the muscle and skin, and transmits into the meridians and Zang-fu organs. Yin can be damaged by heat toxin in the long term. If the spleen fails to perform its transportation, the internal excessive dampness will fight against the drug poison to cause accumulation of heat toxin with dampness in the muscle and skin.

TCM Differentiation and Treatment:

Pattern	Signs and Symptoms	Treatment Principle	Acupuncture	Formula
	Papules, macules and or wheals of the skin, fresh red or purple red color, and even purple spots, blood blisters, acute onset, accompanied by high fever, itching, warmth, extremely dry mouth and lips, thirst, constipation, scanty urine. T: crimson without coating or, scanty coating P: rapid	Clear heat, relieve toxicity, cool blood, reduce rash	LI4 (he gu), LI11 (qi chi), BL40 (wei zhong)	
	Red macules, blisters, bullas, or skin erosion, swelling, or early exfoliative dermatitis, pruritus, vexation, fever, dizziness, headache, dry mouth or greasy taste in the mouth, constipation or loose stool, yellow and brown urine. T: red, thin and whitish or yellowish coating P: slippery or rapid pulse.	Clear heat, drain damp, cool blood, relieve toxicity	LI11 (qu chi), BL40 (wei zhong), ST40 (feng long), SP9 (yin ling quan)	
	Late stage of serious drug rash, manifested by flushed color in skin rash, dryness on the surface with skin peeling, accompanied by low fever, thirst, lassitude, vexation, dry stool, yellow urine. T: red, scanty coating P: thready and rapid pulse.	Nourish Yin, relieve toxicity, drain heat	LI11 (qu chi), BL40 (wei zhong), BL23 (shen shu)	

Eczema (shi chuang)

Definition:
Eczema is a Western medical term referring to an allergic inflammatory skin condition characterized by itchy, polymorphic skin lesions of symmetrical (although mild case may be one-sided) distribution. Eczema is typically recurrent and tends to develop into a chronic condition. Different manifestations include: redness, skin swelling, itching and dryness, crusting, flaking, cracking, oozing, and/or bleeding. It can be localized or cover entire body, and occurs regardless of season or age. Patients congenitally susceptible to allergic reactions are most commonly affected, and some tend to be more affected in winter.

Red Flags:
- Secondary bacterial infection may require Western medical treatment

Western Medicine Relevant Diseases:
Atopic dermatitis (AD), or eczema, is a chronic, pruritic inflammatory skin disease of unknown origin that usually starts in early infancy, but also affects a substantial number of adults. AD is commonly associated with elevated levels of immunoglobulin E (IgE). That it is the first disease to present in a series of allergic diseases—including food allergy, asthma, and allergic rhinitis, in order—has given rise to the "atopic march" theory, which suggests that AD is part of a progression that may lead to subsequent allergic disease at other epithelial barrier surfaces.

Common environmental triggers include: foods (milk, eggs, soy, wheat, nuts, fish), airborne allergens, staphylococcus aureus, topical products, sweating, and fabrics.

In the acute phase, lesions are red, edematous, scaly patches or plaques that may be weepy. Occasionally vesicles are present. In the chronic phase, scratching and rubbing create skin lesions that appear dry and lichenified.

Distribution of lesions is age specific. In infants, lesions characteristically occur on the face, scalp, neck, and extensor surfaces of the extremities. In older children and adults, lesions occur on flexural surfaces such as the neck, and the antecubital and popliteal fossae.

Intense pruritus is a key feature. Itch often precedes lesions, and itch worsens with allergen exposures, dry air, sweating, local irritation, wool garments, and emotional stress.

Etiology and Pathogenesis:
Eczema is the result of obstruction of the channels and connections by wind, heat, or dampness.
- Acute eczema is often caused by damp heat
- Chronic eczema is related to prolonged illness and injury to the blood – results in internal wind and dryness, with depletion of moisture and nourishment of the superficial tissues

TCM Differentiation and Treatment:

Pattern	Signs and Symptoms	Treatment Principle	Acupuncture	Formula
Acute (Damp Heat)	Local skin very itchy and red (maybe burning and itchy), rapid eruption of growing patches of rashes and blisters, scratching may cause yellow-sticky oozing and crusting (and may become infected/form scars), may have ABD pain, constipation, diarrhea, dark urination, fever, headache. T: Yellow, greasy coating P: Slippery, rapid pulse	Clear heat, resolve damp		
Chronic (Blood Deficiency)	Roughness, thickening, lichenification of skin, dark brown color/pigmentation, itching, flaking, crusting, bleeding, split, chapping, scratch so much they bleed, chronic, recurring over an extended period of time. Other possible symptoms: dizziness, fatigue, weakness. T: pale P: wiry, thready, forceless	Nourish Blood, moisten dryness, extinguish wind		

Erysipelas (dan du)

Definition:
Acute, infectious disease spread through direct contact. It has a characteristic fresh, red color, abrupt inflammation of the skin/mucus membranes, and is well demarcated with slightly raised area and advancing borders. It is common on the face and lower legs.

Red Flags:
- Acute, fast spreading disease that requires Western medical diagnosis and primary treatment, as it can develop into septicemia.

Western Medicine Relevant Diseases:
Erysipelas is a superficial form of cellulitis (bacterial skin infection) typically caused by streptococci.

Erysipelas causes a shiny, painful, red, raised patch on the skin. The edges have distinct borders and do not blend into the nearby normal skin. The patch feels warm and firm to the touch. It occurs most frequently on the legs and face. People often have a high fever, chills, and a general feeling of illness (malaise).

Doctors base the diagnosis on the characteristic appearance of the rash. Antibiotics given by mouth, such as penicillin, can cure the infection. For a severe infection, intravenous penicillin is needed. Fungal foot infections may be an entry site for infection and may require treatment with antifungal drugs to prevent recurrence.

Etiology and Pathogenesis:
- external injury/skin break allows invasion of toxins (bites, skin disorders give chance for pathogens to invade via the wound) -- fire enters blood level and accumulates (in local involved area) and heat manifests in skin level -- toxins cause blood heat that stagnates in the superficial tissues resulting in the characteristic redness of the skin

TCM Differentiation and Treatment:

Pattern	Signs and Symptoms	Treatment Principle	Acupuncture	Formula
	Rash mainly on head, appearing as cloud shaped patches that are bright red in color, slightly raised above the skin surface, and clearly defined. Affected areas are hot to the touch, painful, and drained of color when pressed, quickly becoming red again when released. The rash spreads quickly and then fades to dull red, with flaky skin. May have aversion to wind, fever, thirst, constipation, dark urine. T: red, yellow coat P: floating, rapid	Dispel wind, clear heat, cool blood, resolve toxins	LI11 (qu chi), SP10 (xue hai), ST41 (jie xi), BL40 (wei zhong), BL12 (feng men) + fever DU14 (da zhui)	
	Rash mainly on lower limbs, may blister, fever, irritability, thirst chest oppression vomiting, loss of appetite, dark urine. T: yellow, greasy coat P: soft, rapid	Clear heat, drain damp, cool blood, resolve toxins	LI4 (he gu), ST36 (ZSL), SP10 (xue hai), LI11 (qu chi), SP9 (yin ling quan)	

Furuncle (jie)

Definition:
This is an acute suppurative disease in the superficial position of the muscle and skin, mostly caused by invasion of dampness and heat in summer and autumn, or by infection due to scratch after primary attack of heat rash, or by accumulation of heat toxins in zang-fu organs. It is characterized by a local redness and swelling with burning sensation and pain in most cases – usually around a hair follicle. After pus discharge, the wound can heal quickly.

Western Medicine Relevant Diseases:
See description under boil.

Etiology and Pathogenesis:

TCM Differentiation and Treatment:

Pattern	Signs and Symptoms	Treatment Principle	Acupuncture	Formula
Heat Toxin Accumulation	Mostly seen in the patients with internal heat, characterized by furuncles over the whole body, or repeated furuncles not easy to be cured, fever, dry mouth, foul breath, thirst with preference for cold drink, constipation, scanty and brown urine. T: red, yellowish coating P: rapid	Clear heat, dissolve toxins		
Lingering Toxins due to Deficient Constitution	Mostly seen in the patients with deficient constitution, characterized by repeated attack of furuncles with thin pus and difficulty in healing the wound, accompanied by the general symptoms of sallow complexion, low spirit and lassitude, poor appetite, loose stool. T: pale tongue with thin and whitish coating P: soft	Strengthen the spleen, harmonize the stomach, clear away and disperse damp heat		

Goitre (ying)

Definition:
Disorder manifested with swelling, enlargement or nodules by the thyroid cartilage of the neck. Other symptoms include a gradual increase in the size of the swelling, no change in local skin color, and prolonged course of illness.

Red Flags:
Thyroid storm is an acute form of hyperthyroidism that results from untreated or inadequately treated severe hyperthyroidism. It is rare, occurring in patients with Graves disease or toxic multinodular goiter. It may be precipitated by infection, trauma, surgery, embolism, diabetic ketoacidosis, or preeclampsia.
Thyroid storm causes abrupt symptoms of hyperthyroidism with one or more of the following: fever, marked weakness and muscle wasting, extreme restlessness with wide emotional swings, confusion, psychosis, coma, nausea, vomiting, diarrhea, and hepatomegaly with mild jaundice. The patient may present with cardiovascular collapse and shock. *Thyroid storm is a life-threatening emergency requiring prompt treatment.*

Western Medicine Relevant Diseases:
TCM Goitre patterns correspond to a range of thyroid conditions in Western medicine, including simple nontoxic goiter, hyperthyroidism, and hypothyroidism.

- Simple nontoxic goiter

A noncancerous hypertrophy of the thyroid without hyperthyroidism, hypothyroidism, or inflammation. Except in severe iodine deficiency, thyroid function is normal and patients are asymptomatic except for an obviously enlarged, non-tender thyroid.

Simple nontoxic goiter is frequently found at puberty, during pregnancy, and at menopause. The cause at these times is usually unclear. Known causes include:
- Intrinsic thyroid hormone production defects
- Ingestion of foods that contain substances that inhibit thyroid hormone synthesis (goitrogens, e.g., cassava, broccoli, cauliflower, cabbage), as may occur in countries in which iodine deficiency is common
- Drugs that can decrease the synthesis of thyroid hormone

Iodine deficiency is rare in North America but remains the most common cause of goiter worldwide (termed endemic goiter).

In the early stages, the goiter is typically soft, symmetric, and smooth. Later, multiple nodules and cysts may develop.

- Hypothyroidism

Hypothyroidism is under-activity of the thyroid gland that leads to inadequate production of thyroid hormones and a slowing of vital body functions. Primary hypothyroidism results from a disorder of the thyroid gland itself (see Hashimoto thyroiditis below). Other causes include: thyroid inflammation, treatment of hyperthyroidism or thyroid cancer, lack of iodine.

Secondary hypothyroidism occurs when the pituitary gland fails to secrete enough thyroid-stimulating hormone (TSH), which is necessary for normal stimulation of the thyroid. Secondary hypothyroidism is much rarer than primary.

Insufficient thyroid hormones cause body functions to slow. Symptoms are subtle and develop gradually:
- Facial expressions become dull.
- The voice is hoarse and speech is slow.
- Eyelids droop.
- The eyes and face become puffy.
- The hair becomes sparse, coarse, and dry.
- The skin becomes coarse, dry, scaly, and thick.

Many people with hypothyroidism gain weight, become constipated, and are unable to tolerate cold. The pulse may slow, the palms and soles may appear slightly orange (carotenemia), and the side parts of the eyebrows slowly fall out. Some people, especially older people, may appear confused, forgetful, or demented.

Hashimoto thyroiditis (autoimmune) is one of the most common causes of primary hypothyroidism in North America. It is more prevalent among women. Incidence increases with age and in patients with chromosomal disorders. A family history of thyroid disorders is common.

Hashimoto thyroiditis, is sometimes associated with other autoimmune disorders, including Addison disease, type 1 diabetes mellitus, pernicious anemia, connective tissue disorders (e.g. rheumatoid arthritis), and celiac disease. There may be an increased incidence of thyroid tumors, rarely thyroid lymphoma. Pathologically, there is extensive infiltration of lymphocytes with lymphoid follicles and scarring.

Patients complain of painless enlargement of the thyroid or fullness in the throat. Examination reveals a non-tender goiter that is smooth or nodular, firm, and more rubbery than the normal thyroid. Many patients present with symptoms of hypothyroidism, but some present with hyperthyroidism.

- Hyperthyroidism

Hyperthyroidism is over-activity of the thyroid gland that leads to high levels of thyroid hormones and speeding up of vital body functions. Heart rate and blood pressure may increase, heart rhythms may be abnormal, and people may sweat excessively, feel nervous and anxious, have difficulty sleeping, and lose weight without trying. Most people with hyperthyroidism have an enlarged thyroid gland (goiter). The entire gland may be enlarged, or nodules may develop within certain areas. If people have sub-acute thyroiditis, the gland may be tender and painful.

Graves disease is the most common cause of hyperthyroidism. It is an autoimmune disorder where the antibodies stimulate the thyroid to produce and secrete excess thyroid hormones into the blood. This cause of hyperthyroidism is often hereditary and almost always leads to enlargement of the thyroid.

Thyroiditis is inflammation of the thyroid gland. The inflammation can be caused by a viral infection, autoimmune thyroid inflammation that occurs after childbirth and, less often, chronic autoimmune inflammation (Hashimoto). At first, the inflammation causes hyperthyroidism as stored hormones are released from the inflamed gland. Later on, hypothyroidism usually follows because the levels of stored hormones are depleted. Finally, the gland usually returns to normal function.

Toxic multi-nodular goiter (Plummer disease), in which there are many nodules, tends to becomes common with aging but is uncommon in adolescents and young adults.

Other causes of hyperthyroidism include
- Growths within the thyroid that cause the thyroid to produce too much thyroid hormone (toxic thyroid nodules)
- Some drugs
- Overstimulation due to an overactive pituitary gland

Etiology and Pathogenesis:
The basic pathogenesis of goiter is Qi stagnation and phlegm accumulation. These may lead to blood stasis, or stagnant Qi and accumulated phlegm can turn into fire to injure yin.

TCM Differentiation and Treatment:

Pattern	Signs and Symptoms	Treatment Principle	Acupuncture	Formula
Qi Stagnation and Phlegm Accumulation	Swelling around thyroid cartilage, soft and painless on palpation, subjective distending sensation, stifling chest, sighing, migrating distending pain in chest/hypochondriac region, symptoms vary with emotions. T: thin white coat P: wiry	Move Qi, relieve constraint, resolve phlegm and reduce goiter	SJ13 (nai hui), LI17 (tian ding), SI17 (tian rong), REN22 (tian tu), LR3 (tai chong), LI4 (he gu), ST36 (ZSL), REN17 (shan zhong)	
Phlegm Accumulation and Blood Stasis	Mass surrounding thyroid cartilage, hard or nodular on palpation, gradual onset and slow progress, stifling sensation in the chest, poor appetite. T: white greasy coat P: wiry or choppy	Invigorate Blood, resolve phlegm, reduce goiter	SJ13 (nai hui), LI17 (tian ding), SI17 (tian rong), REN22 (tian tu), LR3 (tai chong), LI4 (he gu), ST36 (ZSL), REN17 (shan zhong) + BL17 (ge shu), SP10 (xue hai), REN9 (shui fen)	
Yin Deficiency with Fire Blazing	Goiter with symptoms of emaciation, hunger, dry mouth, dry throat, palpitations, excessive perspiration, five palm heat, tidal fever, insomnia, irregular menstruation. T: red, little coat P: rapid, thready	Moisten Yin, drain fire, break masses	SJ13 (nai hui), ST11 (qi she), PC5 (jian shi), LR3 (tai chong), KD3 (tai xi), SP6 (SYJ) +PC6 (nei guan), HT7 (shen men) for palpitations	

Points for protruding exophthalmos + BL10 (tian zhu), GB20 (feng chi), BL1 (jing ming), BL2 (zan zhu), SJ23 (si zhu kong)
Excess sweating + SP6 (SYJ), KD7 (fu liu), LI4 (he gu)

Hemorrhoid (zhi)

Definition:
Small, fleshy protrusions from the anus are known as hemorrhoids. Hemorrhoids generally occur in adults and present with pain, itching and bleeding of the anus.

Red Flags:
- Surgery may be needed if treatments do not work

Western Medicine Relevant Diseases:
In Western medicine, hemorrhoids are dilated veins of the hemorrhoidal plexus in the anal canal. Symptoms include irritation and bleeding. Thrombosed haemorrhoids (pooled blood in a haemorrhoid) are painful.

Increased pressure in the veins of the anorectal area leads to hemorrhoids. This pressure may result from pregnancy, frequent heavy lifting, or repeated straining during defecation (e.g., due to constipation). Hemorrhoids may be external or internal. In a few people, rectal varices result from increased blood pressure in the portal vein, and these are distinct from hemorrhoids.

External hemorrhoids are located below the dentate line and are covered by squamous epithelium. Internal hemorrhoids are located above the dentate line and are lined by rectal mucosa. Hemorrhoids typically occur in the right anterior, right posterior, and left lateral zones. They occur in adults and children.

Etiology and Pathogenesis:
Hemorrhoids can develop from prolonged sitting, standing, or walking with heavy loads. They can also develop from:
- Diet (overindulgence in hot, spicy, greasy foods) – blocks Qi and creates damp heat
- Chronic dysentery or constipation
- Frequent pregnancy and delivery

These factors lead to disharmony of Qi and Blood of intestines and anus causing stagnation and damp heat formation. With excessive bleeding, Qi and Blood deficiency can result.

TCM Differentiation and Treatment:

Pattern	Signs and Symptoms	Treatment Principle	Acupuncture	Formula
	Hemorrhoid surface is fresh red or purple, anal bleeding with stools, blood is fresh red on surface of stool only, or drops of blood in toilet (or blood may spray out if serious), pain and itching, may cause constipation. T: red, yellow/thick/greasy coating P: rapid pulse (slippery)	Clear heat, resolve damp, move stasis	BL32 (ci liao), BL35 (hui yang), DU1 (chang qiang), UB57 (cheng shan), Erbai -if anus area very swollen and painful, add BL54 (zhi bian), BL58 (fei yang) -if bleeding a lot, use SP10 (xue hai), BL24 (qi hai shu) -if constipation, ST25 (tian shu), BL25 (da chang shu), ST37 (shang ju xu)	
	Sallow complexion, low voice, fatigue, poor appetite, inner hemorrhoids have dropped and protrude from anus, pale bleeding from anus, heavy sensation in anus. T: pale P: weak	Raise Qi, tonify Spleen	DU20, (bai hui) REN8 (shen que), BL28 (pang guang shu), BL17 (ge shu), BL57 (cheng shan)	

Herpes Zoster (she chuan chuang)

Definition:
Herpes zoster, also known as shingles, is an acute viral inflammatory disease of the skin with red blister-like lesions appearing in bands. In most cases, the rash is present over the lumbar and costal regions, and resembles the shape of a snake (it is also called Snake Cinnabar in TCM). In the beginning stage, patients may suddenly feel sharp, burning pain along certain areas, like a belt or a track. They may also have fatigue, fever, and poor appetite. Small vesicles the size of mung or soybeans develops and grows into blisters that appear in small groups. The skin between the blisters remains normal and the fluid in the blisters is initially clear. After 5-7 days, the fluid becomes turbid. The blisters dry after about 2 weeks, and crust. Pain may linger.

Red Flags:
- Western medical assessment and treatment is critical
- Condition is contagious (at blister phase only)
- Immediate treatment with antiviral drugs may reduce severity and reduce recovery time

Western Medicine Relevant Diseases:
Herpes zoster is infection that results when varicella-zoster virus reactivates from its latent state in a posterior dorsal root ganglion. Symptoms usually begin with pain along the affected dermatome, followed in 2 to 3 days by a vesicular eruption. Treatment is antiviral drugs given within 72 h after skin lesions appear.

Chickenpox and herpes zoster are caused by the varicella-zoster virus; chickenpox is the acute invasive phase of the virus, and herpes zoster (shingles) represents reactivation of the latent phase.

Herpes zoster inflames the sensory root ganglia, the skin of the associated dermatome, and sometimes the posterior and anterior horns of the gray matter, meninges, and dorsal and ventral roots. Herpes zoster frequently occurs in elderly and HIV-infected patients and is more severe in immune-compromised patients because cell-mediated immunity in these patients is decreased.

Pain develops in the involved site, followed in 2 to 3 days by a rash, usually crops of vesicles on an erythematous base. The site is usually one or more adjacent dermatomes in the thoracic or lumbar region, although a few satellite lesions may also appear. Lesions are typically unilateral and pain may be severe. Lesions usually continue to form for about 3 to 5 days.

Herpes zoster may travel to other regions of the body, including the face.

Many patients, particularly the elderly, have persistent or recurrent pain in the involved distribution (postherpetic neuralgia), which lasts for months or years or permanently. Infection in the trigeminal nerve is particularly likely to lead to severe, persistent pain. The pain of postherpetic neuralgia may be sharp and intermittent or constant and may be debilitating.

Etiology and Pathogenesis:
- Wind fire accumulate in the Shao Yang and Jue Yin skin and muscle layers
- Stagnation of fire in the Liver channel with latent damp-heat in the Spleen channel + invasion of external fire-toxins – causes Liver fire to flare up and damp heat to vaporize giving rise to blister-like skin lesions

TCM Differentiation and Treatment:

Pattern	Signs and Symptoms	Treatment Principle	Acupuncture	Formula
Wind Fire	Begins with burning pain and red color before the rash/blisters erupt; groups of red rashes and blisters develop very fast along lines, if more serious, will see blood blisters. Additional symptoms: bitter mouth, dizzy, irritability, red face, yellow scanty urination, stools hard and dry, feel thirsty. P: wiry and rapid	Clear and drain, release wind, harmonize and treat blood	LR14, (qi men) LR8 (qu quan), GB44 (zu qian yin), SJ3 zhong zhu), SP6 (SYJ), SP10 (xue hai), PC4 (xi men), HT7 (shen men), SJ6 (zhi gou) + local encirclement with careful sterilization	

Damp Toxin	Large blisters that may break with yellow, sticky excretions, rash bright red, appetite poor, bloating T: yellow, thick, greasy with red body P: pulse	Clear and drain fire and damp toxin	LI11 (qu chi), LR3 (tai chong), ST44 (nei ting), SP4 (gong sun), GB43 (xia xi), SJ5 (wei guan), SP6 (SYj), SP10 (xue hai), DU14 (da zhui) + local encirclement with careful sterilization	

4 Stages of Shingles:

Phlegmon (fa)

Definition:
Refers to an acute suppurative infection occurring between the muscle and skin with characteristic patches of local red and painful swelling.

Red Flags:

Western Medicine Relevant Diseases:
Phlegmon patterns are similar to cellulitis in Western medicine. `Cellulitis is acute bacterial infection of the skin and subcutaneous tissue most often caused by streptococci or staphylococci. Symptoms and signs are pain, rapidly spreading erythema, and edema; fever may occur, and regional lymph nodes may enlarge.

Etiology and Pathogenesis:
In TCM, this disease is caused by obstruction of qi and blood due to: internal accumulation of pathogenic damp, heat and fire; or, by infection due to traumatic injury.

TCM Differentiation and Treatment:

Pattern	Signs and Symptoms	Treatment Principle	Acupuncture	Formula
Wind Fire and Stagnated Heat Syndrome	Mostly seen in hand phlegmon, manifested by red swelling, burning pain with unclear margin on the dorsum of the hand, accompanied by aversion to cold, fever, headache, aching sensation in the body. T: red, thin and yellowish coating P: superficial and rapid pulse	Expel wind, clear heat, dissolve toxin, diminish swelling	DU14 (da zhui), LI4 (he gu), LI11 (qu chi), SJ5 (wei guan), GB20 (feng chi)	
Damp Fire Accumulation Syndrome	Mostly seen in hip and foot phlegmon, manifested by local red swelling and burning pain. The swelling is worse in the center, with unclear margin, or wet ulceration. It is accompanied by aversion to cold, headache, aching sensation in the bone, appetite, brown urine. T: red, yellow and greasy coating P: slippery and rapid	Clear heat, dissolve toxin, harmonize ying-nutrient system and remove dampness.	SP9 (yin ling quan), LI4 (he gu), SJ5 (wei guan), LI11 (qu chi), ST40 (feng long)	
Qi and Blood Deficiency	Decaying flesh has dropped after ulceration, but swelling remains. Or, the wound is in slightly red color with thin discharged pus, accompanied by sallow complexion, low spirit, lassitude, poor appetite, pale tongue, teeth marks on the tongue margin. T: thin and whitish coating P: thready and feeble Therapeutic Methods: Regulate and replenish qi and blood.	Regulate and replenish Qi and Blood	SP6 (SYJ), SP10 (xue hai), ST36 (ZSL), REN4 (guan yuan), REN6 (qi hai), BL20 (pi shu), BL17 (ge shu)	

Prostatic Hyperplasia (qian lie xian zeng sheng zheng)

Definition:
Non-cancerous enlargement of the prostate gland that causes urinary difficulty.

Red Flags:
- Refer all cases of blood in urine, severe pain, or complete urinary blockage.

Western Medicine Relevant Diseases:
Benign prostatic hyperplasia (BPH) is a non-cancerous enlargement of the prostate gland that can make urination difficult.

BPH becomes increasingly common after age 50. The exact cause is not known, but involves changes caused by hormones. As the prostate enlarges, it gradually compresses the urethra and blocks the flow of urine. When men with BPH urinate, the bladder may not empty completely. As a result, urine remains in the bladder, making men susceptible to urinary infections and bladder stones. Prolonged obstruction can weaken the bladder and damage the kidneys.

With BHP, men may initially have difficulty starting urination. Urination may also feel incomplete. Because the bladder does not empty completely, men have to urinate more frequently, often at night. Also, the need to urinate may become more urgent. The volume and force of the urinary flow may diminish noticeably, and urine may dribble at the end of urination.
In severe cases, urine flow out of the bladder can be blocked completely, making urination impossible and usually leading to a full feeling and severe pain in the lower abdomen.

Etiology and Pathogenesis:
- External Damp – penetrates channels in legs and flows to settle in Bladder -- Damp heat accumulates; or, excessive consumption of sweets, sugar, dairy and greasy food lead to formation of Damp heat
- Aging or chronic illness weaken Kidney -- Kidney Yang deficiency leads to loss of control over lower orifices; Kidney Yin deficiency leads to failure to form urine
- Obstruction in the Bladder – obstruction by stasis, masses, or calculi causes urinary retention

TCM Differentiation and Treatment:

Pattern	Signs and Symptoms	Treatment Principle	Acupuncture	Formula
	Frequent and hesitant urination, or dribbling drops, dark and hot urine, itching and pain in the urethra, distending fullness or pain in the lower abdomen, possible hematuria, dry mouth, constipation. T: red, yellow and greasy coat P: rapid pulse	Clear heat, drain dampness, unblock obstruction and promote urination	BL28 (pang guang shu), REN3 (zhong ji), SP6 (SYJ), SP9 (yin ling quan)	
	Frequent urination, dribbling urine, intermittent attack, aggravated by fatigue, lingering duration, accompanied by dizziness, tinnitus, soreness and weakness in the low back and knee, emaciation. T: red, scanty coating P: thready and rapid	Tonify the Kidney, nourish Yin, drain empty fire	BL23 (shen shu), KD3 (tai xi), REN3 (zhong ji), REN6 (qi hai), SP6 (SYJ), REN4 (guan	
	Forceless urination, or hesitant dribbling urine, frequent nocturnal urination, pale complexion, SOB, lassitude, cold sensation in the limbs, aversion to cold, accompanied by impotence. T: pale, thin and white coat P: deep and thready	Warm the Yang, augment the Qi, tonify the Kidney and promote urination	BL23 (shen shu), BL20 (pi shu), DU20 (bai hui), yuan), REN3 (zhong ji), KD10 (yin gu), ST36 (ZSL), SP6 (SYJ), DU4 (ming men),	

	Hesitant, dribbling urine, or fine urine stream like a thread that must be forced out, maybe hematuria, distending fullness and pain in the lower abdomen T: purple or red P: hesitant	Clear stasis and obstruction, promotion urination	REN3 (zhong ji), BL28 (pang guang shu), SP6 (SYJ), BL63 jin men), LR6 (zhong du), LR3 (tai chong)	

Prostatitis (qian lie xian yan)

Definition:
Prostatitis is a Western medical term (see description below).

Red Flags:
- See red flags for BPH
- Bacterial infection may need antibiotic treatment

Western Medicine Relevant Diseases:
Prostatitis is pain and swelling, inflammation, or both of the prostate gland. It can result from unknown causes, or from a bacterial infection that spreads to the prostate from the urinary tract or from bacteria in the bloodstream. Bacterial infections may develop slowly and tend to recur (chronic bacterial prostatitis) or develop rapidly (acute bacterial prostatitis). Some people develop chronic prostatitis in the absence of bacterial infection. This type may or may not involve inflammation. Occasionally, prostatitis without bacterial infection causes inflammation but no symptoms.

In all types of prostatitis that cause symptoms, many of the symptoms are caused by spasm of the muscles in the bladder and pelvis, especially in the perineum. Pain develops in the perineum, the lower back, and often the penis and testes. Men also may need to urinate frequently and urgently, and urinating may cause pain or burning. Pain may make obtaining an erection or ejaculating difficult. Constipation can develop, making defecation painful.

With acute bacterial prostatitis, symptoms tend to be more severe. Some symptoms tend to occur more often, such as fever and chills, difficulty urinating, and blood in the urine. Bacterial prostatitis can result in a collection of pus (abscess) in the prostate or inflammation of the epididymis.

Etiology and Pathogenesis:
- Poor diet (indulgence in spicy foods, alcohol) or external damp – leads to internal damp heat that transmits downward to Bladder
- Aging or over-indulgence in sex – drain Kidney essence
- External invasion of pathogenic heat and toxins

TCM Differentiation and Treatment:

Pattern	Signs and Symptoms	Treatment Principle	Acupuncture	Formula
Heat Toxin Accumulation	Acute prostatitis, burning pain in the urethra, dysuria, purulent blood in urine, pain in the perineum and abdomen, chills, fever, thirst with desire for drinks, tenesmus, constipation. T: red, yellow coat P: wiry and rapid	Drain heat and toxin, regulate urination, stop pain		
Downward Transmission of Damp Heat	Frequency and urgency of urination, burning pain in the urethra, descending distension and pain in the perineum, discharge of turbid fluid, hematuria, chills, fever, bitter and greasy taste in the mouth, yellow urine, constipation. T: red, yellow and greasy coat P: slippery and rapid	Drain damp heat, regulate urination, stop pain		
Kidney Yin Deficiency	Dribbling after urination, discharge of white turbid substance, scanty and brown urine, burning pain with urination, insomnia, dream-disturbed sleep, dizziness, blurred vision, sore back and knees, premature ejaculation, seminal emission, 5 palm heat, dry mouth and throat. T: red, scanty or peeled coat P: thready and rapid	Tonify Kidney Yin, regulate urination, stop pain		

| Kidney Yang Deficiency | Frequent urination, dribbling urine, pain in the perineum, low spirit, sore back, lassitude, spasm in lower abdomen, cold sensation in the hands and feet, lusterless complexion, poor appetite, impotence, premature ejaculation.
T: pale tongue with teeth marks on the margin, thin and whitish coating
P: thready and feeble | Tonify Kidney Yang, regulate urination, stop pain | | |

Scrofula (luo li)

Definition:
Chronic infectious disease appearing mostly on the neck. Characteristic arrangement of lumps, like pearls threaded on a string.

Red Flags:
- Primary Western medical care required

Western Medicine Relevant Diseases:
In Western medicine, scrofula includes a tuberculosis found outside the lung: tuberculous lymphadenitis. This typically involves the lymph nodes in the posterior cervical and supraclavicular chains. Infection in these areas is thought to be due to contiguous spread from intra-thoracic lymphatics. Mediastinal lymph nodes are also commonly enlarged as a part of primary pulmonary disease.
Cervical tuberculous lymphadenitis is characterized by progressive swelling of the affected nodes. In advanced cases, nodes may become inflamed and tender; the overlying skin may break down, resulting in a draining fistula.

Etiology and Pathogenesis:

TCM Differentiation and Treatment:

Pattern	Signs and Symptoms	Treatment Principle	Acupuncture	Formula
Liver Qi Stagnation	Typically during initial and intermediate stages of scrofula, swelling of one or several cervical lymph nodes to the size of a bean, no change in color of skin, mass is firm and moveable. During intermediate stage, gradual increase in size of nodules, and adhesion to the skin. Mental depression, hypochondriac distension/bloating/pain, bloating, poor appetite. T: normal, or sides red P: wiry	Sooth Liver and relieve constraint	GB41 (zu ling qi), LV13 (zhang men), PC6 (nei guan), GB34 (yang ling quan), ST36 (ZSL), REN12 (zhong wan), SJ10 (tian jing)	
Kidney Yin Deficiency	Emaciation, night sweats, tidal fever, fatigue, irritability. T: red P: thin, rapid	Nourish Yin, clear fire	SJ10 (tian jing), bai lao, HT3 (shai hai), UB20 (pi shu), UB23 (shen shu), HT6 (yin xi), UB43 (gau huang shu), Jiehexue -if cough, LU7 (lie que); if cough with blood, LU6 (zong kui), BL13 (fei shu)	

Sebaceous Cyst (zhi liu)

Definition:
An elevated lesion containing fluid or viscous material appearing as a nodule in the superficial layers of the skin.

Western Medicine Relevant Diseases:
This pattern includes a type of cutaneous cyst known as an epidermal inclusion cyst (epidermoid cyst), one of the most common types of cysts. These cysts seldom cause discomfort unless they have rupture, causing a rapidly enlarging, painful reaction and abscess. Epidermal inclusion cysts are often surmounted by a visible pore; their contents are white, cheesy, and malodorous. They are most commonly found on the face, neck, or torso.

Etiology and Pathogenesis:
- Stagnation of damp heat in the channels and collaterals

TCM Differentiation and Treatment:

Pattern	Signs and Symptoms	Treatment Principle	Acupuncture	Formula
Damp Heat Stagnation	Closed fluid filled sac, non-painful, slow growing, on face, neck or trunk. T: red, greasy coat P: rapid, slippery	Drain damp heat, dissipate stasis.		

Shank Ulcer (lian chuang)

Definition:
Skin lesion that may be composed of a number of separate, normally shallow ulcerations that may be circular, oblong, or irregular in shape with either distinct or indistinct borders. The granulation tissue looks pale and is covered by a layer of fatty fibroid tissue. he lesions are productive and there may be necrosis of the surface with adjacent areas feeling hard and tense. In some cases, the muscular membrane is also involved. Subjective symptoms range from light pain or itching, to severe pain along the borders of the affected area. Shank ulcers have a long, protracted course.

(from Flaws, *Handbook of Traditional Chinese Dermatology*)

Red Flags:

Western Medicine Relevant Diseases:
Shank ulcer patterns include any lower limb ulcers in Western medicine, for example, those resulting from diabetes mellitus or ulceration of varicose veins.
Poor circulation to the skin can lead to ulcers and infections and causes wounds to heal slowly. People with diabetes are particularly likely to have ulcers and infections of the feet and legs. Too often, these wounds heal slowly or not at all, and amputation of the foot or part of the leg may be needed.

People with diabetes often develop bacterial and fungal infections, typically of the skin. When the levels of glucose in the blood are high, white blood cells cannot effectively fight infections. Any infection that develops tends to be more severe and takes longer to resolve.

Etiology and Pathogenesis:
- External invasion of damp heat – penetrates interior – transforms into internal damp heat
- Diet (too much alcohol, sweets, greasy food) – transforms into internal damp heat
  - In both above cases, damp heat sinks downward affecting yang ming vessels (full of Qi and Blood) – brews and steams – flesh becomes putrid – Qi and Blood are blocked – stasis results
- Over-taxation, aging, chronic illness, or congenital deficiencies:
  - lead to weak Spleen Qi – damages Qi and Blood formation and Spleen T&T fails – damp develops and flows downward blocking channels and depriving the flesh of nutrients
- Insect bites, animal bites, injury – lead to Qi and Blood stagnation – flesh cannot be nourished

TCM Differentiation and Treatment:

Pattern	Signs and Symptoms	Treatment Principle	Acupuncture	Formula
Damp Heat Accumulation	Initially, areas swollen, red, and painful. Ulcer eventually opens and becomes itchy with a discharge of watery pus. In the advanced stage, may have sunken sore with rancid pus, necrotic tissue, distension and heaviness in the legs, fatigue and weakness.	Clear heat, damp, and resolve toxins	Local points, SP9 (yin ling quan), BL40 (wei zhong), LI11 (qu zhi), ST36 (ZSL), SP6 (SYJ)	
Spleen Deficiency and Damp	Grey-white ulcer with watery, thin, clear pus. Worse in evening. Weak limbs, fatigue. T: pale P: slow	Tonify Spleen Qi, drain damp, resolve ulcer	SP6 (SYJ), SP9 (yin ling quan), SP3 (tai bai), ST36 (ZSL), ST40 (feng long)	
Blood Stasis and Qi Stagnation	Color around ulcer is dark purple, chronic discharge from ulcer, pain worse with standing or walking, dark veins in legs. T: purple P: choppy	Move Qi and Blood, resolve ulcer	SP10 (xue hai), SP6 (SYJ), LI4 (he gu), BL17 (ge shu)	

Tinea (xian)

Definition:

Western Medicine Relevant Diseases:
In Western medicine, tinea (tinea corporis) is a dermatophyte (fungal) infection of the face, trunk, and extremities that causes pink-to-red annular (O-shaped) patches and plaques with raised scaly borders that expand peripherally and tend to clear centrally. A rare variant form appears as nummular (circle- or round-shaped) scaling patches studded with small papules or pustules that have no central clearing. Common causes are *Trichophyton mentagrophytes*, *T. rubrum*, and *Microsporum canis*.

Etiology and Pathogenesis:
- Invasion of wind, damp and heat pathogens in the superficial layers disturbing Qi and Blood

TCM Differentiation and Treatment:

Pattern	Signs and Symptoms	Treatment Principle	Acupuncture	Formula
Wind Damp Heat Invasion	Acute eruption of vesicles that may join to form larger bullae, and may rupture and discharge thick exudates (or not break). Itching may be mild to severe.	Expel wind, clear damp heat	BL40 (wei zhong), LI11 (qu chi), SP9 (yin ling quan), GB20 (feng chi)	

Neurodermatitis (niu pi xian)

Definition:
Niu pi xian, or "ox-hide tinea", is named because the thick leathery skin of affected areas resembles the skin of an ox's neck. It typically presents with itching, followed by developing clusters of round flattened papules that may be light brown in color. With continued development, the papules form large patches, the skin thickens, dries out, and becomes wrinkled. Scratching leads to peeling of the dried skin and more itching.

Western medicine relevant conditions:
Lichen simplex chronicus (neurodermatitis) is caused by chronic scratching of an area of skin. The act of scratching triggers more itching, beginning a vicious circle of itching-scratching-itching. Sometimes the scratching begins for no apparent reason. Other times scratching starts because of a contact dermatitis, parasitic infestation, or other condition, but the person continues to scratch long after the inciting cause is gone.

The underlying pathophysiology is unknown but may involve alterations in the way the nervous system perceives and processes itchy sensations. Skin that tends toward eczematous conditions is more prone to lichenification.

Lichen simplex chronicus is characterized by pruritic, dry, scaling, hyperpigmented, lichenified plaques in irregular, oval, or angular shapes. It involves easily reached sites, most commonly the legs, arms, neck, upper trunk, and anal region.

(from http://www.merckmanuals.com/professional/dermatologic-disorders/dermatitis/contact-dermatitis)

Etiology and pathogenesis:

TCM Differentiation and Treatment:

Pattern	Signs and Symptoms	Treatment Principle	Acupuncture	Formula
External Wind, Heat and Damp	Relatively short duration, affected area presenting papules, redness, ulceration, moistness, and scabs. T: red, yellow greasy coat P: soft, rapid	Clear wind, clear heat, drain damp	SP9, SP3, LU9, GB20, LI4, plus ashi points and points based on location	
Blood deficiency and wind-dryness	Extended duration of illness, with thickening, dryness, and peeling of the skin in affected areas; insomnia, dizziness, and vertigo. T: pale, thin coat P: weak, thready	Nourish Blood, dispel wind, moisten dryness	LI11, SP10, SP6, BL17, ST36, ashi points Itching disturbing sleep + KD6, HT7	

Urticaria (yin zhen)

Definition:
Urticaria is a dermatological condition often seen in clinic. These rashes appear in patches, and tend to be raised, bumpy, bright red or pale white in color. They may be very itchy and may spread with itching. Urticaria can appear and disappear quickly without scarring and can occur at any age. Episodes are either acute (lasting approximately one week) or chronic, recurring overall months or years.

Red Flags:
- Emergency care is required for the following:

Western Medicine Relevant Diseases:
Urticaria consists of migratory, well-circumscribed, erythematous, pruritic plaques on the skin.

Urticaria also may be accompanied by angioedema, which results from mast cell and basophil activation in the deeper dermis and subcutaneous tissues and manifests as edema of the face and lips, extremities, or genitals. Angioedema can occur in the bowel and present as colicky abdominal pain. Angioedema can be life-threatening if airway obstruction occurs because of laryngeal edema or tongue swelling.

Urticaria results from the release of histamine, bradykinin, kallikrein, and other vaso-active substances from mast cells and basophils in the superficial dermis, resulting in intra-dermal edema caused by capillary and venous vasodilation and occasionally caused by leukocyte infiltration.

The process can be immune mediated or non-immune mediated.

Immune-mediated mast cell activation includes
- Type 1 Hypersensitivity reactions, in which allergen-bound IgE antibodies bind to high-affinity cell surface receptors on mast cells and basophils
- Autoimmune disorders, in which antibodies to an IgE receptor functionally cross-link IgE receptors and cause mast cell degranulation

Non immune-mediated mast cell activation includes
- Direct non-allergic activation of mast cells by certain drugs
- Activation by physical or emotional stimuli; mechanism is poorly understood but possibly involves the release of neuropeptides that interact with mast cells

A presumptive trigger (e.g., drug, food ingestion, insect bite or sting, infection) occasionally can be identified.

Chronic urticaria most often results from
- Idiopathic causes
- Autoimmune disorders

Chronic urticaria often lasts months to years, eventually resolving without a cause being found.

Etiology and Pathogenesis:
- Wind attack and failure of Wei Qi allows for wind cold or wind heat invasion at skin level
- Prolonged illness – leads to Qi and Blood deficiency – give rise to internal wind
- Diet – food intolerances, improper food intake -- give rise to Stomach and Intestine heat (damp heat)

TCM Differentiation and Treatment:

Pattern	Signs and Symptoms	Treatment Principle	Acupuncture	Formula
Wind Attack	Rash worse after exposure to wind, fever, thirst, slight cough, slight aversion to wind +Wind Heat will have red colored patchy rash, rapid floating pulse +Wind Cold will have white colored patchy rash, floating tight pulse	Release wind, harmonize the Ying	LI15 (jian yu), LI5 (yang xi), SP6 (SYJ), LU7 (lie que), LI11 (qu chi) -Du14 (da zhui) if fever -LI11 (qu chi) for heat	
Stomach and Intestine Accumulated Heat	Red patchy rash, epigastric/ABD pain, constipation or diarrhea, poor appetite, possible nausea and vomiting. T: yellow greasy coat P: rapid, slippery	Clear Heat, Harmonize the Ying	LI11 (qu chi), ST36 (ZSL), SP9 (yin ling quan), SP10 (xue hai), SP6 (SYJ), ST25 (tian shu)	
Qi and Blood Deficiency	Recurring rash over several months or even years, worse when fatigued. T: pale P: deep, thready	Supplement Qi and Blood	LI11 (qu chi), SP10 (que hai), SP6 (SYJ), ST36 (ZSL), BL17 (ge shu), BL20 (pi shu)	

Varicose Veins (jin liu)

Definition:
Veins that have become enlarged and twisted, most commonly found on the leg.

Red Flags:
- Rupture of varicose veins requires urgent medical attention

Western Medicine Relevant Diseases:
Varicose veins are dilated superficial veins in the lower extremities. Usually, no cause is obvious. The etiology is usually unknown, but varicose veins may result from primary venous valve insufficiency with reflux or from primary dilation of the vein wall due to structural weakness. In some people, varicose veins result from chronic venous insufficiency and venous hypertension. Most people have no obvious risk factors. Varicose veins are common within families, suggesting a genetic component. Varicose veins are more common among women because estrogen affects venous structure, pregnancy increases pelvic and leg venous pressures, or both.

Varicose veins may initially be tense and palpable but are not necessarily visible. Later, they may progressively enlarge, protrude, and become obvious; they can cause a sense of fullness, fatigue, pressure, and superficial pain or hyperesthesia in the legs. Varicose veins are most visible when the patient stands.

Etiology and Pathogenesis:
- Poor diet (overconsumption of sweet and damp forming foods) – weakens Spleen – Spleen is unable to hold (Spleen rules muscle and connective tissue)
- Poor diet, aging, illness, overweight, pregnancy, standing for long periods, emotional stress – may lead to stagnation of Qi and Blood -- blood cannot circulate – Blood stasis leads to varicose veins

TCM Differentiation and Treatment:

Pattern	Signs and Symptoms	Treatment Principle	Acupuncture	Formula
	Symptoms include tight varicose veins, local redness, swelling, hotness and pain, red color skin around the veins, scorching pain, thirst with no desire to drink, foul breath, restlessness T: red, tender and puffy tongue with yellow greasy coating P: slippery and rapid pulse.		SP6 (SYJ), ST36 (ZSL), SP3 (tai bai), DU20 (bai hui)	
	Varicose veins like messy ropes, local aching, tightness, heaviness and distension, oily and bright surrounding skin, body heaviness and tiredness, heavy head, symptoms worse in the afternoons T: dark purple and enlarged with turbid greasy coating P: deep and rapid		SP9 (yin ling quan), ST40 (feng long), BL40 (wei zhong), LI4 (ge shu), LR3 (tai chong), ST36 (ZSL)	
	Varicose veins shaped like earthworms, soft on palpation, mild continuous pain, gray or sallow skin color, local cold and damp sensation, dizziness, symptoms worse with stress, sallow complexion T: pale, enlarged with white greasy coating P: moderate and weak		Ren4 (guan yuan), Ren6 (qi hai), SP6 (SYJ), ST36 (ZSL), Ren8 (shen que)	

Warts (you)

Definition:
Small, benign growths, often found on hands, and common in teenage years. Top is slightly raised, with flat surface, smooth and slippery. Can range in size from millet to soya bean and color from light brown to flesh color. Warts are normally painless, but may be slightly itchy.

Western Medicine Relevant Diseases:
Warts are common, benign, epidermal lesions caused by human papillomavirus infection. They can appear anywhere on the body in a variety of morphologies.

Etiology and Pathogenesis:
- Wind and heat invading and accumulating in the skin
- Liver Qi stagnation – failed nourishment in meridian

TCM Differentiation and Treatment:

Pattern	Signs and Symptoms	Treatment Principle	Acupuncture	Formula
Wind Heat	Warts of short duration, often accompanied by aversion to wind, fever. T: thin yellow coat P: floating, rapid	Expel wind, clear heat, resolve toxins, disperse warts		
Liver Qi Stagnation	Warts of long duration, distention of hypochondrium, bitter taste, irritability. P: wiry	Sooth Liver, disperse warts		

Obstetrics and Gynecology (Fu Ke)

Abdominal Masses (Zheng Jia)

Definition:
Refers to a gynecological condition characterized by the occurrence of lumps or masses in the lower abdomen. These may be accompanied by pain, distention, vaginal bleeding or discharge. *Zheng* describes masses with defined form and fixed location, with pain in a specific area (i.e. substantial masses related to Blood stasis). *Jia* refers to masses without a distinct form, which change location and are movable on palpation (i.e. non-substantial masses related to Qi stagnation).

Red Flags:
- Western medical diagnosis is essential to determine cause of masses

Western Medicine Relevant Diseases:
In Western medicine, masses may be due to many different conditions, including:

1. _____: Uterine fibroids are common, benign uterine tumors of smooth muscle origin. Fibroids frequently cause abnormal uterine bleeding, pelvic pain and pressure, urinary and intestinal symptoms, and pregnancy complications. Most fibroids in the uterus are subserosal, followed by intramural, then submucosal. Occasionally, fibroids occur in the broad ligaments, fallopian tubes, or cervix. What causes fibroids to grow in the uterus is unknown. High levels of estrogen and possibly **progesterone** seem to stimulate their growth. Fibroids may become larger during pregnancy—when levels of these hormones increase—and fibroids tend to shrink after menopause—when levels decrease drastically. Fibroids can cause abnormal uterine bleeding. If fibroids grow and degenerate (i.e. outgrow their blood supply), or if pedunculated fibroids twist, severe acute or chronic pressure or pain can result. Urinary symptoms can result from bladder compression, and intestinal symptoms can result from intestinal compression. Fibroids may increase risk of infertility. During pregnancy, they may cause recurrent spontaneous abortion, premature contractions, or abnormal fetal presentation or make cesarean delivery necessary.

2. _____: is a clinical syndrome characterized by mild obesity, irregular menses or amenorrhea, and signs of androgen excess (e.g., hirsutism, acne). Typically, ovaries contain many 2- to 6-mm follicular (and sometimes larger) cysts. Ovaries may be enlarged with smooth, thickened capsules or may be normal in size. This syndrome involves anovulation or ovulatory dysfunction and androgen excess of unclear etiology. Polycystic ovary syndrome has several serious complications: Estrogen levels may be elevated, increasing risk of endometrial hyperplasia and, eventually, endometrial cancer. Androgen levels are often elevated, increasing the risk of metabolic syndrome and causing **hirsutism**. Hyperinsulinemia due to insulin resistance may be present and may contribute to increased ovarian production of androgens. Over the long-term, androgen excess increases the risk of cardiovascular disorders, including hypertension.

   Symptoms typically begin during puberty and worsen with time. Typical symptoms include mild obesity, slight hirsutism, and irregular menses or amenorrhea. However, in up to half of women with PCOS, weight is normal, and some women are underweight. Body hair may grow in a male pattern. Some women have other signs of virilization, such as acne and temporal balding. Areas of thickened, darkened skin may appear in the axillae, on the nape of the neck, in skin-folds, and on knuckles and/or elbows; the cause is high insulin levels due to insulin resistance.

3. _____: benign ovarian masses include functional cysts and tumors; most are asymptomatic. There are 2 types of functional cysts: follicular cysts (develop from graafian follicles); corpus luteum (develop from the corpus luteum). They may hemorrhage into the cyst cavity, distending the ovarian capsule or rupturing into the peritoneum. Most functional cysts are < 1.5 cm in diameter; few exceed 5 cm. Functional cysts usually resolve spontaneously over days to weeks. Functional cysts are uncommon after menopause. Benign ovarian tumors usually grow slowly and rarely become malignant. They include: benign cystic teratomas (also called dermoid cysts because although derived from all 3 germ cell layers, they consist mainly of ectodermal tissue); fibromas (these slow-growing tumors are usually < 7 cm in diameter); and, cystadenomas (most commonly serous or mucinous). Most functional cysts and benign tumors are asymptomatic. Sometimes they cause menstrual abnormalities. Hemorrhagic corpus luteum cysts may cause pain or signs of peritonitis, particularly when they rupture. Occasionally, severe abdominal pain results from adnexal torsion of a cyst or mass, usually > 4 cm. Ascites and rarely pleural effusion may accompany fibromas.

4. _____: does not usually cause masses, but may do so when there is build up of scar tissue. Endometriosis is the presence of endometrial tissue outside the uterus on structures such as the ovaries, ligaments, or colon. See menstrual hematemesis and epistaxis for more detail.

5. _____: causes ABD mass only when it is invasive and has grown beyond the cervix. Cervical cancer is usually a squamous cell carcinoma caused by human papillomavirus infection; less often, it is an adenocarcinoma. Cervical neoplasia is asymptomatic; the first symptom of early cervical cancer is usually irregular, often postcoital vaginal bleeding. Diagnosis is by a screening cervical Papanicolaou test and biopsy. Staging is clinical. Treatment usually involves surgical resection for early-stage disease or radiation therapy plus chemotherapy for locally advanced disease. f the cancer has widely metastasized, chemotherapy is often used alone.

Etiology and Pathogenesis:
- Emotional strain – stagnation of Liver Qi – stasis of Liver Blood (Liver channel plays a critical role in movement of Qi in lower abdomen and Liver Blood is important for circulation of Blood in this area, in women)
- Diet – irregular eating or excess cold and raw foods – lead to cold in lower abdomen – cold contracts and interferes with circulation of Qi and Blood – may lead to stasis
- External cold – can invade the lower abdomen – impairs circulation – leads to Blood stasis; or, external damp may invade the channels and settle in the lower abdomen leading to phlegm and masses

TCM Differentiation and Treatment:

Pattern	Signs and Symptoms	Treatment Principle	Acupuncture	Formula
Qi Stagnation	Movable masses that come and go, ABD distension and pain that comes and goes with masses, hypochondrium distention and fullness, depression, moodiness, irritability. T: sides may be slightly red P: wiry	Soothe the Liver, eliminate stagnation, move Qi and dissolve masses	GB34 (yang ling quan), REN6 (qi hai), LR3-LI4 (4 gates), SJ6 (zhi gou), PC6 (nei guan), SP6 (SYJ), LU7-KD6 (Ren Mai)	
Blood Stasis	Lower ABD masses that are hard and fixed, pain with palpation, dull complexion, heavy menstruation, pay be lengthened menstrual cycle. T: dark, purplish, possible macules P: deep, choppy	Move Qi and Blood, dispel stasis	GB34 (yang ling quan), LR3 (tai chong), SP6 (SYJ), SP10 (xue hai), BL17 (ge shu), LU7-KD6 (ren mai), REN6 (qi hai), SP4 (gong sun) – PC6 (nei guan)	
Phlegm Damp	Lower ABD masses that are soft in texture and possibly painful, heavy vaginal discharge that is white/thick/sticky, chest and costal region discomfort. T: greasy P: slippery	Move Qi, resolve phlegm damp, resolve masses	REN6 (qi hai), BL22 (san jiao shu), LI4 (he gu), ST40 (feng long), SP9 (yin ling quan), REN3 (zhong ji), BL34 (xia liao)	

Amenorrhea (bi jing)

Definition:
Refers to either primary amenorrhea where menstruation has not begun by 18 years of age, or secondary amenorrhea where the menstrual cycle has been interrupted for 3 months or longer. This does not include the cessation of menstruation due to congenital underdevelopment or malformation of reproductive organs, during breastfeeding or pregnancy, menopause, immediately after first menses, or an interruption of 1 or 2 cycles after a sudden change in environments.

Red Flags:
- Referral for Western medical assessment and diagnosis for amenorrhea is important.

Girls should see a doctor within a few weeks if:
- They have no signs of puberty (such as breast development or a growth spurt) by age 13.
- Pubic hair has not appeared by age 14.
- Periods have not started by age 16 or by 2 years after girls develop secondary sexual characteristics.

If women of childbearing age have had menstrual periods that have stopped, they should do a home pregnancy test. If the test is negative and if they have headaches or changes in vision, they should see a doctor within a week (could indicate tumour of pituitary or hypothalamus).
Otherwise, they should see a doctor within a few weeks if:
- They are not pregnant and have missed 3 menstrual periods.
- They have fewer than 9 periods a year.
- The pattern of periods suddenly changes.

Western Medicine Relevant Diseases:
In Western medicine, menstrual periods are regulated by a complex hormonal system. Each month, this system produces hormones in a certain sequence to prepare the body for pregnancy. When there is no pregnancy, the sequence ends with the uterus shedding it's lining, producing a menstrual period. The hormones are produced by the hypothalamus, the pituitary gland (luteinizing hormone and follicle-stimulating hormone), and the ovaries, which produce estrogen and progesterone. Other hormones, such as thyroid hormones and prolactin (produced by the pituitary gland), can affect the menstrual cycle.

The most common reason for no menstrual periods is a malfunction of any part of this hormonal system. Less commonly, the hormonal system is functioning normally, but another problem prevents periods from occurring. For example, menstrual bleeding may not occur because the uterus is scarred or because a birth defect, fibroid, or polyp blocks the flow of menstrual blood out of the vagina.

The disorders that cause primary amenorrhea are relatively uncommon, but the most common are:
- A genetic disorder (e.g. Turner syndrome – only in girls and is when an x chromosome is missing)
- A birth defect of the reproductive organs that blocks the flow of menstrual blood

The most common causes of secondary amenorrhea are:

The hypothalamus may malfunction for several reasons:
- Stress or excessive exercise (as done by competitive athletes, particularly women who participate in sports that involve maintaining a low body weight)
- Poor nutrition (as may occur in women who have an eating disorder or who have lost a significant amount of weight)
- Mental disorders (such as depression or obsessive-compulsive disorder)
- Radiation therapy or an injury

The pituitary gland may malfunction because:
- It is damaged.
- Levels of prolactin are high, as may result from a pituitary tumor.

The thyroid gland may cause amenorrhea due to either hypothyroidism or hyperthyroidism.

Less common causes of secondary amenorrhea include chronic disorders (particularly of the lungs, digestive tract, blood kidneys, or liver), some autoimmune disorders, cancer, HIV infection, radiation therapy, head injuries, a hydatidiform mole (overgrowth of tissue from the placenta), Cushing's syndrome, and malfunction of the adrenal glands. Scarring of the uterus (usually due to an infection or surgery), polyps, and fibroids can also cause secondary amenorrhea.

(red flags and above from: http://www.merckmanuals.com/home/women-s-health-issues/menstrual-disorders-and-abnormal-vaginal-bleeding/absence-of-menstrual-periods)

Etiology and Pathogenesis:
- Emotional stress – Liver Qi stagnation – Blood stasis – obstructs uterus – Penetrating Vessel Qi cannot flow to produce menses
- Excessive physical work or exercise – weaken Spleen – Spleen fails to make Blood
- Hereditary weakness, too many children with births close together, or overwork – deficiency of Kidney Essence and Liver Blood – emptiness of Penetrating and Directing Vessels
- Diet – poor nourishment leads to depletion of Qi and Blood
- Overwork – deficiency of Liver and Kidney Yin
- Poor diet or Spleen deficiency – lead to dampness that obstructs the Uterus so Blood cannot flow

TCM Differentiation and Treatment:

Pattern	Signs and Symptoms	Treatment Principle	Acupuncture	Formula
Liver and Kidney Deficiency	Often primary amenorrhea, or may develop from scanty where the menstrual discharge gradually decreases; accompanying symptoms: weak constitution, low backache, weak legs, dizziness, vertigo, tinnitus, depression, mentally tired. T: pale P: deep, weak	Tonify Kidneys, nourish Liver, regulate periods	BL18 (gan shu), BL23 (shen shu), BL52 (zhi shi), REN4 (guan yuan), REN6 (qi hai), LU7-KD6 (ren mai), LR8 (qu quan), SP6 (SYJ), ST36 (ZSL)	
Qi and Blood Deficiency	Menstruation gradually stops after several months of decreasing periods with light and pale discharge of menstrual blood, dizziness, poor vision, numbness and tingling, poor memory, insomnia, palpitations, anxiety, depression, dull complexion, dry skin, dry hair, dry eyes, fatigue. T: pale P: weak, choppy, or fine	Nourish Blood, tonify Qi, regulate menstruation	REN4 (guan yuan), BL20 (pi shu), ST36 (ZSL), SP6 (SYJ), SP10 (xue hai), BL17 (ge shu), BL18 (gan shu)	
Yin Deficiency	Gradual decrease in menstrual discharge until menstruation no longer occurs, five center heat, flushed cheeks, dry mouth and throat, night sweating, bone steaming fever, dry cough. T: red with little coat	Nourish Yin, clear heat, regulate periods	LU7-KD6 (ren mai), BL18 (gan shu), BL23 (shen shu), BL17 (ge shu), SP6 (SYJ), KD2 (ran gu), LR2 (xing jian), LR8 (qu quan)	

	P: rapid, thready			
Qi Stagnation and Blood Stasis	Secondary amenorrhea, irritability, moodiness, ABD distension and pain, depression, dark complexion. T: purple P: wiry	Soothe Liver, move Qi and Blood	SP4-PC6 (chong mai), REN6 (qi hai), ST30 (qi chong), LR3 (tai chong), SP6 (SYJ), KD6 (zhao hai), SP10 (xue hai)	
Phlegm Damp	Secondary amenorrhea, prolonged cycle gradually developing to no periods, obesity, vaginal discharge, lassitude, feeling of heaviness, chest oppression, nausea. T: swollen, greasy coat P: slippery	Resolve Dampness, move Qi, resolve Phlegm, restore periods	SP6 (SYJ), SP9 (yin ling quan), ST28 (shui dao), REN6 (qi hai), GB41-SJ5 (dai mai), REN9 (shui fen), ST40 (feng long), SP8 (di ji), ST36 (ZSL)	

Bleeding during pregnancy, unstable pregnancy (tai lou, tai dong bu an)

Definition:
Tai lou refers to slight, intermittent uterine bleeding during pregnancy. *Tai dong bu an* refers to frequent fetal movement, ABD pain, bearing down sensations, and possible slight vaginal bleeding. Both conditions warn of possible miscarriage.

Red Flags:

Western Medicine Relevant Diseases:
During the first 20 weeks of pregnancy, 20 to 30% of women have vaginal bleeding. In about half of these women, the pregnancy ends in a miscarriage. The amount of bleeding can range from spots of blood to a massive amount. Passing large amounts of blood is always a concern, but spotting or mild bleeding may also indicate a serious disorder.

The most common cause of vaginal bleeding during early pregnancy is miscarriage. There are different degrees of miscarriage. A miscarriage may be possible (threatened abortion) or certain to occur (inevitable abortion). All of the contents of the uterus (fetus and placenta) may be expelled (complete abortion) or not (incomplete abortion). The contents of the uterus may be infected before, during, or after the miscarriage (septic abortion). The fetus may die in the uterus and remain there (missed abortion). Any type of miscarriage can cause vaginal bleeding during early pregnancy.

The most dangerous cause of vaginal bleeding is ectopic pregnancy. Another possibly dangerous, but less common cause is rupture of a corpus luteum cyst. After an egg is released, the structure that released it (the corpus luteum) may fill with fluid or blood instead of breaking down and disappearing as it usually does. If an ectopic pregnancy or a corpus luteum cyst ruptures, bleeding may be profuse, leading to shock.

During late pregnancy (after 20 weeks), 3 to 4% of women have vaginal bleeding. Such women are at risk of losing the baby or of hemorrhaging. Sometimes so much blood is lost that blood pressure becomes dangerously low (causing shock) or small blood clots form throughout the bloodstream (called disseminated intravascular coagulation).

The most common cause of bleeding during late pregnancy is the start of labor. Usually, labor starts with a small discharge of blood mixed with mucus from the vagina. This discharge, called the bloody show, occurs when small veins are torn as the cervix begins to dilate, enabling the fetus to pass through the vagina. The amount of blood in the discharge is small.

More serious but less common causes include:

In placental abruption, the placenta detaches from the uterus too soon. What causes this detachment is unclear, but it may occur because blood flow to the placenta is inadequate. Sometimes the placenta detaches after an injury. Placental abruption is the most common life-threatening cause of bleeding during late pregnancy.

In placenta previa, the placenta is attached to the lower rather than the upper part of the uterus. When the placenta is lower in the uterus, it may partly or completely block the cervix. Bleeding may occur without warning, or it may be triggered when a practitioner examines the cervix.

In vasa previa, the blood vessels that provide blood to the fetus (through the umbilical cord) grow across the cervix, blocking the fetus's passageway. When labor starts, these small blood vessels may be torn, depriving the fetus of blood. Because the fetus has a relatively small amount of blood, loss of even a small amount can be serious, and the fetus may die.

Rupture of the uterus may occur during labor. It almost always occurs in women whose uterus has been damaged and contains scar tissue. Such damage may occur during a cesarean delivery or surgery or result from an infection or a severe abdominal injury.

Bleeding may also result from disorders unrelated to pregnancy.

(From http://www.merckmanuals.com/home/women-s-health-issues/symptoms-during-pregnancy/introduction-to-symptoms-during-pregnancy)

Etiology and Pathogenesis:
- Overwork, excessive physical work – weakens Kidney Yin or Kidney Yang – may lead to weakening of the Directing and Penetrating Vessels
- Chronic illness, or poor diet – a long chronic illness or a diet lacking in nourishment – may lead to Qi and Blood deficiency, failing to nourish the fetus
- Emotional issues – worry, anger, frustration may lead to Liver Qi stagnation – may turn to Liver Fire and Blood Heat (could also be caused by a diet of spicy foods and alcohol, or warm febrile disease)
- Trauma - may injure the Directing and Penetrating Vessels

TCM Differentiation and Treatment:

Pattern	Signs and Symptoms	Treatment Principle	Acupuncture	Formula
Kidney Deficiency	Threatened miscarriage in early pregnancy, lumbar soreness, scanty vaginal bleeding, dizziness, tinnitus, vertigo, exhaustion, bearing down sensation, frequent urination. T: pale P: deep, weak	Tonify Kidney, boost Qi, calm the fetus	BL23 (shen shu), KD3 (tai xi), DU4 (ming men), DU20 (bai hui), BL20 (pi shu), ST36 (ZSL), KD5 (shui quan)	
Qi and Blood Deficiency	Threatened miscarriage, scanty vaginal bleeding that is thin and pale, tiredness, weakness, pale complexion, palpitations, SOB. T: pale P: weak	Tonify and raise Qi, nourish Blood, consolidate Directing and Penetrating Vessels, calm the fetus	ST36 (ZSL), REN12 (zhong wan), BL20 (pi shu), BL17 (ge shu), BL18 (gan shu), BL23 (shen shu), LR8 (qu quan)	
Blood Heat	Threatened miscarriage early in the term, scanty vaginal bleeding that is bright red, feeling of heat, thirst, mental restlessness, insomnia, dark urine. T: red with yellow coat P: rapid, overflowing	Clear heat, cool Blood, calm the fetus	LR2 (xing jian), LI11 (qu chi), SP10 (xue hai), BL17 (ge shu), SP1 (yin bai), KD2 (ran gu), LR3 (tai chong)	
Traumatic Injury	Threatened miscarriage following a fall or trauma, ABD pain, scanty vaginal bleeding.	Tonify Qi, harmonize Blood, consolidate Directing and Penetrating Vessels, calm the fetus	DU20 (bai hui), REN12 (zhong wan), PC6 (nei guan), SP10 (xue hai), - LU7-KI6 (ren mai), DU3 (yao tang guan), DU20 (bai hui), REN12 (zhong wan)	

Dysmenorrhea (tong jing)

Definition:
A disorder characterized by cramping pains in the lower abdomen preceding, during or following menstruation. Pain may extend to the lower back and sacral region, and may cause nausea, vomiting, or even fainting.

Red Flags:
The following findings merit referral:
- Unremitting pain
- Fever
- Evidence of peritonitis (chills, fever, abd. tenderness/distension, extreme thirst, fluid in abdomen, decresed urine/BM, vomit)

Western Medicine Relevant Diseases:
In Western medicine, dysmenorrhea is uterine pain around the time of menses. Pain may occur with menses or precede menses by 1 to 3 days. Pain tends to peak 24 hours after onset of menses and subside after 2 to 3 days. It is usually sharp but may be cramping, throbbing, or a dull, constant ache; it may radiate to the legs. Headache, nausea, constipation or diarrhea, lower back pain, and urinary frequency are common; vomiting occurs occasionally.

Dysmenorrhea can be primary (more common) or secondary (due to pelvic abnormalities).

Primary dysmenorrhea:
Symptoms cannot be explained by structural gynecologic disorders. Pain is thought to result from uterine contractions and ischemia, probably mediated by prostaglandins and other inflammatory mediators produced in secretory endometrium and possibly associated with prolonged uterine contractions and decreased blood flow to the myometrium.

Contributing factors may include the following:
- Passage of menstrual tissue through the cervix
- A narrow cervix
- A malpositioned uterus
- Lack of exercise
- Anxiety about menses

Primary dysmenorrhea begins within a year after menarche. The pain usually begins when menses start (or just before) and persists for the first 1 to 2 days; this pain, described as spasmodic, is superimposed over constant lower abdominal pain, which may radiate to the back or thighs. Patients may also experience malaise, fatigue, nausea, vomiting, diarrhea, low back pain, or headache.

Risk factors for severe symptoms include: early age at menarche, long or heavy menstrual periods, smoking, or a family history of dysmenorrhea. Symptoms tend to lessen with age and after pregnancy.

Secondary dysmenorrheal:
Symptoms are due to pelvic abnormalities. Almost any abnormality or process that can affect the pelvic viscera can cause dysmenorrhea.

Common causes include: endometriosis, uterine adenomyosis, and fibroids. Less common causes include congenital malformations, ovarian cysts and tumors, pelvic inflammatory disease, pelvic congestion, intrauterine adhesions, psychogenic pain, and intrauterine devices (IUDs).

(from http://www.merckmanuals.com/professional/gynecology-and-obstetrics/menstrual-abnormalities/dysmenorrhea)

Etiology and Pathogenesis:
- Emotional strain – anger, frustration, resentment – may lead to Liver Qi stagnation – causes Blood to stagnate in uterus (or may turn to Liver Fire and Blood Heat)
- Cold and dampness – excessive exposure to cold and dampness – may cause cold to invade the uterus – cold contracts and causes Blood stasis
- Overwork, chronic illness – leads to deficiency of Qi and Blood – malnourishment of Penetrating and Directing vessels
- Excessive sexual activity, childbirth – weakens Liver and Kidneys – leads to emptiness of Penetrating and Directing vessels so that they cannot move Qi and Blood

TCM Differentiation and Treatment:

Pattern	Signs and Symptoms	Treatment Principle	Acupuncture	Formula
	Cold and pain of the lower ABD, either before or during menstruation; pain worse with pressure, better with heat; scanty menstrual discharge that is dark and may contain blood clots; aversion to cold, possible body aches and pain. T: white coat (possibly greasy) P: deep, tight	Warm the vessels, clear cold and dampness, move Qi and Blood, relieve pain	ST28 (shui dao), ST29 (gui lai), SP8 (di ji), REN3 (zhong ji), BL32 (ci liao), SP6 (SYJ), SP9 (yin ling quan), ST40 (feng long)	
	Distending pain in lower ABD before or during menstruation, pain worse with pressure, period may be hesitant to start, distension in hypochondriac region/breasts, irritability; if more Qi stagnation, then bloating and distension; if more Blood stagnation, sharper pain, relieved when clots move out. T: sides may be red P: wiry, or choppy	Soothe Liver, move Qi and Blood, dispel stagnation, relieve pain	SP4-PC6 (chong mai), REN6 (qi hai), LR3-LI4 (4 gates), GB34 (yang ling wuan), KD13 (qi xue), ST29 (gui lai), SP8 (di ji), SP10 (xue hai)	
	Lower ABD pain before menstruation, worse with pressure, possible burning or distending pain in low back/sacrum, menstrual discharge thick and dark red, thick yellowish leucorrhea, concentrated urine, possible mild fever. T: red with greasy yellow coat P: rapid, slippery	Clear heat, resolve damp, stop pain	SP6 (SYJ), REN3 (zhong ji), BL32 (ci liao), BL22 (san jiao shu), ST40 (feng long), SP9 (yin ling quan), ST28 (shui dao), SP8 (di ji), LI11 (qu chi), LR5 (li gou)	
	Dull, achy lower ABD pain either during or following menstruation, pain better with pressure, empty bearing down sensation in the lower ABD, scanty menstrual discharge that is light in color and thin in texture, tiredness, fatigue, dull complexion, loss of appetite or diarrhea. T: pale P: weak	Tonify Qi, nourish Blood, relieve pain	SP6 (SYJ), ST36 (ZSL), REN4 (guan yuan), REN6 (qi hai), BL20 (pi shu), BL32 (ci liao)	
	Cold and pain of lower ABD either during or following menstruation, pain better with heat and pressure, small volume of dark menstrual discharge, weak aching lower back and knees, copious clear urine. T: white, moist coat P: deep	Warm channels and uterus, supplement Yang, stop pain	BL23 (shen shu), REN4 (guan yuan), REN6 (qi hai), ST36 (ZSL), SP6 (SYJ), REN3 (zhong ji), SP8 (di ji), BL32 (ci liao)	
	Achy, dull lower ABD pain either before or following menstruation, better with pressure, thin light-colored menstrual discharge, sore low back, general fatigue, dizziness, and possible tidal fever. T: pale (or narrow, red if KD Yin Xu) P: weak, thready	Tonify Liver and Kidney, relieve pain	BL18 (gan shu), BL23 (shen shu), REN4 (guan yuan), ST36 (ZSL), LU7-KI6 (ren mai), BL32 (ci liao)	

Infertility (bu yun)

Definition:
Refers to women of childbearing age who have normal sexual activity, are not using contraception, have a male partner with normal reproductive function, and who have been trying to conceive for at least 2 years, but have not become pregnant. Primary infertility means that the woman has never conceived. Secondary infertility means that the woman has had a previous pregnancy. Infertility from congenital abnormalities is not included.

Red Flags:
- Refer for Western medical assessment

Western Medicine Relevant Condition:
In Western medicine, infertility is usually defined as the inability of a couple to conceive after 1 yr of unprotected intercourse. Frequent, unprotected intercourse results in conception for 50% of couples within 3 mos, for 75% within 6 mos, and for 90% within 1 yr.

Infertility in women can be caused by:
- Decreased ovarian reserve or ovulatory dysfunction
- Tubal dysfunction and pelvic lesions
- Abnormal cervical mucus
- Unidentified factors

Couples wishing to conceive are encouraged to have frequent intercourse when conception is most likely—during the 6 days, and particularly the 3 days before ovulation.

(from http://www.merckmanuals.com/professional/gynecology-and-obstetrics/infertility/overview-of-infertility)

TCM Differentiation and Treatment:

Pattern	Signs and Symptoms	Treatment Principle	Acupuncture	Formula
Kidney Yang Deficiency	Prolonged menstrual cycles, period may be scanty or heavy, backache, dizziness, feel cold, depression, frequent urination. T: pale, swollen, wet P: deep, weak	Tonify and warm Kidney Yang, strengthen the uterus	KD13 (qi xue), KD3 (tai xi), BL23 (shen shu), BL52 (zhi shi), REN4 (guan yuan), DU4 (ming men), LU7-KD6 (ren mai), REN8 (shen que), SP6 (SYJ), ST36 (ZSL), zi gong xue	
Kidney Yin Deficiency	Long-term infertility, periods early, scanty, blood, 5-palm heat, night sweating, dizziness, tinnitus. T: red without coat P: rapid, thready	Nourish Kidney Yin and Essence	REN 4 (guan yuan), BL23 (shen shu), KD2 (ran gu), KD3 (tai xi), SP6 (SYJ), zi gong xue, LU7-KD6 (ren mai)	
Liver Stagnation	Irregular periods, pre-menstrual tension, painful periods, breast distension, irritability. T: slightly red sides P: wiry	Move Qi, soothe Liver, eliminate stagnation, regulate periods	LR3 (tai chong), GB34 (yang ling quan), SJ6 (zhi gou), PC6 (nei guan), REN6 (qi hai), REN4 (guan yuan), KD14 (si man), SP4-PC6 (chong mai)	
Cold in Uterus	Primary infertility, delayed cycle, scanty period, small clots, painful period, better with heat, feel cold during period, pale face, sore back. T: pale, thick white coat P: weak, tight	Warm and tonify Kidney Yang, warm uterus, scatter cold	REN2 (qu gu), REN4 (guan yuan), DU4 (ming men), KD7 (fu liu), BL23 (shen shu), DU4 (ming men)	
Obstruction of Phlegm-Damp	Inability to conceive, overweight, prolonged menstrual cycles, possible amenorrhea, thick sticky vaginal discharge, pale complexion, dizziness, nausea. T: white greasy coat P: slippery	Drain damp, dissolve phlegm, move Qi, regulate menstruation	REN3 (zhong ji), SP6 (SYJ), ST40 (feng long), BL20 (pi shu), zi gong xue, BL32 (ci liao), SP9 (yin ling quan)	
Blood Stasis	Irregular, painful periods, dark clotted blood, irritability, mental restlessness, pain worse on palpation. T: dark purple P: wiry or choppy	Invigorate Blood, eliminate stasis, regulate menstruation	REN3 (zhong ji), SP6 (SYJ), SP10 (xue hai), BL17 (ge shu), LR3 (tai chong), SP8 (di ji), ST30 (qi chong), zi gong xue, SP4-PC6 (chong mai)	

Insufficient breastmilk (que ru)

Definition:
Refers to patterns with decreased secretion of milk after childbirth.

Red Flags:
- Refer to breast feeding specialist if mother is considering stopping breast feeding in early days due to apparent breast milk insufficiency
- Refer immediately if signs of dehydration in infant

Western Medicine Relevant Condition:
Difficulties in supplying milk to the infant are most commonly related to the irregular or incomplete removal of milk. In the human mammary gland, lactation is under autocrine control, in which the frequency and degree of milk removal appears to regulate an inhibitory peptide present in the milk. In other words, if the milk is not removed, this inhibitory peptide accumulates and subsequently decreases the synthesis of milk. If the milk is frequently removed, this inhibitory peptide does not accumulate, and milk synthesis increases.

Because the milk supply is directly related to its removal and ongoing synthesis, factors that hinder milk removal affect milk production. Factors that could disrupt the complete removal of milk are numerous. For example, stress and fatigue in both parents may have an impact on the mother's milk production.

Examples of primary lactation failure include conditions in the mother such as anatomic breast abnormalities or hormonal aberrations. Insufficient mammary glandular tissue, postpartum hemorrhage with Sheehan syndrome (often after high labu blood loss – hypopituitarism), theca-lutein cyst (type of ovarian cyst), polycystic ovarian syndrome, and some breast surgeries have been implicated as possible causes of lactation failure.

(from http://www.medscape.com/viewarticle/565620_4 and http://www.merckmanuals.com/professional/pediatrics/care-of-newborns-and-infants/breastfeeding)

Etiology and Pathogenesis:
- Excessive blood loss during childbirth – leads to depletion of Qi and Blood – insufficient Qi to express the breast milk and insufficient Blood to transform into milk
- Post-partum emotional disturbances – cause Liver Qi stagnation – obstructs channels and flow of milk

TCM Differentiation and Treatment:

Pattern	Signs and Symptoms	Treatment Principle	Acupuncture	Formula
Qi and Blood Deficiency	Insufficient or absent lactation after childbirth, watery milk, no feeling of distension in the breasts, sallow complexion, dry skin, poor appetite, tiredness. T: pale P: weak	Tonify Qi and Blood, promote lactation		
Liver Qi Stagnation	Absent or scanty lactation, distension, hardness and pain of breasts, hypochondrial distension, irritability, epigastric distension. T: red on sides P: wiry	Soothe Liver, eliminate stagnation, move Qi, promote lactation		

Inter-menstrual Bleeding

Definition:
Menstrual bleeding that occurs consistently at about the mid-point of the menstrual cycle (approximately 12-16 days). May last 2-3 days or longer, and may be spotting or like a small period. Slight one-sided lower abdominal pain is also possible.

Red Flags:

Western Medicine Relevant Condition:
Western medicine categorizes inter-menstrual bleeding as abnormal uterine bleeding (AUB). AUB is bleeding that, after examination and ultrasonography, cannot be attributed to the usual causes (structural gynecologic abnormalities, cancer, inflammation, systemic disorders, pregnancy, complications of pregnancy, use of oral contraceptives or certain drugs). Bleeding may be anovulatory or ovulatory.

During an anovulatory cycle, the corpus luteum does not form. Thus, the normal cyclical secretion of **progesterone** does not occur, and estrogen stimulates the endometrium unopposed. Without **progesterone**, the endometrium continues to proliferate, eventually outgrowing its blood supply; it then sloughs incompletely and bleeds irregularly and sometimes profusely or for a long time. When this abnormal process occurs repeatedly, the endometrium can become hyperplastic, sometimes with atypical or cancerous cells.

In ovulatory AUB, **progesterone** secretion is prolonged; irregular shedding of the endometrium results, probably because estrogen levels remain low, near the threshold for bleeding (as occurs during menses). In obese women, ovulatory AUB can occur if estrogen levels are high, resulting in amenorrhea alternating with irregular or prolonged bleeding.

Anovulation is most often:
- Secondary to polycystic ovary syndrome
- Idiopathic (sometimes occurring when gonadotropin levels are normal)
- Sometimes anovulation results from hypothyroidism.

During perimenopause, AUB may be an early sign of ovarian insufficiency or failure; follicles are still developing but, despite increasing levels of follicle-stimulating hormone (FSH), do not produce enough estrogen to trigger ovulation.

Ovulatory AUB may occur in:
- Polycystic ovary syndrome
- Endometriosis, which does not affect ovulation

Other causes are a short follicular phase and luteal phase dysfunction (due to inadequate **progesterone** stimulation of the endometrium); a rapid decrease in estrogen before ovulation can cause spotting.

(from http://www.merckmanuals.com/professional/gynecology-and-obstetrics/menstrual-abnormalities/dysfunctional-uterine-bleeding-dub)

Etiology and Pathogenesis:
- Overwork, too many children too close together injures Liver and Kidney Yin – may lead to Empty Heat which agitates the Blood
- Irregular diet – excessive consumption of greasy foods or dairy – weakens Spleen and leads to Damp – mixes with Heat
- Traumas, abdominal operations, post-partum stasis of blood – stasis of Blood leads to obstruction – new Blood that is formed has no place to go and leaks out
- Excessive physical exercise – weakens Spleen and Kidney Yang – Qi cannot hold Blood

TCM Differentiation and Treatment:

Pattern	Signs and Symptoms	Treatment Principle	Acupuncture	Formula
Liver and Kidney Yin Deficiency	Bleeding is scanty, scarlet red without clots, no ABD pain, dizziness, tinnitus, night-sweating, backache, dark urine. T: red without coat P: fine, rapid	Nourish Yin, Tonify Liver and Kidneys, clear heat, stop bleeding	LU7-KD6 (ren mai), REN4 (guan yuan), REN7 (yin jiao), KD5 (shui quan), LI11 (qu chi), SP10 (xue hai), SP8 (di ji)	
Damp Heat	Bleeding may be heavy or scanty, sticky viscous blood, no clots, fatigue, sore joints, chest oppression, poor appetite, vaginal discharge. T: sticky yellow coat P: slippery	Clear damp heat, stop bleeding	SP6 (SYJ), SP9 (yin ling quan), REN9 (shui fen), REN3 (zhong ji), GB4--SJ5, (dai mai), SP1 (yin bai), ST28 (shui dao), SP8 (di ji)	
Blood Stasis	Bleeding may be scanty or profuse, dark blood with clots, ABD pain, mental restlessness. T: purple P: wiry	Move Qi and Blood, eliminate stasis, stop bleeding	SP4-PC6 (chong mai), REN6 (qi hai), ST29 (gui lai), SP10 (xue hai), KD14 (si man), BL17 (ge shu), SP6 (SYJ), SP1 (yin bai)	
Spleen and Kidney Yang Deficiency	Bleeding may be scanty or profuse, pale blood without clots, no ABD pain, dizziness, tinnitus, backache, loose stools, tiredness, depression, feel cold, frequent urination. T: pale, swollen P: weak, deep	Strengthen Spleen and Kidneys, tonify Yang, warm Uterus, contain Blood	BL20 (pi shu), BL23 (shen shu), REN4 (guan yuan), REN6 (qi hai), REN12 (zhong wan), ST36 (ZSL), SP6 (SYJ), SP8 (di ji)	

Irregular menstruation (yue jing bu tiao)

Definition:
Refers to periods that come at an irregular cycle, sometimes early and sometimes late. Specifically, the period must come over 7 days earlier or later than usual, more than 3 times in succession. The duration of the period remains normal. (Note: does not include *Beng Lou*)

Red Flags:
- Refer for Western medical assessment

Western Medicine Relevant Condition:
The hormonal interactions that control menstruation occur in the following sequence:

Di

Hormones produced by other glands such as the adrenal glands and the thyroid gland, can affect the functioning of the ovaries and menstruation.

Patterns of irregular menstruation may involve disturbances in this cycle. See also Abnormal Uterine Bleeding (Inter-menstrual bleeding).

Etiology and Pathogenesis:
- Emotional stress – Liver Qi stagnation – obstructs Directing and Penetrating Vessels – also, Blood stagnates and Sea of Blood cannot fill the uterus
- Overwork, too many children too close together – leads to Kidney deficiency – Sea of Blood cannot fill the uterus

TCM Differentiation and Treatment:

Pattern	Signs and Symptoms	Treatment Principle	Acupuncture	Formula
Liver Qi Stagnation	Irregular periods, often with scanty bleeding, some clots, ABD and breast distension, pre-menstrual tension, depression, sighing, irritability. T: may be slightly red sides P: wiry	Soothe Liver, move Qi, eliminate stagnation, regulate periods	LR3 (tai chong), SJ6 (zhi gou), PC6 (nei guan), LR14 (qi men), REN4 (guan yuan), REN6 (qi hai), SP4 (gong sun)	
Kidney Yang Deficiency	Irregular periods that are scanty with pale blood, no clots, backache, dizziness, tinnitus, feel cold. T: pale and swollen P: weak, deep	Tonify and warm Kidneys, regulate periods	BL23 (shen shu), REN4 (guan yuan), KD3 (tai xi), LU7-KD6 (ren mai), ST36 (ZSL), SP6 (SYJ)	

Leukorrhagia (dai xia)

Definition:
Includes discharge that is excessive, or has changes in color, texture, and odor. Slight vaginal discharge that increases in volume and viscosity at mid-cycle is normal.

Red Flags:
- Fever, pelvic pain
- Irregular pattern of bloody discharge (or change in color of discharge), volume, or smell (possible STD)
- Vaginal discharge after menopause

Western Medicine Relevant Condition:
Vaginal itching (pruritus), discharge, or both result from infectious or noninfectious inflammation of the vaginal mucosa (vaginitis), often with inflammation of the vulva (vulvovaginitis). Symptoms may also include irritation, burning, erythema, and sometimes dysuria and dyspareunia. Symptoms of vaginitis are one of the most common gynecologic complaints.

Some vaginal discharge is normal, particularly when estrogen levels are high. However, irritation, burning, and pruritus are never normal.

Normally in women of reproductive age, *Lactobacillus* sp is the predominant constituent of normal vaginal flora. Colonization by these bacteria keeps vaginal pH in the normal range (3.8 to 4.2), thereby preventing overgrowth of pathogenic bacteria. Also, high estrogen levels maintain vaginal thickness, bolstering local defenses.

Factors that predispose to overgrowth of bacterial vaginal pathogens include:
- Use of antibiotics (which may decrease lactobacilli)
- Alkaline vaginal pH due to menstrual blood, semen, or a decrease in lactobacilli
- Poor hygiene
- Frequent douching
- Diabetes mellitus
- An intravaginal foreign object

Vaginitis usually involves infection with GI tract flora (nonspecific vulvovaginitis). Vaginitis is usually infectious. The most common types are: bacterial vaginosis, candidal vaginitis, trichomonal vaginitis. Sometimes another infection (such as an STD) causes a discharge. These infections often also cause pelvic inflammatory disease. Vaginitis may also result from foreign bodies (e.g. a forgotten tampon). Inflammatory non-infectious vaginitis is uncommon.

Other causes of discharge include cancers and, in women who are incontinent or bedbound, and vulvitis.

Conditions that predispose to vaginal or vulvar infection include
- Fistulas between the intestine and genital tract (which allow intestinal flora to seed the genital tract)
- Pelvic radiation or tumors (which break down tissue and thus compromise normal host defenses)

Noninfectious vulvitis accounts for up to 30% of vulvovaginitis cases. It may result from hypersensitivity or irritant reactions to various agents, including hygiene sprays or perfumes, menstrual pads, laundry soaps, bleaches, fabric softeners, and sometimes spermicides, vaginal creams or lubricants, latex condoms, vaginal contraceptive rings, and diaphragms.

(from http://www.merckmanuals.com/professional/gynecology-and-obstetrics/symptoms-of-gynecologic-disorders/vaginal-itching-and-discharge)

Etiology and Pathogenesis:
- Irregular diet, excessive physical work – excessive consumption of dairy foods, greasy foods and sugar may lead to Damp infusing downward; excessive physical work weakens the Spleen which fails to transform and transport leading to Damp accumulation
- Emotional strain leads to Liver Qi stagnation – Liver invades Spleen and impairs transformation and transportation leading to damp
- Overwork leads to Liver and Kidney Yin deficiency – weakness of Directing and Girdle Vessels which cannot hold Yin fluids
- Invasion of external Damp – settles in genital system

TCM Differentiation and Treatment:

Pattern	Signs and Symptoms	Treatment Principle	Acupuncture	Formula
	Excess vaginal discharge that is white or slightly yellow, sticky, without smell, and persistent; dull complexion, tiredness, depression, cold limbs, loose stools. T: pale P: weak, slippery	Tonify Spleen Qi, raise Yang, resolve damp	REN12 (zhong wan), ST36 (ZSL), SP3 (tai bai), SP6 (SYJ), SP9 (yin ling quan), BL22 (san jiao shu), DU20 (bai hui), REN6 (qi hai)	
	Profuse, white, dilute vaginal discharge; dizziness, tiredness, backache, frequent urination, feel cold. T: pale and wet P: deep, weak	Tonify and warm Kidneys, stop discharge	BL23 (shen shu), REN4 (guan yuan), KD13 (qi xue), ST36 (ZSL), SP6 (SYJ), KD3 (tai xi), DU20 (bai hui)	
	White vaginal discharge that is dilute and odorless, dizziness, tinnitus, 5-palm heat, feeling of heat in the evening. T: red without coat P: floating empty	Nourish Yin, tonify Kidneys, clear heat, stop discharge	REN4 (guan yuan) KD13 (qi xue), LU7-KD6 (ren mai), SP6 (SYJ), KD3 (tai xi), DU20 (bai hui)	
	Profuse yellow or brown discharge that is sticky, foul odor, loose stools. T: sticky yellow coat P: slippery	Clear heat, drain damp	GB41 (zu lin qi), SJ5 (wei guan), REN3 (zhong ji), REN2 (qu gu), GB26 (dai mai), SP9 (yin ling quan), SP6 (SYJ), BL32 (ci liao)	

Lochiorrhea (chan hou e lu bu jue)

Definition:
Refers to postpartum patterns where the vaginal discharge of the lochia continues for a period of more than 20 days after delivery and continues to be red, rather than changing to a yellow, serous discharge.

Red Flags:
- Refer for Western medical assessment to rule out infection

Western Medicine Relevant Condition:
Lochia refers to the bloody discharge from the placental site. For the first 3-4 days after delivery, the lochia is red. Its color then becomes lighter and eventually serous. The final lochia discharge is mostly white blood cells. Lochia that remains red and abundant for longer than normal indicates delayed involution of the uterus, which may be due to retention of a piece of placenta within the uterus, or to infection.

Etiology and Pathogenesis:
- Pre-existing Qi deficiency of mother, loss of blood and consumption of Qi during childbirth, or lack of sufficient post-natal rest and recuperation – lead to Qi deficiency and Qi not holding blood
- Yin deficiency, internal heat, invasion of heat, or stagnation of Liver Qi turning to heat – Chong and Ren may be damaged by heat – blood escapes the Vessels
- Following childbirth – uterine network vessels are subject to blood stasis and internal obstruction (from e.g. invasion by cold, or retention of placenta) – blood flowing outside the vessels may lead to continuous discharge of lochia

TCM Differentiation and Treatment:

Pattern	Signs and Symptoms	Treatment Principle	Acupuncture	Formula
Qi Deficiency	Continuous discharge of large volume of light red thin odorless lochia, bearing down sensation in lower ABD, tiredness, fatigue, dislike speaking, pale complexion. T: pale P: weak	Supplement Qi, contain Blood		
Blood Stasis	Dribbling discharge of small volume of dark lochia with blood clots, pain in lower ABD, worse with pressure. T: dark purple P: wiry, deep, or choppy	Move Qi and Blood, resolve stasis, stop lochiorrhea		
Blood Heat	Discharge of large volume of red, thick, foul smelling lochia, flushed complexion, dry mouth and throat. T: red P: rapid	Clear heat, nourish yin, stop lochiorrhea		

Menstrual breast aching (jing xing ru fang zhang tong)

Definition:
Refers to breast distension and aching before, during, or after the period. This can vary from mild to severe, with swelling, hardness and pain.

Red Flags:
- Refer for Western medical assessment if nodules or masses do not disappear after menstrual cycle, or if there are signs of breast infection

Western Medicine Relevant Condition:
In Western medicine, menstrual breast aching is attributed to changes in hormones during the menstrual cycle. Changes in the levels estrogen and progesterone can cause breast pain. Levels of these hormones increase just before or during a menstrual period and during pregnancy. When these levels increase, they cause the milk glands and ducts of the breasts to enlarge and the breasts to retain fluid. The breasts then become swollen and sometimes painful. Such pain is usually felt throughout the breasts, making them tender to touch. Pain related to the menstrual period may come and go for months or years.

See "breast lump" in external medicine section for other causes of breast pain with masses.

Etiology and Pathogenesis:
- Emotional stress – Liver Qi stagnation – stagnant Liver Qi invades the Stomach – this affects the breast because the Liver channel influences the nipple and the Stomach channel the breast
- Overwork, too many children – cause Liver and Kidney Yin deficiency – breast vessels cannot be nourished

TCM Differentiation and Treatment:

Pattern	Signs and Symptoms	Treatment Principle	Acupuncture	Formula
	Breast distension, aching, and pain before or during period, irritability, depression, sighing, chest oppression. T: thin white coat, or red sides of tongue P: wiry	Soothe Liver, move Qi, release constraint and stop pain	LR14 (qi men), ST18 (ru gen), LR3 (tai chong), SJ6 (zhi gou), GB21 (jian jing), GB34 (yang ling quan), PC6 (nei guan)	
	Breast distension and discomfort late in period or after period, malar flush, mental restlessness, insomnia, 5 palm heat, dry eyes/throat/mouth, night sweating. T: red, peeled coat P: thin, rapid	Nourish Kidney and Liver, nourish Yin, clear heat, stop pain	LU7-KD6 (ren mai), REN4 (guan yuan), REN7 (yin jiao), KD3 (tai xi), SP6 (SYJ), LR3 (tai chong), KD2 (ran gu), REN17 (dan zhong), ST18 (ru gen)	

Menstrual edema (jing xing fu zhong)

Definition:
Edema related to the menstrual cycle may affect the face, hands, lower legs and abdomen. It usually occurs before the period.

Red Flags:
- Refer in cases of edema that do not diminish following the menstrual cycle
- See red flags for edema in internal medicine

Western Medicine Relevant Condition:
Western medicine attributes menstrual edema to hormonal changes in the body, in particular a reduction in levels of progesterone that may cause fluid retention.

Etiology and Pathogenesis:
- Excessive physical work – weakens the Spleen and may affect the Kidneys – deficient Spleen and Kidney Yang fails to transform, transport and excrete fluids which accumulate causing edema
- Emotional stress – leads to stagnation of Liver Qi – if Liver Qi does not flow freely, it fails to promote Qi and fluids moving freely all over the body

TCM Differentiation and Treatment:

Pattern	Signs and Symptoms	Treatment Principle	Acupuncture	Formula
Spleen and Kidney Yang deficiency	Edema before or during the period, backache, tiredness, loose stools, chilliness, heavy period. T: pale, swollen P: deep, weak	Tonify Kidneys and Spleen, warm Yang, transform fluids		
Qi Stagnation	Swelling and edema before the period of the ABD, breasts, hands or ankles, irritability, pre-menstrual tension. T: red sides P: wiry	Move fluids, move Qi, soothe Liver		

Menstrual headache (jing xing tou tong)

Definition:
Headaches that are linked to menstrual cycle and may occur before, during or after the period.

Red Flags:
- See red flags of headache in internal medicine

Western Medicine Relevant Condition:
Western medicine attributes menstrual headaches to hormonal changes in the body, in particular the drop in estrogen just before the menstrual cycle begins.

Etiology and Pathogenesis:
- Excessive physical work or sports – may injure the Spleen and lead to Qi and Blood deficiency – Blood deficiency is aggravated after the period because of the relative stage of emptiness of the Penetrating Vessel
- Emotional stress – may lead to Liver Qi stagnation which may turn to Fire – Fire flares upward (even more so during periods, when the Qi of the Penetrating Vessel may rebel upwards); or, Liver Qi stagnation turns to Liver Blood Stasis

TCM Differentiation and Treatment:

Pattern	Signs and Symptoms	Treatment Principle	Acupuncture	Formula
	Dull H/A on the vertex during or after the period, dizziness, palpitations, insomnia, blurred vision, tiredness, dull complexion. T: pale P: choppy or fine	Nourish Blood	LU7-KD6 (ren mai) OR SP4-PC6 (chong mai), REN4, (guan yuan) ST36 (ZSL), SP6 (SYJ), LR8 (qu quan), BL20 (pi shu), BL18 (gan shu)	
	Severe throbbing H/A in the temples, eyes, or side of head before or during period, heavy flow, dizziness, bitter taste, thirst, dry signs, red eyes, tinnitus, irritability. T: red with yellow coat P: wiry	Clear Liver, drain fire, nourish Yin, subdue wind	LR2 (xing jian), GB43 (xia xi), LI4-LR3 (4 gates), LI11 (qu chi), SJ5 (wei guan), KD3 (tai xi), SP6 (SYJ)	
	Stabbing H/A before period in temples, eyes, or sides of head, dark menstrual blood with clots, painful periods, ABD pain. T: purple P: wiry or choppy	Invigorate Blood, resolve stasis	SP4-PC6 (chong mai), SP10 (xue hai), BL17 (ge shu), ST29 (gui lai), SP6 (SYJ), KD14 (si man), LR3 (tai chong), DU20 (bai hui)	

Menstrual hematemesis and epistaxis (jing xing tu niu)

Definition:
Epistaxis or hematemesis may occur before, during or after the period. These symptoms are usually associated with Qi rebelling upward and are strongly related to a Penetrating Vessel pathology.

Red Flags:
- Refer for severe epistaxis or hematemesis to rule out any potentially serious underlying conditions, such as gastrointestinal bleeding
- Refer for emergency care if bleeding is serious or there are signs of shock

Western Medicine Relevant Condition:
From a Western perspective, these symptoms may indicate endometriosis, but they may also occur in the absence of such a disease.

In endometriosis, functioning endometrial tissue is implanted in the pelvis outside the uterine cavity. Endometriosis is usually confined to the peritoneal or serosal surfaces of pelvic organs, commonly the ovaries, broad ligaments, posterior cul-de-sac, and uterosacral ligaments. Less common sites include the fallopian tubes, serosal surfaces of the small and large intestines, ureters, bladder, vagina, cervix, surgical scars, and, more rarely, the lung, pleura, and pericardium.

Bleeding from peritoneal implants is thought to initiate sterile inflammation, followed by fibrin deposition, adhesion formation, and, eventually, scarring, which distorts peritoneal surfaces of organs, leading to pain and distorted pelvic anatomy.

The most widely accepted hypothesis for the pathophysiology of endometriosis is that endometrial cells are transported from the uterine cavity during menstruation and subsequently become implanted at ectopic sites. Retrograde flow of menstrual tissue through the fallopian tubes is common and could transport endometrial cells intra-abdominally; the lymphatic or circulatory system could transport endometrial cells to distant sites (e.g., the pleural cavity).

Symptoms include dysmenorrheal, dyspareunia, masses and infertility. Interstitial cystitis with suprapubic or pelvic pain, urinary frequency, and urge incontinence is common. Intermenstrual bleeding is possible.

Symptoms can vary depending on location of implants.
- Large intestine: Pain during defecation, abdominal bloating, diarrhea or constipation, or rectal bleeding during menses
- Bladder: Dysuria, hematuria, suprapubic or pelvic pain (particularly during urination), urinary frequency, urge incontinence, or a combination
- Ovaries: Formation of an endometrioma (a 2- to 10-cm cystic mass localized to an ovary), which occasionally ruptures or leaks, causing acute abdominal pain and peritoneal signs
- Adnexal structures: Formation of adnexal adhesions, resulting in a pelvic mass or pain
- Extrapelvic structures: Vague abdominal pain (sometimes)

(from http://www.merckmanuals.com/professional/gynecology-and-obstetrics/endometriosis/endometriosis)

Etiology and Pathogenesis:
- Emotional stress – may cause Liver Qi to stagnate – leads to Liver Fire – if Qi rebels upward due to a Penetrating Vessel pathology, it carries Fire with it and Fire agitates Blood
- Overwork, stress, constitutional deficiency, or chronic illness – weaken both Lung and Kidney Yin – Yin deficiency gives rise to Empty Heat – this rises during menstruation due to exuberance of the Penetrating Vessel -- may damage the Lung

TCM Differentiation and Treatment:

Pattern	Signs and Symptoms	Treatment Principle	Acupuncture	Formula
Liver Qi Stagnation turned to Fire	Hematemesis or epistaxis before or during period, heavy period, red face, irritability, premenstrual tension, feeling of heat, red eyes, thirst. T: red sides P: wiry and rapid	Clear the Liver, drain Fire, subdue rebellious Qi, stop bleeding		
Lung and Kidney Yin Deficiency	Hematemesis or epistaxis during or after period, scanty period, dry throat, dry cough, night-sweating, dizziness, tinnitus, 5 palm heat, irregular periods. T: red without coat P: fine, rapid	Nourish Yin, nourish Lungs, cool Blood, clear empty heat, stop bleeding		

Menstrual mental disorder (jing xing qing zhi yi chang)

Definition:
Includes the emotional and physical symptoms occurring before a period. These may include: depression, sadness, irritability, anxiety, lethargy, aggressiveness, cravings, crying, and outbursts of anger. The symptoms can vary from mild to serious.

Red Flags:
- See red flags of depression in internal medicine section

Western Medicine Relevant Condition:
In Western medicine, these patterns correspond to premenstrual syndrome (PMS). PMS is characterized by irritability, anxiety, depression, edema, breast pain, and headaches, occurring during the 7 to 10 days before and usually ending a few hours after onset of menses. The cause is unclear.

Possible causes or contributing factors include:
- Multiple endocrine factors (e.g., hypoglycemia, other changes in carbohydrate metabolism, hyperprolactinemia, fluctuations in levels of circulating estrogen and progesterone, abnormal responses to estrogen and progesterone, excess aldosterone or ADH). Estrogen and progesterone can cause transitory fluid retention, as can excess aldosterone or ADH.
- A genetic predisposition.
- Serotonin deficiency. Serotonin deficiency is thought to contribute because women who are most affected by PMS have lower serotonin levels and because SSRIs (which increase serotonin) sometimes relieve symptoms of PMS.
- Possibly magnesium and calcium deficiencies.

Type and intensity of symptoms vary widely. The most common symptoms are irritability, anxiety, agitation, anger, insomnia, difficulty concentrating, lethargy, depression, and severe fatigue. Fluid retention causes edema, transient weight gain, and breast fullness and pain. Pelvic heaviness or pressure and backache may occur. Some women have dysmenorrhea.

Other nonspecific symptoms may include headache, vertigo, paresthesias of the extremities, syncope, palpitations, constipation, nausea, vomiting, and changes in appetite. Acne and neurodermatitis may also occur. Existing skin disorders may worsen, as may respiratory problems (e.g., allergies, infection) and eye problems (e.g., visual disturbances, conjunctivitis).

Some women have severe PMS symptoms that occur regularly and only during the 2nd half of the menstrual cycle; symptoms end with menses or shortly after. Mood is markedly depressed, and anxiety, irritability, and emotional instability are pronounced. Suicidal thoughts may be present. Interest in daily activities is greatly decreased. This is called Premenstrual Dysphoric Disorder (PMDD). In contrast to PMS, **PMDD** causes symptoms that are severe enough to interfere with routine daily activities or overall functioning. PMDD is a severely distressing, disabling, and often under-diagnosed.

(from http://www.merckmanuals.com/professional/gynecology-and-obstetrics/menstrual-abnormalities/premenstrual-syndrome-pms)

TCM Differentiation and Treatment:

Pattern	Signs and Symptoms	Treatment Principle	Acupuncture	Formula
Liver Qi Stagnation	ABD and breast distension, irritability, clumsiness, moodiness, depression, hypochondrial pain and distension. T: in chronic cases, sides may be red P: wiry	Soothe the Liver, eliminate stagnation, calm the mind	LR3 (tai chong), LI4 (he gu), GB34 (yang ling quan), GB41 (zu lin qi), SP6 (SYJ), SJ6 (zhi gou), PC6 (nei guan)	
Phlegm Fire Harassing Upwards	Agitation, depression, slightly manic behavior, aggressiveness, chest oppression, red face, blood shot eyes. T: red with sticky yellow coat P: slippery rapid	Clear heat, resolve phlegm, calm the mind	PC7 (da ling), ST40 (feng long), LI11 (qu chi), SP9 (yin ling quan), SP4-PC6 (chong mai), REN12, (zhong wan) BL20 (pi shu), PC5 (jian shi)	
Liver and Kidney Yin Deficiency	Slight breast distension, irritability, sore back and knees, dizziness, blurred vision, poor memory, insomnia, dry eyes and throat, 5 palm heat. T: red without coat P: fine, rapid	Nourish Liver and Kidney Yin, move Liver Qi	LR8 (qu quan), REN4 (guan yuan), SP6 (SYJ), LR3 (tai chong), BL18 (gan shu), BL23 (shen shu)	

Menstrual oral ulcer (jing xing kou mei)

Definition:
The appearance of mouth and/or tongue ulcers at period time.

Western Medicine Relevant Condition:
Due to the hormonal changes (particularly the increase in progesterone) that occur during the menstrual cycle, some women experience oral changes that can include bright red swollen gums, swollen salivary glands, development of canker sores, or bleeding gums.

(from http://www.webmd.com/oral-health/hormones-oral-health#1)

Etiology and Pathogenesis:
- Overwork, too many children too close – leads to Kidney Yin deficiency – may lead to empty heat which rises to the mouth and tongue producing ulcers
- Irregular diet – too much hot-spicy and greasy food causes formation of Damp Heat in the Stomach – during period time, rebellious Qi of the Penetrating Vessel may rise up and Stomach Fire or Damp heat will ascend with it

TCM Differentiation and Treatment:

Pattern	Signs and Symptoms	Treatment Principle	Acupuncture	Formula
	Tongue ulcers during or after the period, 5-palm heat, night-sweating, feeling heat in the evening, dizziness, tinnitus, dry mouth. T: red without coat P: fine, rapid	Nourish Kidney Yin, clear Empty Heat	KD3 (tai xi), REN4 (guan yuan), LU7-KD6, (ren mai) HT5 (tong li), KD2 (ran gu)	
	Mouth ulcers during or before period, foul breath, thirst, dry stools, irritability. T: red with yellow coat P: rapid	Clear heat, drain fire	ST44 (nei ting), LI11 (qi chi), LI4, (he gu) SP4-PC6 (chong mai), ST25 (tian shu)	

Metrorrhagia and metrostaxis (beng lou)

Definition:
Beng means flooding, and indicates a period that starts with a sudden flood, often before the regular time. *Lou* means trickling, and indicates a period that continues to trickle after proper time. *Beng lou* should be distinguished from heavy periods, which are defined as heavy blood loss during proper period time of 5-7 days, with periods at regular intervals.

Red Flags:
- Refer for Western medical evaluation to rule out more serious conditions, particularly organic disorders
- Refer for emergency care if there are signs of hemorrhagic shock
- Refer for premenarchal and postmenopausal vaginal bleeding

Western Medicine Relevant Conditions:
In Western medicine, menorrhagia means menses that are excessive and metrorrhagia means bleeding occurring irregularly between menses. Menorrhagia and metrorrhagia could be due to a wide range of conditions.

Most abnormal vaginal bleeding involves:
- Hormonal abnormalities in the hypothalamic-pituitary-ovarian axis
- Structural, inflammatory, or other gynecologic disorders (e.g., tumors)
- Bleeding disorders (uncommon)

Hormonal abnormalities include: thyroid and adrenal gland dysfunction, pituitary tumors, anovulatory cycles, PCOS, obesity, and vasculature imbalance.

Structural gynecologic disorders include: myomas, cancer (e.g. of cervix or uterus), endometrial hyperplasia, endometriosis, fibroids, and polyps.

Other gynecological disorders include: vaginitis, cervicitis, foreign body in the vagina, injury of the cervix or vagina.

(from http://emedicine.medscape.com/article/255540-overview#a9 and http://www.merckmanuals.com/professional/gynecology-and-obstetrics/symptoms-of-gynecologic-disorders/vaginal-bleeding)

Etiology and Pathogenesis:
- Emotional strain – leads to stagnation of Qi and this may turn to Fire – Fire affects Liver Blood and may cause Blood Heat – makes Blood reckless and causes it to burst from vessels; emotional strain may also cause Qi stagnation that leads to Blood Stasis – prevents new blood from taking its place and new blood leaks out
- Overwork and excessive sexual activity – weaken Liver and Kidney Yin – give rise to Empty Heat that makes the blood run reckless
- Physical overwork, chronic illness – weaken the Spleen which fails to control Blood
- Childbirth – post partum blood stasis, or invasion of cold or heat

TCM Differentiation and Treatment:
*Treatment note: stop bleeding; treat root cause of bleeding; and then work on restoring organ health.

Pattern	Signs and Symptoms	Treatment Principle	Acupuncture	Formula
	Uterine bleeding with thick, deep red discharge, flushed complexion, irritable, dry mouth, thirst, dark urine, constipation. T: red, yellow coat P: forceful, rapid	Clear Heat, cool Blood, stop bleeding.	SP1 (yin bai), SP6 (SYJ), SP10 (xue hai), LI11 (qu chi), SP4-PC6 (chong mai)	
	Uterine bleeding with dark discharge containing clots, lower ABD pain worse with pressure and better when clots move out, ABD distension, dark complexion; period may be hesitant, starting and stopping. T: dark, possible stasis macules P: choppy, wiry	Move Blood, eliminate stasis, stop bleeding.	SP4-PC6 (chong mai), LR3 (tai chong), SJ6 (zhi gou), LR1 (shang yang), SP8 (yi ji), ST30 (qi chong), SP10 (xue hai), SP1 (yin bai)	
	Uterine bleeding with thin, light colored discharge, pale complexion, fatigue, SOB, loss of appetite, loose stools, possible chilliness. T: pale, swollen P: deep, weak	Tonify Spleen Qi to hold Blood, nourish Blood, regulate period	REN4 (guan yuan), REN6 (qi hai), DU20 (bai hui), ST36 (ZSL), SP6 (SYJ), BL20 (pi shu), SP1 (yin bai)	
	Trickling of blood after period time, late cycle, fresh red and watery blood, dizziness, tinnitus, weak knees, feeling of heat in evening, night sweats, hot flashes, malar flush, restlessness. T: red without coat P: rapid, thready	Nourish Yin, strengthen Kidneys, stop bleeding	REN6 (qi hai), BL23 (shen shu), REN4 (guan yuan), KD3 (tai xi), ST36 (ZSL), SP6 (SYJ), KD2 (ran gu), KD13 (qi xue), LU7-KD6 (ren mai)	
	Prolonged bleeding with a trickle for a long time after the proper period, periods coming late, blood pale, feel cold, sore back, cold limbs, pale complexion, weak knees, pale urine. T: pale and swollen P: deep and weak	Tonify and warm Kidneys, consolidate Directing and Penetrating Vessels, stop bleeding	REN6 (qi hai), BL23 (shen shu), REN4 (guan yuan), ST30 (qi chong), KD7 (fu liu), ST36 (ZSL), SP6 (SYJ), KD13 (qi xue)	

Miscarriage (zhui tai, xiao chan, hua tai)
(see also bleeding during pregnancy, unstable pregnancy)

Definition:
In TCM, habitual miscarriage usually means that miscarriage has occurred on at least three occasions.

Western Medicine Relevant Condition:
Working with Western medical professionals is recommended. Determining the cause of habitual miscarriage may require extensive medical evaluation of both partners.

Causes of recurrent pregnancy loss may be maternal, fetal, or placental.

Common maternal causes include:

Placental causes include pre-existing chronic disorders that are poorly controlled (e.g. chronic hypertension).

Fetal causes are usually:
- Chromosomal or genetic abnormalities
- Anatomic malformations

(from http://www.merckmanuals.com/professional/gynecology-and-obstetrics/abnormalities-of-pregnancy/spontaneous-abortion)

Etiology and Pathogenesis:
- Most common underlying cause is Kidney deficiency, or other related factors, such as Spleen deficiency, Penetrating and Directing vessels not being firm, and Qi sinking.
- Etiology should consider whether due to fetus or mother:
    - Due to the fetus: weak original Qi from parents to old or ill while conceiving, so fetus cannot develop
    - Due to mother: many factors possible, including e.g. weak constitution, weak Kidneys, excess sex, emotional problems, warm disease, accident or trauma, emotional shock, or drugs.

TCM Differentiation and Treatment:

Treatment note: Prevention is key. Before pregnancy, focus on building constitution and treating any underlying conditions (this may take up to 1 year). During pregnancy, focus on calming the fetus.

Pattern	Signs and Symptoms	Treatment Principle	Acupuncture	Formula
Kidney Yang Deficiency	Hx of miscarriages early in pregnancy, backache, depression, feeling cold, cold feet, frequent pale urination, history of infertility. T: pale P: deep, weak	Tonify and warm the Kidneys, warm the Uterus, consolidate Penetrating and Directing Vessels	BL20 (pi shu), BL23 (shen shu), DU20 (bai hui), REN6 (qi hai), DU4 (ming men), KD3 (tai xi), ST36 (ZSL), jing gong	
Kidney Yin Deficiency	Hx of miscarriages early in pregnancy, history of infertility, dizziness, tinnitus, night sweating, backache, malar flush. T: red without coat P: floating empty	Nourish Kidney Yin, nourish Blood, consolidate Penetrating and Directing Vessels	KD3 (tai xi), LU7-KD6 (ren mai), REN7 (yin jiao), REN6 (qi hai), DU20 (bai hui), ST36 (ZSL), DU4 (ming men), BL23 (shen shu)	
Spleen Qi Deficiency	Hx of miscarriages, tiredness, loose stools, depression, poor appetite. T: pale P: weak	Tonify Spleen, raise Qi, consolidate Directing Vessel.	DU20 (bai hui), REN6 (qi hai), REN12 (zhong wan), ST36 (ZSL), SP6 (SYJ), KD3 (tai xi), BL23 (shen shu), BL20 (pi shu)	
Blood Deficiency	Hx of miscarriages, dizziness, blurred vision, Hx of scanty periods, insomnia, depression, dry hair and skin, tingling of limbs. T: pale and thin P: choppy or fine	Nourish Blood, nourish Kidneys, consolidate Directing Vessel	LU7-KD6 (ren mai) OR SP4-PC6 (chong mai, LR8 (qu quan), BL18 (gan shu), BL20 (pi shu), BL23 (shen shu), BL17 (ge shu), ST36 (ZSL), SP6 (SYJ), DU20 (bai hui), REN6 (qi hai)	

Morning Sickness (ren chen e zu)

Definition:
Morning sickness refers to patterns of nausea and vomiting during pregnancy. Other symptoms include dizziness, and aversion to food. This may be an early sign of pregnancy, although not all women experience it. It ranges from mild nausea to severe vomiting and may last for the first three months or the entire pregnancy. It can occur at any time of day.

Red Flags:

Western Medicine Relevant Condition:
The pathophysiology of nausea and vomiting during early pregnancy is unknown, although metabolic, endocrine, GI, and psychological factors probably all play a role. Estrogen may contribute because estrogen levels are elevated in patients with hyperemesis gravidarum. Hyperemesis gravidarum is persistent, severe pregnancy-induced vomiting that causes significant dehydration, often with electrolyte abnormalities, ketosis, and weight loss.

Etiology and Pathogenesis:
- Spleen and Stomach deficiency – during pregnancy, Qi and Blood accumulate in the Chong-Ren to nourish the fetus – Chong Ren more easily rebels – weak Spleen and Stomach cannot control this (SP Xu could also lead to formation of Phlegm aggravating nausea)
- Liver Qi stagnation – less Blood in Liver during pregnancy – Liver Qi becomes stronger + increased stress leads to Liver Qi stagnation – Liver may attack Spleen and Stomach

TCM Differentiation and Treatment:

Pattern	Signs and Symptoms	Treatment Principle	Acupuncture	Formula
Spleen and Stomach deficiency	Nausea and vomiting, or vomiting undigested food or clear mucus, bland sense of taste, fullness and distension of epigastrium and ABD, tiredness. T: pale, moist coat P: slippery	Fortify Spleen, control rebellion, stop vomit	ST36 (ZSL), REN12 (zhong wan), SP4-PC6 (zhong mai), PC6 (nei guan)	
Liver and Stomach disharmony	Vomiting of acid or bitter fluids, fullness of chest, costal pain, belching, frequent sighing, distended sensation of the head, dizziness, depression, thirst, bitter taste. T: slightly yellow coat P: wiry, slippery	Soothe Liver, harmonize Stomach, control rebellion, stop vomit	PC6, (nei guan) LR3 (tai chong), ST36 (ZSL), REN12 (zhong wan), REN17 (dan zhong), GB34 (yang ling quan)	

Perimenopausal syndrome (jue jing qian hou zhu zheng)

Definition:
Refers to patterns occurring just prior to or following the onset of menopause in women. Symptoms are numerous and include: hot flashes marked by flushed complexion and sweating, dizziness, blurred vision, tinnitus, palpitations, insomnia, and irritability. In more severe cases, there can be depression and anxiety.

Red Flags:
- Western medical evaluation is recommended to rule out any organic diseases

Western Medicine Relevant Condition:
Menopause is the term given to the changes that occur in women around the age of 50, when the ovaries cease to respond to follicle stimulating hormone and luteinizing hormone, resulting in a lack of ovulation, cessation of the menstrual cycle, and declining estrogen and progesterone levels. Perimenopause refers to the several years (duration varies greatly) before and the first year after the last menses. It is typically the most symptomatic phase.

The decreased levels of hormones lead to changes such as thinning of the mucosa, loss of elasticity, and decreased glandular secretions in the vagina and cervix. The changes in hormone levels in the early stage of menopause frequently lead to systemic signs such as periodic sweating, headaches, irritability, and insomnia.

Neuropsychiatric changes (e.g., poor concentration, memory loss, depressive symptoms, anxiety) may also accompany menopause. Recurrent night sweats can contribute to insomnia, fatigue, irritability, and poor concentration by disrupting sleep.

(from http://www.merckmanuals.com/professional/gynecology-and-obstetrics/menopause/menopause)

Etiology and Pathogenesis:
These patterns are fundamentally due to a decline of Kidney Essence, which can take the form of Kidney Yin deficiency, Kidney Yang deficiency, or a combination of both.
- Emotional stress – worry, anxiety and fear weaken the Kidneys and lead to Yin deficiency – Kidney Yin fails to nourish Heart Yin and both may lead to empty heat
- Overwork, too many children too close together – may lead to Kidney Yin deficiency

TCM Differentiation and Treatment:

Pattern	Signs and Symptoms	Treatment Principle	Acupuncture	Formula
	Dizziness, tinnitus, malar flush, night sweating, hot flashes, 5 palm heat, sore back, dry mouth, dry hair, dry skin, itching, constipation. T: red without coat P: floating empty or fine rapid	Nourish Kidney Yin, clear empty heat, calm the mind	LU7-KD6 (ren mai), KD3 (tai xi), KD10 (yin gu), REN4 (guan yuan), SP6 (SYJ), HT6 (yin xi), KD7 (fu liu), LI4 (he gu)	
	Hot flashes but cold hands and feet, night sweating in the early morning, pale face, depression, chilliness, backache, edema of ankles. T: pale P: fine, deep	Tonify and warm the Kidneys, tonify Yang, strengthen the Spleen	BL23 (shen shu), BL52 (zhi shi), KD3 (tai xhi), LU7-KD6 (ren mai) OR SI3-BL62 (du mai), REN6 (qi hai) REN15 ((jiu wei), KD7 (fu liu)	
	Hot flashes, palpitations, insomnia, night sweating, blurred vision, dizziness, tinnitus, anxiety, mental restlessness, backache, malar flush, feeling of heat in the evening, dry mouth, dry throat, poor memory, dry stools. T: red body, redder tip P: rapid fine or floating empty	Nourish Kidney Yin, calm the mind, clear empty heat	LU7-KD6 (ren mai), KD3 (tai xi), REN4 (guan yuan), SP6 (SYJ), KD13 (qi xue), HT6 (yin xi), KD7 (fu liu), HT8 (shao fu), PC7 (da ling), REN15 (jiu wei), DU24 (shen ting)	

Postpartum abdominal pain (chan hou fu tong)

Definition:
Refers to post-partum abdominal pains that may occur during 6 weeks after delivery.

Red Flags:
- Refer if there are signs of post-partum infection, such as severe or worsening pain and high fever.

Western Medicine Relevant Condition:
Western Medicine attributes most postpartum abdominal pain to uterine contractions or infection.

For approximately 2 weeks after delivery, the uterus will contract. These contractions are irregular and often painful. Contractions are intensified by breastfeeding. Breastfeeding triggers the production of the hormone **oxytocin that** stimulates the flow of milk and uterine contractions. Normally, after 5 to 7 days, the uterus is firm and no longer tender but is still somewhat enlarged, extending to halfway between the pubic bone and the navel. By 2 weeks after delivery, the uterus returns to close to its normal size.

Postpartum infections may be:
- Directly related to delivery (occurring in the uterus or the area around the uterus)
- Indirectly related to delivery (occurring in e.g. the kidneys or bladder)

Etiology and Pathogenesis:
- Excessive blood loss during childbirth – leads to Blood deficiency and loss of nourishment, and possible Blood stasis
- Exposure to cold (blood is deficient after labor and cold can easily invade), irregular diet – may create internal Cold which could also lead to Blood stasis
- Emotional stress – leads to stagnation of Qi, which can cause ABD pain – and, may also lead to Blood stasis
- Post partum retention of blood – stagnates and forms Blood stasis

TCM Differentiation and Treatment:

Pattern	Signs and Symptoms	Treatment Principle	Acupuncture	Formula
	Dull ABD pain after childbirth, better with pressure, scanty uterine bleeding that is pale in color, dizziness, vertigo, tiredness, blurred vision, constipation, dry skin. T: pale P: choppy	Tonify Qi, nourish Blood, stop pain	REN6 (qi hai), REN4 (guan yuan), ST36 (ZSL), SP6 (SYJ), LR8 (qu quan), BL17 (ge shu)	
	Cold pain in lower ABD, worse with pressure, better with warmth, pale and possible clotted discharge of lochia. T: dull, dark P: deep, tight	Warm Yang, unblock constriction and relieve pain	REN4 (guan yuan), REN6 (qi hai), BL23 (shen shu), DU4 (ming men), BL32 (ci liao)	
	ABD pain after childbirth that is worse with pressure, discharge of dark and clotted lochia, possible masses in lower ABD, dark complexion. T: purple P: choppy, wiry	Move Qi and Blood, resolve stasis, stop pain	SP4-PC6 (chong mai), ST30 (qi chong), KD14 (si man), SP10 (xue hai), BL17 (ge shu), SP6 (SYJ), LR3 (tai chong), ST29 (gui lai)	

Postpartum convulsion (chan hou jing zheng)

Definition:
Convulsions after childbirth are characterized by rigidity of the spine, tremors of the limbs, lockjaw, and opisthotonus.

Red Flags:
- Emergency care required
- Lockjaw, opisthotonos, sweating with cold limbs, and weak breathing are all signs of very serious and life-threatening condition

Western Medicine Relevant Condition:
In Western medicine, these patterns correspond to tetanus infection, which is now a rare occurrence after childbirth. In the past, tetanus was caused by poor hygienic conditions during and after delivery.

(Maciocia, *Obstetrics and Gynecology in Chinese Medicine*)

Etiology and Pathogenesis:

TCM Differentiation and Treatment:

Pattern	Signs and Symptoms	Treatment Principle	Acupuncture	Formula
Blood and Yin Deficiency with Empty Wind	Profuse loss of blood during childbirth, tremor of limbs, rigidity of spine, pale complexion or malar flush. T: no coat P: choppy or floating empty	Nourish Blood and Yin, extinguish wind	LR8 (qu quan), BL18 (gan shu), KD3 (tai xi), SP6 (SYJ), REN4 (guan yuan)	
Exterior invasion of Toxin	Shivering and fever soon after childbirth, headache, stiff neck, rigidity of spine, lockjaw, convulsions, opisthotonos in severe cases. T: red with yellow coat P: wiry, full	Resolve toxin, drain fire, extinguish wind	LI11 (qu chi), SP10, (xue hai) LR3 (tai chong), LR2 (xing jian), DU16 (feng fu), GB20 (feng chi), DU8 (jin suo), DU14 (da zhui), SP9 (yin ling quan)	

Postpartum dizziness (chan hou xue yun)

Definition:

Red Flags:
- Acute condition requires emergency medical care

Western Medicine Relevant Condition:
In Western medicine, these patterns correspond to either shock following hemorrhage or to septic shock following an infection. Both conditions require emergency medical care and specialized treatment.

(Maciocia, *Obstetrics and Gynecology in Chinese Medicine*)

Etiology and Pathogenesis:
- Excessive blood loss during delivery or constitutional Qi and Blood deficiency – Qi and Blood fail to nourish the Heart – collapse
- Cold attack during delivery causes Qi blockage/stasis – Qi rises and disturbs the heart

TCM Differentiation and Treatment:

Pattern	Signs and Symptoms	Treatment Principle	Acupuncture	Formula
Deficiency pattern – Collapse of Qi with deficiency of Blood (flaccid syndrome)	Excessive blood loss during/following delivery, acute onset vertigo, dizziness, blurred vision, pale complexion, palpitations, restlessness, cold extremities, cold sweat, possible loss of consciousness. T: pale P: empty	Supplement Qi and Blood, rescue collapse	DU20 (bai hui), DU26 (shui gou), SP6 (SYJ), ST36 (ZSL), REN4 (guan yuan), REN6 (qi hai), REN8 (shen que) moxa	
Excess pattern – Blood Stasis (tense syndrome)	Retention of lochia or passage of small amount of lochia after childbirth, lower ABD pain worse with pressure, discomfort in chest, rapid breathing, possible loss of consciousness, clenched fists, trismus, dark complexion, purple lips. T: purple P: choppy	Move Qi and Blood, rescue collapse	DU20 (bai hui), DU26 (shen ting), SP6 (SYJ), SP10 (xue hai), BL17 (ge shu), SP4 (gong sun)	

Postpartum fever (chan hou fa re)

Definition:
Refers to fever during the 6 weeks after delivery that does not abate on its own and which is accompanied by other symptoms and signs. This may be a mild fever with slight chills, or one that is very high. Slight fever one or two days after childbirth with no other symptoms disappears gradually over a few days is often normal and may not indicate any pathology. Also, a slight fever that appears 3-4 days after childbirth and in between breastfeeding is not pathological and should disappear within a few days.

Red Flags:
- Refer for cases of persistent or worsening fever during the postpartum period to rule out infection

Western Medicine Relevant Condition:
Fever in the postpartum period is a relatively common occurrence. In Western medicine, postpartum fever is defined as a temperature of 38.7 degrees C (101.6 degrees F) or greater for the first 24 hours or greater than 38.0 degrees C (100.4 degrees F) on any two of the first 10 days postpartum.

The most common cause of postpartum fever is endometritis, which is inflammation in the lining of the uterus, in this case from infection. Given that the source of the infections is both from the genitourinary tract as well as from the skin flora, the infection is usually polymicrobial, requiring the administration of antibiotics.

Other significant causes of postpartum fever include urinary tract infection/pyelonephritis, surgical wound infection (e.g. in the case of surgical delivery), septic thrombophlebitis and mastitis.

(from http://www.medscape.com/viewarticle/804263)

Etiology and Pathogenesis:

TCM Differentiation and Treatment:

Pattern	Signs and Symptoms	Treatment Principle	Acupuncture	Formula
Invasion of External Toxins	High fever and chills, pain in lower ABD, worse with pressure, profuse or scanty lochia that is dark in color with a foul smell, dysphoria, thirst, scanty urine, constipation; in severe cases, convulsions. T: red, yellow coat P: rapid, forceful	Clear heat, drain toxin, cool blood, eliminate stasis	LI11 (qu chi), PC3 (qu ze), KD2 (ran gu), LR3 (tai chong), SP9 (yin ling quan), DU14 (bai hui), Shi Xuan	
Invasion of external Wind	Fever, aversion to cold, H/A, body aches; either cold signs (e.g. no sweating, floating tight pulse), or heat signs (e.g. yellow nasal discharge, sweating, floating rapid pulse).	Nourish Blood, expel Wind Cold or Wind Heat, release exterior	LU7 (ie que), LI4 (he gu), SJ5 (wei guan), LU11 (shao shang), DU14 (bai hui), BL12 (feng men), BL17 (ge shu)	
Blood Stasis	Fever after childbirth, feeling of heat, dark discharge with clots, lower ABD pain worse with pressure, dry mouth. T: reddish purple P: wiry, choppy	Nourish Blood, eliminate stasis	KD14 (si man), ST29 (gui lai), SP6 (SYJ), SP10 (xue hai), SP4-PC6 (chong mai), BL17, (ge shu) LR3 (tai chong), LI11 (qu chi)	
Blood Deficiency	Continuous low grade fever after childbirth, sweating, blurred vision, dizziness, exhaustion, palpitations, insomnia, malar flush, tingling limbs. T: pale P: choppy	Tonify Qi, nourish Blood, subdue floating Yang	REN12 (zhong wan), ST36 (ZSL), SP6 (SYJ), REN4 (guan yuan), LR8 (qu quan), BL17 (ge shu), SJ5 (wei guan)	

Postpartum retention of urine (chan hou pai niao yi chang)

Definition:
Refers to difficulty in urination or retention of urine after childbirth. These are urinary problems without fever or pain (i.e. without a urinary infection).

Red Flags:

Western Medicine Relevant Condition:
The pathophysiology of postpartum urinary retention is not clearly understood but various mechanisms have been suggested:

The bladder is a hormone-responsive organ and its functions may be subject to the fluctuation of hormones during pregnancy and in the postpartum period. The postpartum bladder is hypotonic, remaining so for a number of days post delivery. Pregnancy causes reduced muscle tone in the bladder from the third month with the bladder gradually increasing in capacity as the pregnancy progresses.

This may be as a result of physiological hormonal changes such as elevated progesterone levels during a normal pregnancy. In the absence of the weight of the pregnant uterus limiting the size of the bladder, as well as possible trauma to the bladder, pelvic floor muscles and nerves during delivery, the bladder becomes susceptible to retention.

One of the most common causes of postpartum urinary retention is the use of regional anesthesia due to afferent neural blockade, which suppresses the sensory stimuli from the bladder. As a result, the reflex mechanism that induces micturition is blocked. This may result in reduced contractility of bladder and urinary retention.

Urinary retention may also be the result of nerve injury during delivery. Studies have shown that the pudendal nerve, with afferent nerve branches (S2-4) supplying the bladder, is damaged during pelvic surgery and vaginal delivery.

Another possible explanation of postpartum urinary retention is a transient phenomenon caused by tissue oedema around the urogenital area, resulting in a transient mechanical obstruction to urine outflow. The tissue oedema could be due to a prolonged labor process with compression of the fetal presenting part onto the birth canal or other factors such as instrumental/assisted delivery or extensive vaginal and perineal laceration. Within days of delivery, as the tissue oedema improves, the urinary retention gradually returns to normal.
(from http://www.ogpnews.com/2011/12/post-partum-bladder-care-background-practice-and-complications/444)

Etiology and Pathogenesis:
- Excessive strain during labor taxes Qi and leads to Spleen Qi deficiency. Spleen cannot raise Qi affecting Bladder Qi, which fails to transform and excrete fluids. Excessive strain during labor also taxes Kidneys – deficient Kidney Qi fails to provide Qi to the Bladder to help its function of Qi transformation
- Injury to the Bladder (from prolonged labor or surgical procedures) may give rise to Qi stagnation

TCM Differentiation and Treatment:

Pattern	Signs and Symptoms	Treatment Principle	Acupuncture	Formula
Spleen Qi Deficiency	Slight retention of urine after childbirth, fullness and distension of hypogastrium, tiredness, loose stools, poor appetite, pale complexion, sweating. T: pale P: weak	Tonify Qi, Strengthen Spleen	REN12 (zhong wan), REN6 (qi hai), REN3 (zhong ji), ST36 (ZSL), SP6 (SYJ), BL22 (san jiao shu), BL28 (pang guang shu), DU20 (bai hui), BL20 (pi shu)	
Kidney Qi Deficiency	Retention of urine after childbirth, distension and fullness in hypogastrium, pale complexion, backache, dizziness, tinnitus, feeling cold. T: pale, moist P: deep, weak	Strengthen Kidney Qi, tonify Kidney Yang	BL23 (shen shu), BL28 (pang guang shu), BL22, KD7, REN3 (zhong ji), REN4 (guan yuan), LU7-KD6 (ren mai), DU20 (bai hui), REN8 (shen que)	
Injury to Bladder	History of injury, often blood in urine. P: wiry on left rear position	Western medical care required. As supplement, tonify and firm Qi	Bl28 (pang guang shu), REN3 (zhonj ji), BL32 (ci liao), BL63 (jin men), BL53 (bao huang), DU20 (bai hui)	

Uterine prolapse (yin ting)

Definition:
Prolapse of uterus may happen anytime, but women are especially susceptible after childbirth. Prolapse is due to Spleen or Kidney Qi sinking.

Red Flags:
- Refer for Western medical assessment and support – risk of injury and infection may be high in serious cases; for 3rd and 4th degree conditions, surgery may be necessary

Western Medicine Relevant Condition:
In Western medicine, uterine prolapse is graded based on level of descent:

Symptoms tend to be minimal with 1st-degree uterine prolapse. In 2nd- or 3rd-degree uterine prolapse, fullness, pressure, dyspareunia, and a sensation of organs falling out are common. Lower back pain may develop. Incomplete emptying of the bladder and constipation are possible. Third-degree uterine prolapse manifests as a bulge or protrusion of the cervix or vaginal cuff, although spontaneous reduction may occur before patients present. Vaginal mucosa may become dried, thickened, chronically inflamed, secondarily infected, and ulcerated. Ulcers may be painful or bleed and may resemble vaginal cancer. The cervix, if protruding, may also become ulcerated.

(from http://www.merckmanuals.com/professional/gynecology-and-obstetrics/pelvic-relaxation-syndromes/uterine-and-vaginal-prolapse)

Etiology and Pathogenesis:
Spleen or Kidney deficiency due to the following can easily progress to Qi sinking, which leads to prolapse.
- Long labor with excessive straining
- Too much physical work too early after deliver
- Pregnancies and deliveries too close together

TCM Differentiation and Treatment:

Pattern	Signs and Symptoms	Treatment Principle	Acupuncture	Formula
Spleen Deficiency	Functional prolapse or organic prolapse, heaviness/prolapse sensation, general fatigue, worse with exertion, weakness, possible profuse vaginal discharge.	Tonify Spleen Qi, raise Yang, consolidate organs	DU20 (bai hui), GB28 (wei dao), REN6 (qi hai), SP6 (SYJ), ST36 (ZSL), Ti tuo, Zi gong xue	
Kidney Deficiency	Functional or organic prolapse, heaviness/prolapse sensation, weak and achy back and knees, frequent urination, dry vagina, dizziness, tinnitus. P: deep and weak	Tonify Kidney Qi, consolidate organs	REN4, KD6, DU20, KD12, LR8, Ti tuo, Zi gong	

Pedriatics

Anorexia (yan shi)

Definition:
In TCM, anorexia is a disorder of the Spleen and Stomach that is characterized by prolonged loss of appetite, or refusal to eat. The amount of food intake is less than that of normal children of comparable age. There may be weight loss or poor weight gain, lassitude and tiredness. Anorexia is most common between the ages of one and six years. It begins slowly and has a relatively prolonged course. If it persists for a long time, it may lead to inadequate sources for the generation of Qi and Blood.

Red Flags:
Refer for Western medical evaluation if:

Western Medicine Relevant Conditions:
In Western medicine, childhood anorexia may be attributed to:
- Behavioral issues: an eating problem may develop if a parent or caregiver tries to coerce the child to eat or shows too much concern about the child's appetite or eating habits. The extra attention children with an eating problem receive when parents coax and threaten may inadvertently reward and thus reinforce the child's tendency to refuse eating. Some children may even respond to parental attempts at force-feeding by vomiting.
- Overeating, eating between meals, drinking too much juice, or not exerting enough energy.

Eating disorders, such as anorexia nervosa and bulimia nervosa, typically do not occur until adolescence.

(from http://www.merckmanuals.com/home/children-s-health-issues/behavioral-problems-in-children/eating-problems-in-young-children)

Etiology and Pathogenesis:
The main pathology is impairment of Spleen and Stomach functions of transportation and transformation due to:
- Spleen and Stomach deficiency – either due to weak constitution, or tendency for children to have weak Spleen Qi
- Inadequate feeding – care-givers may lack knowledge of proper nutrition for small children, and may overfeed child excessive amounts of rich or greasy foods, damaging the Spleen and Stomach
- Prolonged illness – any prolonged or serious illness may damage the Spleen and Stomach, impairing their functions

TCM Differentiation and Treatment:

Pattern	Signs and Symptoms	Treatment Principle	Acupuncture	Formula
Spleen Qi Deficiency and Damp	No desire to eat, nausea, chest oppression, full feeling, loose feces or feces with undigested food, sallow or pallid complexion. T: red, thin white coat P: soft, slippery	Tonify Spleen Qi, resolve damp, induce appetite and digestion	REN12 (zhong wan), ST36 (ZSL), SP6 (SYJ), BL20 (pi shu), BL21 (wei shu), REN6 (qi hai), SP9 (yin ling quan)	
Food and Milk Retention	Poor appetite, rejection of food, vomiting of milk or food, sour odor of curdled milk, abdominal distension and discomfort, foul smelling feces. T: coat is thick and greasy P: taut	Promote digestion and eliminate retention	REN12 (zhong wan), ST36 (ZSL), SP6 (SYJ), ST25 (tian shu), REN13 (shang wan)	
Stomach Yin Deficiency	Hunger with no desire to eat, insomnia, constipation, dry skin, dry lips and mouth, hot palms and soles of feet. T: red, cracked, thin, dry P: thin, rapid	Nourish Yin, benefit Stomach, induce appetite and digestion	REN12 (zhong wan), ST36 (ZSL), SP6 (SYJ), BL20 (pi shu), BL21 (wei shu), REN6 (qi hai), KD3 (tai xi), SP4 (gong sun)	
Spleen and Stomach Qi Deficiency	No desire to eat, no desire to speak, lusterless/sallow complexion, emaciation, diarrhea with undigested food. T: swollen, tender, pale P: feeble, slow	Tonify Spleen and Stomach Qi, induce appetite and digestion	REN12 (zhong wan), ST36 (ZSL), SP6 (SYJ), BL20 (pi shu), BL21 (wei shu), REN6 (qi hai)	

Asthma (xiao chuan)

Definition:
Childhood asthma is mainly an allergic disease. It manifests as recurrent bouts of an oppressive feeling of tightness in the chest, wheezing, shortness of breath, coughing, and difficult breathing. During an attack, the child will not be able to calmly rest while lying down, but must sit up to help breathing. In children, there may also be stomach pain associated with an attack.

Red Flags:

Western Medicine Relevant Conditions:
In Western medicine, asthma is a recurring inflammatory lung disorder in which certain triggers (e.g. pollen, mold, smoke, exercise, environmental pollutants) inflame the airways and cause them to temporarily narrow, resulting in difficulty breathing. Although asthma can develop at any age, it most commonly begins in the first 5 years of life.

The pathophysiology of asthma involves:
- Bronchoconstriction
- Airway edema and inflammation
- Airway hyper reactivity
- Airway remodeling

In patients with asthma, certain cells in the airways (e.g. eosinophils and mast cells) release chemical substances. These substances cause the airways to become inflamed and swollen and stimulate the muscle cells in the walls of the airways to contract. Repeated stimulation by these chemical substances increases mucus production in the airways, causes shedding of the cells lining the airways, and enlarges the muscle cells in the walls of the airways. Each of these responses contributes to a sudden narrowing of the airways (an asthma attack). In most children, the airways return to normal between asthma attacks.

It is not completely understood why some children develop asthma, but a number of risk factors are recognized:
- Viral infections
- Inherited and prenatal factors
- Allergen exposure

Etiology and Pathogenesis:
In TCM, asthma is seen as a disease of exterior pathogens triggering latent phlegm trapped in the Lung. Phlegm is the primary etiology, and it results from failure of the Lung to distribute and disseminate fluids adequately, or from failure of the Spleen to transform and transport fluids, or failure of the Kidney to steam and transform fluids. Phlegm forms and accumulates in the Lung. This latent phlegm is then stirred by exterior wind carrying allergens, improper diet, emotional stress, or exertion. Airway obstruction by latent phlegm causes impaired dispersion and descent of Lung Qi, manifesting as asthma. Asthma may be classified as acute (and further classified as acute hot or acute cold), or chronic (due to Lung, Spleen, or Kidney deficiency).

TCM Differentiation and Treatment:

Pattern	Signs and Symptoms	Treatment Principle	Acupuncture	Formula
Hot asthma	Cough with wheezing; thick, yellow phlegm, fever, red face, chest oppression, thirst with desire to drink. T: red, thick yellow coat P: rapid, slippery	Clear heat, transform phlegm, descend Qi, stop asthma	LU5 (chi ze), LU6 (kong zui), LU10 (yu ji), ding chuan, ST40 (feng long), REN22 (tian tu)	
Cold asthma	Cough with rapid breathing, sound of phlegm rattling in throat; clear, watery, white phlegm, cold body, no perspiration, dull complexion, no thirst. T: think or thick white coat P: floating, slippery	Disperse wind-cold, transform phlegm, descend Qi, stop asthma	LU7 (lie que)-LI4 (he gu), ding chuan, BL13 (fei shu)-LU1 (zhong fu), LU5 (chi ze), REN17 (dan zhong), REN22 (tian tu)	
Lung Qi Deficiency	Dull white facial complexion, shortness of breath, dislike of speaking, low voice, fatigue, lack of strength, spontaneous sweat, aversion to cold, easily catches cold, thin white phlegm T: pale with thin coat P: thin, weak	Tonify Lung Qi, drain phlegm strengthen exterior	LU9 (tai yuan), BL13 (fei shu), SP6 (SYJ), ST36 (ZSL), ST40 (feng long)	
Spleen Qi Deficiency	Cough with profuse phlegm, poor appetite, fullness in upper abdomen, sallow complexion, loose stools, emaciation, lack of strength. T: pale with scanty coat P: weak	Tonify Spleen, transform phlegm	LU9 (tai yuan), BL13 (fei shu), BL20 (pi shu), SP6 (SYJ), SP9 (yin ling quan), ST40 (feng long)	
Kidney Qi Deficiency	Dull white facial complexion, cold body, low back pain, profuse urine, loose stools, possible bed-wetting, clear phlegm. T: pale, thin white coat P: deep, weak	Strengthen Kidney, drain phlegm, consolidate Qi	KD3 (tai xi), BL23 (shen shu), LU9 (tai yuan), BL13 (fei shu), REN4 (guan yuan), REN6 (qi hai), ST40 (feng long)	

Intestinal parasitic worms (chang dao chong zheng)

Definition:
Patterns resulting from infection by intestinal parasitic worms.

Red Flags:
- Western medical assessment and treatment required

Western Medicine Relevant Conditions:
- Pinworm infection:

Pinworm infection is caused by the intestinal roundworm *enterobius vermicularis*. Infection occurs after pinworm eggs (ova) are swallowed. The larvae in the eggs hatch in the small intestine, then move to the large intestine. There, the larvae mature within 2 to 6 weeks, and the adult worms mate. After the eggs develop, the adult female worm moves to the rectum and exits through the anus to lay eggs. The eggs are deposited in a sticky, gelatinous substance that sticks to the skin around the anus. From there, eggs can be transferred to fingernails, clothing, bedding, toys, or food. Eggs can survive outside the body up to 3 weeks at normal room temperature.

Eggs are often introduced into the mouth from fingers or from contaminated food. Children may re-infect themselves by transferring eggs from the area around their anus to their mouth. Children who suck their thumbs are at increased risk of infection.

- Roundworm infection:

Trichinosis is infection caused by the roundworm *trichinella spiralis* or another trichinella roundworm. *Trichinella* larvae live in the muscle tissue of animals, typically pigs, wild boars and many other carnivores. Children develop trichinosis if they eat uncooked, undercooked, or under-processed meat from an animal that carries the parasite.

When a person eats meat containing live *Trichinella* cysts, the cyst wall is digested, releasing larvae that quickly mature to adulthood and mate in the intestine. The females then burrow into the intestinal wall and, after several days, begin to produce larvae. The larvae are carried through the body through the lymphatic vessels and bloodstream. The larvae penetrate muscles, causing inflammation. In 1 to 2 months, they form cysts that can live for years in the body.

Certain muscles, such as those in the tongue, around the eyes, and between the ribs, are most often infected. Trichinosis symptoms vary, depending on the stage of infection, number of invading larvae, tissues invaded, and general physical condition of the person. Many people have no symptoms.

Symptoms of trichinosis occur in two stages.
- Stage 1: Intestinal infection develops 1 to 2 days after eating contaminated meat. Symptoms include nausea, diarrhea, abdominal cramps, and a slight fever.
- Stage 2: Symptoms from the larval invasion of muscles usually start after about 7 to 15 days. Symptoms include muscle pain and tenderness, weakness, fever, headache, and swelling of the face, particularly around the eyes. The pain is often most pronounced in the muscles used to breathe, speak, chew, and swallow. A rash that does not itch may develop. In some people, the whites of the eyes become red, and their eyes hurt and become sensitive to bright light.

If many larvae are present, the heart, brain, and lungs may become inflamed. Heart failure, abnormal heart rhythms, seizures, and severe breathing problems may result. Death can occur but is rare.

- Tapeworm infection:

Tapeworm infection of the intestine occurs mainly when people eat raw or undercooked contaminated pork, beef, or freshwater fish or, for the dwarf tapeworm, contaminated food or water. The pork, beef, and fish tapeworms are large, flat worms that live in the intestine of people and can grow 15 to 30 feet in length. Egg-bearing sections of the worm are passed in the stool.

If untreated human waste is released into the environment, the eggs may be ingested by intermediate hosts, such as pigs, cattle, or, in the case of fish tapeworms, small freshwater crustaceans, which are in turn ingested by fish. The eggs hatch into larvae in the intermediate host. The larvae invade the intestinal wall and are carried through the bloodstream to skeletal muscle and other tissues, where they form cysts.

Children acquire the parasite by eating the cysts in raw or undercooked meat or certain types of freshwater fish. The cysts hatch and develop into adult worms, which latch onto the wall of the intestine. The worms then grow in length and begin producing eggs.

Although tapeworms in the intestine usually cause no symptoms, some people experience weight loss, upper abdominal discomfort, diarrhea, and other symptoms. Occasionally, people with a tapeworm can feel a piece of the worm move out through the anus or see part of the ribbon-like tapeworm in stool. The fish tapeworm can cause anemia because it absorbs vitamin B12, which is necessary for red blood cells to mature.

(from http://www.merckmanuals.com/home/infections/parasitic-infections/overview-of-parasitic-infections)

Etiology and Pathogenesis:
- Parasites enter body through contaminated food or water – obstruct intestines – impair Spleen and Stomach transformation and transportation leading to damp heat and food stasis, and causing abdominal distention and pain
- Parasitic worms also consume nutrients injuring both Qi and Blood, and weakening the organs causing emaciation and lack of strength

TCM Differentiation and Treatment:

Pattern	Signs and Symptoms	Treatment Principle	Acupuncture	Formula
Pinworms	Itching of the anus, especially at night, restless sleep, presence of small white worms near anus, possible loss of appetite and emaciation.	Expel worms, relieve itching	Si feng, bai chong wo, ST36 (ZSL), SP6 (SYJ)	
Roundworms	Intermittent pain in the umbilical region, epigastric discomfort, vomiting of worms when severe, possible desire to eat peculiar substances, sallow complexion, emaciation, itching of nostrils, drooling and grinding of teeth in sleep, white patches on face and lips. May be muscle pain and tenderness, especially around mouth, tongue and eyes.	Expel worms, relieve pain and itching strengthen Spleen and Stomach	Si feng, SP15 (da heng), REN6 (qi hai), ST36 (ZSL), bai chong wo	
Tapeworms	Mild abdominal pain or distention and discomfort, itching of the anus, diarrhea and tapeworm segments in the stool, sallow complexion, emaciation, dizzy spells, fatigue, insomnia.	Expel worms, rectify Spleen and Stomach	Si feng, bai chong wo, REN12 (zhong wan), ST36 (ZSL), ST21 (liang men)	

Chickenpox (shui dou)

Definition:
Shui dou means "water blister", which is a characteristic sign of this acute, epidemic virus that causes an itchy macular rash that turns to papules and then fluid filled vesicles.

Red Flags:
- Highly contagious infection

Western Medicine Relevant Conditions:
Chickenpox (varicella) is a highly contagious infection with the varicella-zoster virus that causes a characteristic itchy rash, consisting of small, raised, blistered, or crusted spots. Chickenpox is an infection that mostly affects children.

The disease is spread by airborne droplets of moisture containing the varicella-zoster virus, which is a herpes virus. A person with chickenpox is most contagious just after symptoms start but remains contagious until the last blisters have crusted.

In children with a normal immune system, chickenpox is rarely severe. Most people with chickenpox simply have sores on the skin and in the mouth. However, the virus sometimes infects the lungs, brain, heart, liver, or joints. Such serious infections are more common among newborns and those with a weakened immune system.

A person who has had chickenpox develops immunity and cannot contract it again. However, the varicella-zoster virus remains dormant in the body after an initial infection with chickenpox, sometimes reactivating in later life, causing shingles.

Symptoms begin 10 to 21 days after infection. They include
- Mild headache
- Moderate fever
- Loss of appetite
- A general feeling of illness (malaise)

Younger children often do not have these symptoms, but symptoms are often severe in adults.

About 24 to 36 hours after the first symptoms begin, a rash of small, flat, red spots appears. The spots usually begin on the trunk and face, later appearing on the arms and legs. Some children have only a few spots. Others have them almost everywhere, including on the scalp and inside the mouth.

Within 6 to 8 hours, each spot becomes raised; forms an itchy, round, fluid-filled blister against a red background; and finally crusts. Spots continue to develop and crust for several days. The spots may become infected by bacteria, causing skin infection with redness (cellulitis) or blisters (bullous impetigo) or, rarely, infection of the tissues under the skin. New spots usually stop appearing by the fifth day, the majority are crusted by the sixth day, and most disappear in fewer than 20 days.

Spots in the mouth quickly rupture and form raw sores (ulcers), which often make swallowing painful. Raw sores may also occur on the eyelids and in the upper airways, rectum, and vagina. Spots in the voice box (larynx) and upper airways may occasionally cause severe difficulty in breathing. Lymph nodes at the side of the neck may become enlarged and tender. The worst part of the illness usually lasts 4 to 7 days.

Complications are rare, but include:
- Pneumonia
- Encephalitis
- Heart infection
- Joint inflammation
- Reye's syndrome (swelling of the LR and brain)

Etiology and Pathogenesis:
- Zheng Qi is weaker in children. Epidemic wind heat and damp heat toxins can easily attack and invade through the mouth and nose, leading to chickenpox.

TCM Differentiation and Treatment:

Pattern	Signs and Symptoms	Treatment Principle	Acupuncture	Formula
Pathogens in the Wei level	Sudden onset fever, sneezing, coughing, characteristic chicken pox lesions develop. T: red, white coat P: thin, rapid	Expel wind, clear heat, remove toxins, eliminate damp	LI4 (he gu), SJ5 (wei guan), LU5 (chi ze), SP9 (yin ling quan)	
Heat in the Qi and Ying level	High fever, multiple lesions with turbid liquid, mouth ulcers, thirst, red face and lips, constipation and scanty urine. T: deep red, yellow coat P: full and rapid	Clear heat, cool blood, remove toxins	LI11 (qu chi), LI4 (he gu), ST44 (nei ting), DU14 (da zhui), BL40 (wei zhong), shi xuan	
Severe heat toxin	High fever without relief, swollen and red skin lesions, pus and turbid liquid inside vesicles, red lips, red face, agitation, vexation. T: deep red, thick yellow coat P: rapid and forceful	Clear heat, cool blood, remove toxins	LI11 (qu chi), ST44 (nei ting), DU14 (da zhui), BL40 (wei zhong) (may need hospitalization)	

Common Cold (gan mao)

Definition:
Common condition throughout childhood characterized by nasal congestion, runny nose, sneezing, aversion to cold and fever, possible sore throat, headache and body aches.

Red Flags:
- High fever
- Any fever in a child under 2 months old; mild fever in child between 3 – 36 months
- Crying, stiffness of neck, listlessness, confusion, difficult breathing

Western Medicine Relevant Conditions:
The common cold is a viral infection of the lining of the nose, sinuses, and throat.

Common colds are among the most common illnesses. Many different viruses (rhinoviruses, adenoviruses, coronaviruses, and human metapneumoviruses) cause colds, but rhinoviruses (of which there are more than 100 subtypes) are implicated more often than others. Colds caused by rhinoviruses occur more commonly in the spring and fall. Other viruses cause common cold like illnesses at other times of the year.
Colds spread mainly when people's hands come in contact with nasal secretions from an infected person. These secretions contain cold viruses. When people then touch their mouth, nose, or eyes, the viruses gain entry to the body and cause a cold. Less often, colds are spread when people breathe air containing droplets that were coughed or sneezed out by an infected person. A cold is most contagious during the first 1 or 2 days after symptoms develop.
Symptoms start 1 to 3 days after infection. Usually, the first symptom is a scratchy or sore throat or discomfort in the nose. Later, people start sneezing, have a runny nose, and feel mildly ill. Fever is not common, but a mild fever may occur at the beginning of the cold. At first, secretions from the nose are watery and clear and can be annoyingly plentiful, but eventually, they become thicker, opaque, yellow-green, and less plentiful. Many people also develop a mild cough. Symptoms usually disappear in 4 to 10 days, although the cough often lasts into the second week.

Complications may prolong the disease. Rhinovirus infection often triggers asthma attacks in people with asthma. Some people develop bacterial infections of the middle ear (otitis media) or sinuses. These infections develop because congestion in the nose blocks the normal drainage of those areas, allowing bacteria to grow in collections of blocked secretions.
(from http://www.merckmanuals.com/home/infections/viral-infections/common-cold)

Etiology and Pathogenesis:
- External pathogens enter through the skin and lungs. In the skin, they block Wei Qi and lead to aversion to cold, fever, and body aches. In the Lungs, they block Lung functions of dispersing and descending leading to nasal congestion, cough, and sore throat.

TCM Differentiation and Treatment:

Pattern	Signs and Symptoms	Treatment Principle	Acupuncture	Formula
Wind Cold	Aversion to cold, feel cold, prefer warmth, possible low fever, chills, no sweating, nasal congestion with clear white phlegm, sneezing, possible cough. T: normal with thin white coat P: floating, tight	Release exterior, expel wind, descend and disperse Lung	LU7 (lie que), LI4 (he gu), BL12 (feng men), BL13 (fei shu), DU16 (feng fu), GB20 (feng chi)	
Wind Heat	More fever, less chills, dry mouth, sore throat, cough, thirst, stuffy nose with yellow discharge, pain in face and eyes. T: red, thin yellow coat P: superficial, rapid	Release exterior, expel wind heat, descend and disperse Lung	LI4 (he gu), LU7 (lie que), SJ5 (wei guan), LI11 (qu chi), DU14 (da zhui), GB20 (feng chi), LU10 (yu ji)	
Summer Heat	Fever, dizziness, headache, heaviness, sore limbs, thirst with no desire to drink, sticky taste in mouth, sticky nasal discharge, nausea, abdominal fullness, scanty urine. T: red, greasy yellow coat P: soft, rapid	Clear summer heat, resolve damp, release exterior	LI4 (he gu), LU5 (chi ze), LU6 (kong zui), SP9 (yin ling quan), DU14 (da zhui), SP6 (SYJ), ST36 (ZSL), REN12 (zhong wan)	

Wind Cold with Qi deficiency	Repeat colds, nasal congestion with thin mucus, aversion to wind, low fever, easily sweat, lusterless complexion, fatigue, shortness of breath. T: pale P: weak	Release exterior, tonify Qi	LU7 (lie que), LI4 (he gu), ST36 (ZSL), SP6 (SYJ), BL13 (fei shu), BL20 (pi shu)	
Wind Heat with Yin deficiency	Repeat colds, low fever, dry throat, night sweats, five center heat, nasal congestion. T: bright red P: thin	Release exterior, nourish Yin	Wind heat points plus LU9 (tai yuan)	

Convulsions (jing feng)

Definition:
Convulsions or fright wind (jing feng) refers to patterns presenting the following major symptoms: muscular spasms of the limbs, jaw tetany, opisthotonos, and loss of consciousness. Convulsion is a frequently seen condition in children under five years old, and they become less vulnerable with age.

Red Flags:
When a child has a convulsion, first aid protocol should be followed:
- Lay the child down on one side
- Keep the child away from potential hazards (such as stairs or sharp objects)
- Not put anything in the child's mouth and not try to hold the child's tongue

After the seizure ends:
- Stay with the child until the child is fully awake
- Check whether the child is breathing and, if breathing is not apparent, start resuscitation
- Do not give any food, liquid, or drug by mouth until the child is fully awake
- Check for fever and treat

An ambulance should be called if the seizure lasts more than 5 minutes, if the child is injured during the seizure or has difficulty breathing after the seizure, or if another seizure occurs immediately. All children should be taken to the hospital the first time they have a seizure.

Western Medicine Relevant Conditions:
Seizures are an abnormal, unregulated electrical discharge of nerve cells in the brain or part of the brain. This abnormal discharge can alter awareness or cause abnormal sensations, involuntary movements, or convulsions. Convulsions are violent, involuntary, rhythmic contractions of the muscles that affect a large part of the body. In newborns, seizures may be difficult to recognize. Newborns may smack their lips or chew involuntarily. Their eyes may appear to gaze in different directions. They may periodically go limp. In older infants or young children, one part or all of the body may shake, jerk, or tighten up. The limbs may move without purpose. Children may stare or become confused.

Some causes of seizures in newborns and infants include: temporary disorders such as high fevers, lack of oxygen during birth, a serious infection, brain disorders (e.g. malformations of the brain, hemorrhage within the brain), metabolic disorders, of use of drugs during pregnancy.

A seizure itself does not appear to damage the brain or cause lasting problems unless it continues for more than about an hour (most seizures last only a few minutes). However, many disorders that *cause* seizures can cause lasting problems. For example, they can interfere with the child's development. Whether some types of recurring seizures can affect the developing brain is debated.
(from http://www.merckmanuals.com/home/children-s-health-issues/neurologic-disorders-in-children/seizures-in-children)

Etiology and Pathogenesis:
Infantile convulsions may result from a variety of factors.

TCM Differentiation and Treatment:

Pattern	Signs and Symptoms	Treatment Principle	Acupuncture	Formula
Acute Wind Heat	Sudden onset, fever, headache, cough, red throat, irritability, eyes stare upwards, convulsion of the limbs, possible loss of consciousness. T: red with yellow coat P: floating, rapid	Expel wind, clear heat, stop convulsion	DU26 (shui gou), LR3 (tai chong), LI11 (qu chi), LI4 (he gu), DU14 (da zhui), extra point Er Jian	
Acute Summer Heat	Mainly in high summer or hot weather, high fever, agitation, thirst, possible nausea and vomiting, sudden loss of consciousness, convulsion, eyes stare upwards. T: red with yellow coat P: slippery, rapid	Expel Summer heat, release exterior, stop convulsion	DU26 (shui gou), LR3 (tai chong), LI11 (qu chi), LI4 (he gu), DU14 (da zhui), ST40 (feng long), extra point Er Jian	
Acute Damp Heat (epidemic)	Abrupt onset high fever, loss of consciousness, repeated convulsions, abdominal pain with nausea and vomiting, diarrhea with loose stools and foul odor containing pus and blood. T: red with greasy yellow coat P: slippery, rapid	Cool heat, eliminate Damp, relieve poisons, extinguish wind, stop convulsions	DU26 (shui gou), REN12 (zhong wan), ST40 (feng long), HT7 (shen men), LR3 (tai chong), LI4 (he gu), extra point Er Jian	
Sudden Fright	Abrupt convulsion with loss of consciousness upon sudden fright, hysterical behavior, greenish-blue complexion. T: thin white coat P: deep	Relieve convulsions, quiet the spirit	DU26 (shui gou), HT7 (shen men), KD3 (tai xi), yin tang	
Spleen and Stomach Deficiency	Listlessness, lethargy, sleep with eyes open, sallow, poor appetite, intermittent twitching. T: pale P: deep, weak	Strengthen Spleen and Stomach, calm Liver, stop convulsions	DU26 (shui gou), KD1 (yong quan), BL20 (pi shu), BL21 (wei shu), ST36 (ZSL), DU20 (bai hui), yin tang, LR3 (tai chong)	
Spleen and Kidney Yang Deficiency	Listless, pale, cold limbs, limbs twitching, thin stools, lack of vitality. T: pale P: deep, weak	Warm and tonify Spleen and Kidney Yang, stop convulsions	DU26 (shui gou), KD1 (yong quan), BL20 (pi shu), BL21 (wei shu), ST36 (ZSL), DU20 (bai hui), yin tang, LR3 (tai chong), BL23 (shen shu), REN6 (qi hai)	
Liver and Kidney Yin Deficiency	Spasms and convulsions acute and occasional, low fever, malar flush, emaciation, restlessness, feverish palms and soles, dry stools. T: red with little coat P: rapid, thready	Tonify Liver and Kidney Yin, stop convulsions	BL18 (gan shu), BL23 (shen shu), DU20 (bai hui), KD2 (ran gu), LR3 (tai chong), PC6 (nei guan), LI4 (he gu)	

Remember to use the Yin Qiao Mai if it is nighttime convulsions, and the Yang Qiao Mai if it is daytime convulsions.

Cough (ke shou)

Definition:
Cough is a common symptom of the Lung. In infants, the Lung is a tender organ and infants have weak defensive systems that are easily attacked by external pathogens.

Red Flags:
Emergency Western medical care is required for:

Western Medicine Relevant Conditions:
Cough helps clear materials from the airways and prevent them from going to the lungs. The materials may be particles that have been inhaled or substances from the lungs and/or airways. Most commonly, material coughed up from the lungs and airways is sputum (a mixture of mucus, debris, and cells ejected from the lungs). But sometimes a cough brings up blood. A cough that brings up either is considered productive.

Causes of cough depend on whether the cough has lasted less than 4 weeks (acute) or 4 weeks or more (chronic). The most common cause of an acute cough is an upper respiratory infection due to a virus. The most common causes of chronic cough are: asthma, gastroesophageal reflux, and postnasal drip.

Acute cough may also result from a foreign body (such as a piece of food or a piece of a toy) inhaled into the lungs (aspiration) or less common respiratory infections such as pneumonia, pertussis, or tuberculosis.

Chronic cough may also result from aspiration of a foreign body, hereditary disorders such as cystic fibrosis, a birth defect of the airways or lungs, inflammatory disorders involving the airways or lungs, or may be stress-related.

(from http://www.merckmanuals.com/home/children-s-health-issues/symptoms-in-infants-and-children/cough-in-children)

Etiology and Pathogenesis:
Cough may be acute or chronic, and may be due to exogenous or endogenous causes.
- Exogenous cough – external pathogens (mainly wind) first attack the Lung and the Defensive Qi level. The Lung governs Qi and respiration, and when pathogens attack, they block its Qi movement, impairing the dispersing and descending function and causing cough.
- Endogenous phlegm – the tender Spleen of infants is easily insured, impairing Spleen transportation and transformation, which leads to Phlegm development. Phlegm lodges in the Lung and blocks the dispersion and descent of Lung Qi causing cough.
- Deficiency of Qi and Yin – infant's constitution may be weak, and body may be easily invaded by external pathogens, further damaging Qi and Yin and producing cough

TCM Differentiation and Treatment:

Pattern	Signs and Symptoms	Treatment Principle	Acupuncture	Formula
Wind cold	Cough with itchy throat, hoarse voice, nasal drainage and blockage, aversion to cold, no sweating, fever, headache, phlegm is thin and white. T: normal, thin white coat P: superficial, tight IFV: superficial, red	Release exterior, expel wind-cold, descend Lung Qi, stop cough	LU7 (lie que)-LI4 (he gu), LU1 (zhong fu)-BL13 (fei shu), BL12 (feng men), DU16 (feng fu), LU6 (kong zui), REN22 (tian tu)	
Wind heat	Cough with sore, red throat, fever, aversion to wind, thick yellow mucus, thirst. T: red, thin yellow coat P: superficial, rapid IFV: superficial, deep red	Release exterior, expel wind-heat, descend Lung Qi, stop cough	LU7 (lie que)-LI4 (he gu), SJ5 (wei guan), LI11 (qu chi), LU5 (zhi ze), DU14 (da zui), LU6 (kong zui), REN22 (tian tu)	
Phlegm damp (may also be phlegm damp with heat)	Cough with profuse white phlegm (or yellow with heat), chest tightness, poor appetite, fatigue. T: thick and greasy P: slippery IFV: dark, deep, slow refill	Dry damp, transform phlegm, stop cough	BL13 (fei shu), BL20 (pi shu), LU5 (chi ze), LU6 (kong zui), ST36 (ZSL), ST40 (feng long) + heat signs, add LI11 (qu chi)	
Yin Deficiency	Dry cough without sputum (or scanty), dry throat, thirst, tickle in throat, hoarse voice, five center heat, malar flush, night sweats. T: red, scanty coat P: thin, rapid IFV: thin, red, rapid refill	Nourish Yin, moisten Lung, clear heat, transform phlegm, stop cough	BL13 (fei shu)-LU1 (zhong fu), LU9 (tai yuan), LU7-KD6 (ren mai)	
Qi Deficiency	Long term forceless cough, shortness of breath, no desire to speak, spontaneous sweat, aversion to cold, lack of spirit, pallid complexion. T: pale and tender P: weak IFV: light, deep, quick refill	Tonify Lung and Spleen, dissipate phlegm, stop cough	BL13 (fei shu), BL20 (pi shu), SP6 (SYJ), ST36 (ZSL), LU9 (tai yuan), REN17 (dan zhong)	

Diarrhea (xie xie)

Definition:
Infantile diarrhea is characterized by increased frequency of bowel movements and a loose, watery or poorly formed stool. In children, this is a common disorder. If treatment is delayed or incorrect, diarrhea may turn severe and damage Qi and Yin, leading to malnutrition, and growth and development issues.

Red Flags:
- Dehydration
- Blood or pus in stools
- Bilious vomiting
- Severe abdominal pain
- Symptoms not resolving or worsening
- Petechiae

Western Medicine Relevant Conditions:
In Western medicine, diarrhea is defined as frequent loose or watery bowel movements that deviate from a child's normal pattern. Diarrhea may be accompanied by anorexia, vomiting, acute weight loss, abdominal pain, fever, or passage of blood. If diarrhea is severe or prolonged, dehydration is likely. Even in the absence of dehydration, chronic diarrhea usually results in weight loss or failure to gain weight.

Mechanisms of diarrhea may include the following:
- Osmotic diarrhea results from the presence of non-absorbable solutes in the GI tract, as with lactose intolerance.
- Secretory diarrhea results from substances (e.g., bacterial toxins) that increase secretion of chloride ions and water into the intestinal lumen.
- Inflammatory diarrhea is associated with conditions that cause inflammation or ulceration of the intestinal mucosa (e.g., Crohn's disease, ulcerative colitis). The resultant outpouring of plasma, serum proteins, blood, and mucous increases fecal bulk and fluid content.
- Malabsorption may result from osmotic or secretory mechanisms or conditions that lead to less surface area in the bowel. Conditions such as pancreatic insufficiency and short bowel syndrome and conditions that speed up transit time cause diarrhea due to decreased absorption.

The causes and significance of diarrhea differ depending on whether it is acute (< 2 wk) or chronic (> 2 wk). Most cases of diarrhea are acute.
Acute diarrhea usually is caused by: gastroenteritis, antibiotic use, food allergies, or food poisoning. Most gastroenteritis is caused by a virus; however, any enteric pathogen can cause acute diarrhea.

Chronic diarrhea usually is caused by: dietary factors, infection, celiac disease, inflammatory bowel disease. Chronic diarrhea can also be caused by anatomic disorders and disorders that interfere with absorption or digestion.

TCM Etiology and Pathogenesis:
- Exogenous pathogenic factors, such as Wind, Cold, and Damp, often induce diarrhea. These exogenous factors injure the Spleen and Stomach, disrupting their functions of transportation and transformation, so that the clear and turbid cannot be separated. Both clear and turbid move into the large intestine and diarrhea results.
- Improper diet (e.g. irregular intake of milk or foods, unclean foods, inappropriate foods excessive cold or raw foods) can injure the Spleen and Stomach, impairing their digestive functions leading to diarrhea.
- Constitutional weaknesses, chronic or severe illness may also cause Spleen and Stomach deficiency and diarrhea.

TCM Differentiation and Treatment:

Pattern	Signs and Symptoms	Treatment Principle	Acupuncture	Formula
	Abdominal distention and pain, borborygmus, runny and foul smelling stools, pain better after bowel movements, belching, possibly vomiting undigested food, loss of appetite, restless sleep. T: thick greasy coat P: slippery IFV: pale	Promote digestion, relieve food stagnation, resolve diarrhea	ST25 (tian shu), ST36 (ZSL), ST37 (shang ju xu), SP6 (SYJ), ST44 (nei ting), inner neiting	
	Runny yellow and foul smelling stools, may contain mucus, abdominal pain and fever, thirst, burning sensation of anus, dark scanty urine, lassitude, weakness. T: red with yellow and greasy coat P: rapid, slippery IFV: deep red, thick	Clear heat, expel damp, resolve diarrhea	ST25 (tian shu), ST36 (ZSL), ST37 (shang ju xu), SP6 (SYJ), ST44 (nei ting), inner neiting, SP9 (yin ling quan)	
	Thin and loose feces, pale in color and possibly foamy, no marked foul odor, borborygmus, abdominal pain, fever, aversion to cold, no thirst, ACUTE. T: pale, thin white coat P: floating, tight IFV: light red	Expel wind, eliminate cold, resolve diarrhea	ST25 (tian shu), ST36 (ZSL), ST37 (shang ju xu), REN9 (shui fen), REN12 (zhong wan), SP9 (yin ling quan) + LU7 (lie que), LI4 (he gu), BL12 (feng men)	
	Diarrhea following meals, feces loose and light in color, not foul smelling, sallow complexion, poor appetite, emaciation, lassitude, fatigue, protracted course and frequent occurrence. T: pale P: thin, weak IFV: sallow	Fortify Spleen, boost Qi, promote T&T, resolve diarrhea	ST25 (tian shu), ST36 (ZSL), ST37 (shang ju xu), SP3 (tai bai), SP6 (SYJ), BL20 (pi shu), REN12 (zhong wan), SP4 (gong sun)	
	Prolonged diarrhea, worse in morning, thin stools containing undigested food, feel cold, fatigue, pale complexion, listlessness. T: pale P: deep, thin IFV: pale	Warm and tonify Spleen and Kidney, stop diarrhea	ST25 (tian shu), ST36 (ZSL), ST37 (shang ju xu), BL20 (pi shu), BL23 (shen shu), KD3 (tai xi), SP4 (gong sun), DU4 (ming men), REN4 (guan yuan)	

Enuresis (yi niao)

Definition:
Enuresis is the involuntary discharge of urine during sleep in children over 3 years of age, and particularly in children over 5 years of age. In mild cases, bed-wetting can occur once in several nights, while in more severe cases, bed-wetting occurs once every night or even several times a night.

Red Flags:
Referral in cases where there are:
- Signs or concerns of sexual abuse
- Excessive thirst, polyuria, and weight loss
- Any neurologic signs, especially in the lower extremities
- Physical signs of neurologic impairment

Western Medicine Relevant Conditions:
In Western medicine, nighttime incontinence (nocturnal enuresis, or bed-wetting) is usually not diagnosed until age 7. These age limits are based on children who are developing typically and so may not be applicable to children with developmental delay.

In primary enuresis, children have never achieved urinary continence for ≥ 6 mos. In secondary enuresis, children have developed incontinence after a period of at least 6 mos. of urinary control. An organic cause is more likely in secondary enuresis.

Bladder function has a storage phase and a voiding phase. Abnormalities in either phase can cause primary or secondary enuresis.

In the storage phase, the bladder acts as a reservoir for urine. Storage capacity is affected by bladder size and compliance. Storage capacity increases as children grow. Compliance can be decreased by repeated infections or by outlet obstruction, with resulting bladder muscle hypertrophy.

In the voiding phase, bladder contraction synchronizes with the opening of the bladder neck and the external urinary sphincter. If there is dysfunction in the coordination or sequence of voiding, enuresis can occur. There are multiple reasons for dysfunction. One example is bladder irritation, which can lead to irregular contractions of the bladder and asynchrony of the voiding sequence, resulting in enuresis. Bladder irritation can result from a UTI or from anything that presses on the bladder (e.g., a dilated rectum caused by constipation).

Nocturnal enuresis can be divided into monosymptomatic (occurring only during sleep) and complex (other abnormalities are present, such as diurnal enuresis and/or urinary symptoms).

Organic disorders account for about 30% of cases and are more common in complex compared to monosymptomatic enuresis. The remaining majority of cases are of unclear etiology but are thought to be due to a combination of factors, including:
- Maturational delay
- Uncompleted toilet training
- Functionally small bladder capacity (the bladder is not actually small but contracts before it is completely full)
- Increased nighttime urine volume
- Difficulties in arousal from sleep
- Family history (if one parent had nocturnal enuresis, there is a 30% chance offspring will have it, increasing to 70% if both parents were affected)

The factors contributing to organic causes of nocturnal enuresis include:
- Conditions that increase urine volume (e.g. diabetes mellitus, diabetes insipidus, chronic renal failure, excessive water intake)
- Conditions that increase bladder irritability (e.g. urinary tract infection, pressure on the bladder by the rectum and sigmoid colon
- Structural abnormalities
- Abnormal sphincter weakness (e.g. spina bifida)

(from http://www.merckmanuals.com/professional/pediatrics/incontinence-in-children/urinary-incontinence-in-children)

Etiology and Pathogenesis:

TCM Differentiation and Treatment:

Pattern	Signs and Symptoms	Treatment Principle	Acupuncture	Formula
Kidney Yang Deficiency	Frequent enuresis, increased volume of clear urine, pale complexion, lassitude, weakness, weak and aching back and knees, cold limbs, aversion to cold. T: pale P: slow, weak IFV: pale, deep	Warm and tonify Kidney Yang, stop enuresis	REN3 (zhong ji), REN4 (guan yuan), REN6 (qi hai), BL23 (shen shu), BL28 (pang guang shu), DU4 (ming men)	
Lung and Spleen Qi Deficiency	Frequent enuresis, small volume, spontaneous sweating, lassitude, weak limbs, sallow complexion, anorexia, watery feces, easily catch colds, shortness of breath. T: pale, thin white coat P: weak IFV: light red	Tonify Spleen and Lung, stop enuresis	REN3 (zhong ji), REN4 (guan yuan), REN6 (qi hai), BL13 (fei shu), BL20 (pi shu), BL28 (pang guang shu), DU20 (bai hui), SP6 (SYJ), ST36 (ZSL)	
Damp Heat in Liver Channel	Enuresis and urine that is yellow and decreased in volume, foul smell, dream disturbed sleep, restlessness, irritability, red face, red lips, thirst. T: red P: slippery, rapid IFV: deep red	Clear heat, drain damp, stop enuresis	REN3 (zhong ji), BL28, (pang guang shu), LR8 (qu quan), GB34 (yang ling quan)	

Epilepsy (xian zheng)

Definition:
A recurrent neurological disorder characterized by a sudden, brief episode of altered consciousness. In more severe cases, there may be loss of consciousness, foaming at the mouth, bleating sounds, rolling back of the eyes, and violent involuntary movements of the limbs followed by regained consciousness and no lingering symptoms. These symptoms are the result of liver wind triggering turbid phlegm, which mists the clear orifices and obstructs the channels.

Red Flags:
See convulsions (jing feng).

Western Medicine Relevant Conditions:
In Western medicine, epilepsy is not a specific disorder but refers to a tendency to have recurring seizures that may or may not have an identifiable cause. For more detail, see convulsions (jing feng), and also epilepsy (xian zheng) in internal medicine section.

Etiology and Pathogenesis:
- Liver wind and phlegm are the two main factors in epileptic seizures. Pre-existing phlegm triggered by Liver Wind will travel to the Heart and cover the orifices or travel and obstruct the channels, resulting in seizures.
- Pre-natal exposure to shock and fear (from when a pregnant woman experiences these strong negative emotional stimuli) can cause upset of fetal Qi and Blood and damage the fetal Kidney Essence.
- Head trauma from, e.g. a fall, improper use of obstetric forceps, or difficult labor can result in stagnation of Qi and Blood that results in altered consciousness and seizures.

TCM Differentiation and Treatment:

Pattern	Signs and Symptoms	Treatment Principle	Acupuncture	Formula
Fright	History of fright before onset of convulsions, may scream, cry, fall into trance, tongue may thrust outward, alternating flushed and pale face. T: red, white coat P: wiry, slippery IFV: blue, superficial	Eliminate fright to calm mind		
Phlegm	Profuse saliva and phlegm during onset of convulsions, cough with phlegm, phlegm rattling in throat, staring forward, trance like state, abdominal pain, vomiting. T: white, greasy P: deep, wiry, slippery IFV: thick and yellow	Regulate Qi, transform phlegm, open orifices, resuscitate		
Blood Stasis	Loss of consciousness, one-sided convulsion or general convulsion, dizziness, headache with sharp and fixed pain, stools like rabbit droppings. T: purple spots, no coat P: choppy IFV: deep, slow refill	Move blood stasis, open orifices, stop wind and convulsions		

Erysipelas (chi you dan)

Definition:

Red Flags:
- Refer for Western medical assessment and treatment. Antibiotics may be required.

Western Medicine Relevant Conditions:
- See erysipelas (dan du) in External Medicine section

Etiology and Pathogenesis:
- external injury/skin break allows invasion of toxins (bites, skin disorders give chance for pathogens to invade via the wound) -- fire enters blood level and accumulates (in local involved area) and heat manifests in skin level -- toxins cause blood heat that stagnates in the superficial tissues resulting in the characteristic redness of the skin

TCM Differentiation and Treatment:

Pattern	Signs and Symptoms	Treatment Principle	Acupuncture	Formula
Wind Heat	Rash mainly on face, bright red in color, slightly raised above the skin surface, with marked borders. Affected areas are hot to the touch, painful, and drained of color when pressed, quickly becoming red again when released. May have aversion to wind, fever, thirst, constipation, dark urine. T: red, yellow coat P: floating, rapid	Dispel wind, clear heat, cool blood, resolve toxins	LI4 (he gu), LI11 (qu chi), SJ5 (wei guan), SP10 (xue hai), ST41 (jie xi), BL40 (wei zhong), BL12 (feng men) + fever DU14 (da zhui)	
Damp Heat	Rash mainly on lower limbs, may blister, fever, irritability, thirst chest oppression vomiting, diarrhea, loss of appetite, dark urine. T: yellow, greasy coat P: slippery, rapid	Clear heat, drain damp, cool blood, resolve toxins	LI4 (he gu), ST36 (ZSL), SP10 (xue hai), LI11 (qu chi), SP9 (yin ling quan), BL40 (wei zhong)	

Fetal jaundice (tai huang)

Definition:
Fetal jaundice is a common condition with varying degrees of severity. Jaundice means yellowing of the skin and possibly the whites of the eyes.

Red Flags:

Western Medicine Relevant Conditions:
Jaundice is common in newborns. It occurs when the level of bilirubin in the blood rises. When the bilirubin level gets too high, bilirubin can be deposited in the skin, the whites of the eyes, and other tissues.

Newborns normally have a high red blood cell count at birth, and their red blood cells have a shorter life span than adult red blood cells. The high red blood cell count and shorter life span mean that more of the newborn's red blood cells undergo hemolysis. Aging red blood cells are normally removed by the spleen. Hemoglobin is broken down and recycled. One portion of the hemoglobin molecule is converted into bilirubin, which is carried by the blood to the liver. The liver chemically changes the bilirubin by binding it to another substance, creating conjugated bilirubin. The conjugated bilirubin passes into the bile, which is then excreted into the digestive tract. In adults, bilirubin is further broken down by the bacteria that normally reside in the digestive tract. This form of bilirubin is excreted in the stool and gives stool its typical brown color. However, newborns do not yet have these bacteria or other digestive enzymes needed to process bilirubin. Thus, because newborns produce more bilirubin than older children and adults and eliminate bilirubin at a slower rate than older children and adults, high levels of bilirubin can build up in their blood relatively quickly. This disorder is called hyperbilirubinemia.

Whether jaundice is dangerous depends on what is causing it, how high the bilirubin level is, and how quickly the bilirubin level rises. Some disorders that cause jaundice are dangerous regardless of what the bilirubin level is. However, an extremely high bilirubin level, regardless of cause, is dangerous.

The most serious consequence of a high bilirubin level is kernicterus—a disorder in which bilirubin is deposited in the brain and causes brain damage. Kernicterus occurs only when the level of bilirubin is high. The risk of this disorder is higher for newborns who are premature, seriously ill, or who are given certain drugs. If untreated, kernicterus may lead to unresponsiveness (stupor) or lethargy, loss of muscle tone, a high-pitched cry, poor feeding, and seizures. Later, children can have cerebral palsy, hearing loss, a permanent upward gaze, or other signs of brain damage. Kernicterus is now rare.

The most common causes of jaundice in the newborn are:
- Physiologic jaundice: occurs in most newborns. It develops because the red blood cells in newborns normally break down at a slightly increased rate and because the digestive tract and liver function in newborns are immature.
- Breastfeeding jaundice: is common and occurs in newborns that do not consume enough breast milk (often because the mother's milk has not yet come in well). Newborns who consume less breast milk have fewer bowel movements and thus eliminate less bilirubin.
- Breast milk jaundice: is less common. It occurs when breast milk contains a high level of a substance that slows bilirubin excretion and thus causes the bilirubin level to increase.
- Excessive breakdown of red blood cells: can overwhelm the liver with more bilirubin than it can process. There are several causes of excessive breakdown of red blood cells, such as hemolytic disease.

Etiology and Pathogenesis:
- Damp Heat accumulation during pregnancy is transferred to the fetus. Damp heat accumulates in the Spleen and Stomach, steaming the Liver and Gallbladder, and bile is forced out to the skin.
- Congenital deficiency of the Spleen and Stomach leads to weakness of Spleen Yang. This, in turn, leads to Damp accumulation and disruption of the Liver and Gallbladder.

TCM Differentiation and Treatment:

Pattern	Signs and Symptoms	Treatment Principle	Acupuncture	Formula
Yang jaundice	Brightly colored yellow skin and eyes, deep yellow urine, generalized fever or hot to the touch, possible constipation, spirit clouded, vexation and confusion, fatigue, lack of strength, no desire to eat or drink, abdominal distension and fullness, dry mouth and lips. T: red, greasy coat P: slippery	Clear heat, resolve dampness, resolve jaundice	GB34 (yang ling quan), LR6 (zhong du), SP9 (yin ling quan), ST36 (ZSL), LR3 (tai chong), BL18 (gan shu), BL19 (dan shu), DU9 (zhi yang), SI4 (wan gu)	
Yin jaundice	Dull yellow skin and eyes, fatigue, listlessness, loose stools, abdominal distension, cold limbs, easily vomit after eating. T: pale	Warm middle jiao, resolve damp, tonify Spleen	GB34 (yang ling quan), SP6 (SYJ), SP9 (yin ling quan), ST36 (ZSL), DU9 (zhi yang), BL18 (gan shu), BL19 (dan shu), BL20 (pi shu), SI4 (wan gu)	

Food Retention (ji zhi)

Definition:
Food retention is characterized by overeating, abdominal pain, possibly vomiting, constipation or diarrhea with undigested food, lack of desire to eat.

Western Medicine Relevant Conditions:
In Western medicine, overeating is a concern as it can lead to childhood obesity. Once fat cells form, they do not go away. Thus, obese children are more likely than children of normal weight to be obese as adults. Because childhood obesity can lead to adult obesity, it should be prevented or treated.

(from http://www.merckmanuals.com/home/children-s-health-issues/behavioral-problems-in-children/eating-problems-in-young-children)

Etiology and Pathogenesis:
- When children eat too much or have an improper diet, food stagnates and obstructs the Qi mechanism leading to food stagnation. Weak Spleen Qi may compound this problem.

TCM Differentiation and Treatment:

Pattern	Signs and Symptoms	Treatment Principle	Acupuncture	Formula
Food stagnation	Eating too much followed by constipation or diarrhea with undigested food, strong smelling stools, distended and painful abdomen (worse with pressure), irritability. T: greasy coat P: slippery	Promote digestion, resolve stagnation	ST44 (nei ting), inner neiting, REN12 (zhong wan), REN13 (shang wan), ST36 (ZSL), SJ6 (zhi gou)	
Food stagnation and Spleen Qi deficiency	Large meals (repeatedly) followed by constipation or diarrhea with undigested food, poor appetite, belching, bloating, abdominal distension with pain, sallow complexion, fatigue. T: pale, greasy coat P: thin, slippery	Tonify Spleen, promote digestion, resolve stagnation	As above + SP6 (SYJ), BL20, (pi shu) BL21 (wei shu)	

Malnutrition (gan zheng)

Definition:
This is a chronic condition characterized by emaciation, sallow complexion, poor hair growth, abdominal distension, protrusion of superficial abdominal veins, irregular eating, and listlessness.

Red Flags:
- Refer for Western medical assessment and treatment

Western Medicine Relevant Conditions:
In Western medicine, malnutrition is seen as an imbalance between the nutrients the body needs and the nutrients it gets. Thus, malnutrition also includes over nutrition (consumption of too many calories or too much of any specific nutrient—protein, fat, vitamin, mineral, or other dietary supplement), as well as under nutrition.

Protein-energy under nutrition (also called protein-energy malnutrition) is a severe deficiency of protein and calories that results when people do not consume enough protein and calories for a long time.
In developing countries, protein-energy under nutrition often occurs in children. It contributes to death in more than half of children who die (for example, by increasing the risk of developing life-threatening infections and, if infections develop, by increasing their severity). However, this disorder can affect anyone, regardless of age, if food supplies are inadequate..Protein-energy under nutrition has two main forms: marasmus and kwashiorkor.

Marasmus is a severe deficiency of calories and protein. It tends to develop in infants and very young children. It typically results in weight loss and dehydration. Breastfeeding usually protects against marasmus. Starvation is the most extreme form of marasmus (and under nutrition). It results from a partial or total lack of essential nutrients for a long time.

Kwashiorkor is a severe deficiency more of protein than of calories. Kwashiorkor is less common than marasmus. Kwashiorkor tends to be confined to certain areas of the world where staple foods and foods used to wean babies are deficient in protein even though they provide enough calories as carbohydrates. Examples of such foods are yams, cassava, rice, sweet potatoes, and green bananas. However, anyone can develop kwashiorkor if their diet consists mainly of carbohydrates. People with kwashiorkor retain fluid, making them appear puffy and swollen. If kwashiorkor is severe, the abdomen may protrude.
(from http://www.merckmanuals.com/home/disorders-of-nutrition/undernutrition/undernutrition)

Etiology and Pathogenesis:
The functions of the Spleen and Stomach are immature in the early years of life. Malnutrition involves the dysfunction of these organs, mainly due to: improper diet that lacks the essential nutrients; infection by parasitic worms that consume Qi and Blood; or prolonged illness. Prolonged course of this condition leads to depletion of Qi and Blood and may damage other organs causing secondary patterns.

TCM Differentiation and Treatment:

Pattern	Signs and Symptoms	Treatment Principle	Acupuncture	Formula
Spleen and Stomach Deficiency	Gradual onset, loss of weight, sallow and lusterless complexion, thinning of hair, poor appetite, restlessness, frequent crying, loose stools. With further development: food stagnation, emaciation, abdominal distension with visible veins, scaly skin, brittle hair, listlessness, dry lips and mouth, low grade fever, restless sleep. T: pale, possibly peeled coat P: thin, weak IFV: thin, white	Fortify the Spleen and Stomach, transform stagnation		
Infection by parasitic worms	Above symptoms, plus patients may want to eat strange and inedible materials, abdominal pain, grinding of teeth during sleep. T: pale P: wiry, thready	Move stagnation, expel worms		

Measles (ma zhen)

Definition:
Measles is a communicable pediatric illness with distinguishing features including: fever, cough, runny nose, spots like with sand in the mouth, conjunctivitis, and a red rash. It can occur at any time, but is more prevalent in winter and spring.

Red Flags:
- Measles is a highly infectious disease; complications are rare, but may be serious (see below)

Western Medicine Relevant Conditions:
Measles (rubeola, 9-day measles) is a highly contagious viral infection that causes various symptoms and a characteristic rash. Measles is rarely serious in healthy children, although occasionally it can be fatal or lead to brain damage.

A woman who has had measles or has been vaccinated passes immunity (in the form of antibodies) to her child. This immunity lasts for most of the first year of life. Thereafter, however, susceptibility to measles is high unless vaccination is given. A person who has had measles develops immunity and typically cannot contract it again.

Children become infected with measles by breathing in small airborne droplets of moisture coughed out by an infected person. About 90% of people who are not immune to measles develop the disease after they are exposed to a person with measles. Measles is contagious from several days before until several days after the rash appears.

Measles symptoms begin about 7 to 14 days after infection. The infected child first develops a fever, runny nose, hacking cough, and red eyes. Sometimes the eyes are sensitive to bright light. Before the rash begins, tiny, bright red spots with white or bluish white centers (Koplik spots) may appear inside the mouth. These spots may resemble grains of sand. Then the child develops a sore throat.

A mildly itchy rash appears 3 to 5 days after the start of symptoms. The rash begins in front of and below the ears and on the side of the neck as irregular, flat, red areas that soon become raised. The rash spreads within 1 to 2 days to the trunk, arms, palms, legs, and soles and begins to fade on the face.

At the peak of the illness, the child feels very sick and develops eye inflammation (conjunctivitis), the rash is extensive, and the temperature may exceed 104° F (40° C). In 3 to 5 days, the temperature falls, the child begins to feel better, and any remaining rash quickly fades.

Complications of measles are rare. They include:

(from http://www.merckmanuals.com/home/children-s-health-issues/viral-infections-in-infants-and-children/measles)

Etiology and Pathogenesis:
- Uncomplicated case: Zheng Qi weak (in children) plus attack of seasonal heat toxin (via mouth and nose) leads to invasion of Qi level. As toxins invade Qi level, red rash develops over body (this is the Wei Qi trying to disperse the toxins through the body surface). Once heat toxin is expelled, the rash and fever diminish and the recovery stage begins. There may be injury to Qi and Yin.
- Complicated case: following the rash, there may be complications if the Zheng Qi is insufficient or the toxin is severe and the body is not able to disperse the toxin. This may result in secondary patterns.

TCM Differentiation and Treatment:

Pattern	Signs and Symptoms	Treatment Principle	Acupuncture	Formula
Pathogens in the Wei level	Fever, aversion to cold, stuffy and runny nose, coughing, conjunctivitis, and Koplik spots. T: red with yellow coat P: rapid, superficial	Disperse heat from the exterior	LI4, (he gu) LI11 (qu chi), BL12 (feng men), DU14 (da zhui), SJ5 (wei guan)	
Heat in the Ying Qi level	Rashes begin on face (hairline, ears) and spread to body (rash may be bright to dark red), fever peaks, thirst, bloodshot eyes, cough, irritability. T: dark red, yellow coat P: rapid	Clear heat, cool blood, promote rash eruption	LI11 (qu chi), SP10 (xue hai), shi xuan, DU14 (da zhui), BL40 (wei zhong)	
Yin and Qi deficiency	Rash and fever subside, voice is hoarse, dry cough, thirst, low night fever, malaise, lack of appetite. T: red with dry coat P: thin, slightly rapid	Clear remaining heat toxins, tonify Qi, nourish Yin	SP6 (SYJ), ST36 (ZSL), KD3, (tai xi) SP10 (xue hai), REN4 (guan yuan), REN6 (qi hai), BL20 (pi shu), BL23 (shen shu), LU11 (shao shang)	
Lung blocked by heat toxin	High fever, cough, difficult breathing, phlegm sounds, incomplete rash eruption. T: red, yellow coat P: rapid	Clear heat, remove toxins	LI4 (he gu), LI11 (qu chi), shi xuan, LU1 (zhong fu)-BL13 (fei shu), DU14 (za shui)	
Invasion of throat by heat toxin	Sore and painful swollen throat, hoarse voice, difficult breathing, incomplete rash eruption, dark purple rash. T: dark red, yellow coat P: rapid	Clear heat toxin, ease throat, relieve pain	LI4 (he gu), LI11 (qu chi), shi xuan, LU1 (zhong fu)-BL13 (fei shu), DU14 (za shui), REN23 (lian quan)	
Heat toxin invading Heart and Liver	Dense rashes that are not erupting, dark purple rash, restlessness, convulsions, tremors, delirium, possible coma. T: scarlet red, dry P: wiry, slippery, rapid	Clear heat toxins, resuscitate	Hospitalize	

Mumps (zha sai)

Definition:
Mumps is an acute, contagious disease that presents with fever, swelling, and tenderness of the parotid glands. It may be contracted in any of the seasons, but is more prevalent in winter and spring.

Red Flags:
- Measles is an infectious disease; complications are rare, but may be serious (see below)

Western Medicine Relevant Conditions:
Mumps (epidemic parotitis) is a contagious viral infection that causes painful enlargement of the salivary glands. Children become infected with mumps by breathing in small airborne droplets of moisture coughed out by an infected person or by having direct contact with objects contaminated by infected saliva. Although the infection may occur at any age, most cases occur in children 5 to 10 years old.

Mumps symptoms begin 12 to 24 days after infection. However, about one quarter of people do not develop symptoms. Most children develop chills, headache, poor appetite, a general feeling of illness (malaise), and a low to moderate fever. These symptoms are followed in 12 to 24 hours by swelling of the salivary glands, which is most prominent on the second day and lasts 5 to 7 days.

Some children simply have swelling of the salivary glands without the other symptoms. The swelling results in pain when chewing or swallowing, particularly when swallowing acidic liquids, such as citrus fruit juices. The glands are tender when touched. At this stage, the temperature usually rises to 103 or 104° F (about 39.5 or 40° C) and lasts 1 to 3 days.

Mumps may affect organs other than the salivary glands.

About 30% of men who become infected after puberty develop orchitis. Once healed, the affected testis may be smaller, but testosterone production and fertility are usually unaffected. In women, oophoritis is less commonly recognized, is less painful, and does not impair fertility.

Mumps leads to meningitis in 1 to 10% of people. Meningitis causes headache, vomiting, and a stiff neck. Mumps also causes encephalitis in 1 out of 1,000 to 5,000 people. Encephalitis causes drowsiness, coma, or seizures.

Pancreatitis may occur toward the end of the first week of infection. This disorder causes abdominal pain, severe nausea, and vomiting. These symptoms disappear in about a week, and the person recovers completely.

Other complications, such as swelling of the liver, kidneys, or heart muscle, are extremely rare.

(from http://www.merckmanuals.com/home/children-s-health-issues/viral-infections-in-infants-and-children/mumps)

Etiology and Pathogenesis:
- Wind heat seasonal epidemic pathogens are the main etiological factor in mumps. These toxins invade the body through the mouth and nose, after which they combine with phlegm fire to congest the Shaoyang channels and obstruct the flow of Qi and Blood. This results in swelling, hardness, and pain under the ears and above the parotid glands.
- Since the Gallbladder and Liver channel are externally and internally related (and the Liver channel encircles the genitals) severe seasonal heat toxins can invade the Liver channel causing swelling of the genitals.
- Toxins may also move inward to affect the Heart and Liver, causing convulsions and loss of consciousness.

TCM Differentiation and Treatment:

Pattern	Signs and Symptoms	Treatment Principle	Acupuncture	Formula
	Mild fever, aversion to cold, mild and diffuse swelling with pain near parotid glands, no redness, pain worse with chewing, red and painful throat, thirst. T: red with thin yellow coat P: rapid, floating	Dispel wind, clear heat, resolve toxin, relieve swelling	ST6 (jia che), SJ17 (yi feng), SI17 (tian rong), LI4 (he gu), SJ5 (wei guan), DU14 (da zhui), LI11 (qu chi)	
	Heat, pain, redness and swelling near parotid glands, difficulty chewing, high fever, headache, irritability, thirds, red and painful throat, scanty urine, dry stools, vomiting. T: red with yellow coat P: rapid, slippery	Clear heat, resolve toxin, soften and resolve masses	LI4 (he gu), LI11 (qu chi), DU14 (da zhui), ST6 (jia che), SJ17 (yi feng), SI17 (tian rong), LU11 (shao shang), LI1 (shang yang)	
	Above symptoms plus headache, stiff neck, convulsions, possible loss of consciousness. T: red, yellow coat P: rapid, full	Clear heat, remove toxin, resuscitate	Hospitalize	
	High fever, pain in parotid area decreasing, pain and swelling of testes/ovaries, lower abdominal pain, thirst. T: red, yellow coat P: rapid, full	Clear heat from Liver, Gallbladder, dispel mass, relieve pain	SP6 (SYJ), SP10 (xue hai), LR2 (xing jian), GB44 (zu qiao yin)	

Pneumonia (fei yan ke sou)

Definition:
Pneumonia is a common disorder of pulmonary system during infancy, mainly caused by exogenous pathogenic factors and marked by fever, chills, productive cough, difficult breathing, flaring nostrils, and chest pain. In severe cases, there may be pale complexion and cyanotic lips.

Red Flags:
- See red flags of common cold
- Breathing difficulties, cyanotic complexion

Western Medicine Relevant Conditions:
Pneumonia is acute inflammation of the lungs caused by infection. Causes, symptoms, treatment, preventive measures, and prognosis differ depending on whether the infection is bacterial, mycobacterial, viral, fungal, or parasitic; whether it is acquired in the community, hospital, or other health care–associated location; and whether it develops in a patient who is immuno-competent or immuno-compromised.

Streptococcus pneumoniae is the most common pathogen in all age groups, settings, and geographic regions. However, pathogens of every sort, from viruses to parasites, can cause pneumonia.

The airways and lungs are constantly exposed to pathogens in the external environment; the upper airways and oropharynx in particular are colonized with so-called normal flora. Micro-aspiration of these pathogens from the upper respiratory tract is a regular occurrence, but these pathogens are readily dealt with by lung host defense mechanisms. Pneumonia develops when
- Defense mechanisms are compromised
- Macro-aspiration leads to a large inoculum of bacteria that overwhelms normal host defenses
- A particularly virulent pathogen is introduced

Occasionally, infection develops when pathogens reach the lungs via the bloodstream or by contiguous spread from the chest wall or mediastinum.

Upper airway defenses include salivary IgA, proteases, and lysozymes; growth inhibitors produced by normal flora; and fibronectin, which coats the mucosa and inhibits adherence.

Nonspecific lower airway defenses include cough, mucociliary clearance, and airway angulation preventing infection in airspaces. Specific lower airway defenses include various pathogen-specific immune mechanisms, including IgA and IgG opsonization, antimicrobial peptides, anti-inflammatory effects of surfactant, phagocytosis by alveolar macrophages, and T-cell–mediated immune responses. These mechanisms protect most people against infection.

Numerous conditions alter the normal flora (eg, systemic illness, under nutrition, hospital or nursing home exposure, antibiotic exposure) or impair these defenses (eg, altered mental status, cigarette smoke, nasogastric or endotracheal intubation). Pathogens that then reach airspaces can multiply and cause pneumonia.

(from http://www.merckmanuals.com/professional/pulmonary-disorders/pneumonia/overview-of-pneumonia)

Etiology and Pathogenesis:
- Wei Qi is not fully developed and the viscera are delicate in infants and children, therefore they are susceptible to the invasion of pathogenic factors. Exogenous pathogenic factors (mainly wind) invade the Wei Qi either through the skin or through the mouth and nose, affecting the dispersing and descending functions of the lung, and giving rise to the stagnation of the lung qi.
- If wind and cold are transmitted into the interior, they may transform into heat, or exogenous wind heat may be transmitted into the interior. This will lead to excessive internal pathogenic heat and phlegm (transformed from the scorching body fluid). Phlegm and heat will bind and obstruct the lung, bringing about the symptoms of fever, cough, and shortness of breath.
- If the pathogenic factors are excessive and the healthy qi is deficient, other zang organs may be affected.
- At the late stage of pneumonia, there may be lung heat due to yin deficiency or qi deficiency of the lung and spleen.

TCM Differentiation and Treatment:

Pattern	Signs and Symptoms	Treatment Principle	Acupuncture	Formula
	Aversion to cold, slight fever, no sweating, cough, shortness of breath, lack of thirst, thin white phlegm. T: white coat P: floating, tight	Unbind Lung, release exterior, transform phlegm	BL12 (feng men), BL13 (fei shu), LU9 (tai yuan), ST40 (feng long), LU7 (iie que), ST36 (ZSL)	
	Aversion to cold, fever, profuse sweating, shortness of breath, cough with sticky yellow phlegm, thirst and desire to drink, scanty urine, constipation. T: red, yellow coat P: floating, rapid	Unbind Lung, release exterior, clear heat, transform phlegm	BL12 (feng men), BL13 (fei shu), LU5 (chi ze), DU14 (da zhui), SP9 (yin ling quan)	
	High fever, shortness of breath, nasal flaring, discomfort, restlessness, dry mouth, red face, cyanotic lips. T: red, greasy yellow coat P: rapid, slippery	Unbind Lung, clear heat, transform phlegm	BL13 (fei shu), LU9 (tai yuan), ST40 (feng long), SP9 (yin ling quan), LU5 (chi ze), DU14 (da zhui)	
	Suddenly pale, cyanotic lips, listless, sweating, cold limbs, difficult breathing. T: light purple, watery P: rapid, thin	Warm and tonify Heart Yang	REN4 (guan yuan), REN6 (qi hai), PC6 (nei guan), DU4 (ming men), DU20 (bai hui), BL13 (fei shu), BL15 (xin shu), REN8 (shen que)	
	Dry cough, no phlegm (or scanty), low grade fever, night sweats, malar flush. T: red, dry, no coat P: thin, rapid	Nourish Yin, clear heat, moisten Lung, stop cough	LU7-KD6 (ren mai), LU1 (zhong fu), BL13 (fei shu), LU9 (tai yuan) (SYJ), SP6 (SYJ)	
	Weak cough, phlegm, low fever, spontaneous sweat, poor digestion, loose stool, pale complexion. T: pale, greasy white coat P: thin, weak	Tonify Lung and Spleen, stop cough	BL13 (fei shu), BL20 (pi shu), SP6 (SYJ), ST36 (ZSL), LU9 (tai yuan), LU1 (zhong fu), REN17 (dan zhong)	

Purpura (zi dian)

Definition:
Purpura is a non-infectious condition characterized by reddish purple spots like bruises, typically on the face and buttocks. Often accompanied by gastrointestinal symptoms, swollen and sore joints, and possible kidney issues.

Western Medicine Relevant Conditions:
In Western medicine, purpura simplex is increased bruising that results from vascular fragility. Purpura refers to purplish cutaneous or mucosal lesions caused by hemorrhage. Small lesions (< 2 mm) are termed petechiae, and large lesions are termed ecchymoses or bruises.
Purpura simplex is extremely common. The cause and mechanism are unknown. Purpura simplex may represent a heterogeneous group of disorders or merely a variation of normal.

The disorder usually affects women. Bruises develop on the thighs, buttocks, and upper arms in people without known trauma. The history usually reveals no other abnormal bleeding, but easy bruising may be present in family members. Serious bleeding does not occur.

The platelet count and tests of platelet function, blood coagulation, and fibrinolysis are normal.

(from http://www.merckmanuals.com/professional/hematology-and-oncology/bleeding-due-to-abnormal-blood-vessels/purpura-simplex)

Etiology and Pathogenesis:

TCM Differentiation and Treatment:

Pattern	Signs and Symptoms	Treatment Principle	Acupuncture	Formula
Wind Heat impairing collaterals	Abrupt onset, fever, aversion to wind, cough, sore throat, purpura on low legs/buttocks, abdominal pain, join pain, possible blood in urine. T: red, yellow coat P: superficial, rapid	Expel wind, clear Heat, cool Blood, relieve collaterals	LI4 (he gu), SJ5 (wei guan), DU14 (da zhui), BL14 (jue yin shu), BL40 (wei zhong), SP10 (xue hai)	
Bleeding due to Blood Heat	Abrupt onset, purple red purpura, dry mouth, preference for cold drinks, fever, red face, blood in stool, nosebleed. T: red, yellow coat P: full, rapid	Clear heat, remove toxin, cool Blood, stop bleeding	BL17 (ge shu), BL40 (wei zhong), SP6 (SYJ), SP10 (xue hai), LI11 (qu chi), HT8 (shao fu), PC8 (lao gong), shi xuan	
Qi cannot hold and circulate Blood	Scanty and scattered purpura that is slightly red in color, recurring purpura, worse with exertion, dizziness, palpitations, fatigue, poor appetite, pale and lusterless complexion. T: pale P: thin and forceless	Strengthen Spleen and Heart, supplement Qi, control Blood	BL17 (ge shu), BL20 (pi shu), SP6 (SYJ), SP10, (xue hai) ST36 (ZSL), REN6 (qi hai), HT7 (shen men)	
Fire Flaring due to Yin Deficiency	Recurring purpura, bleeding from nose and gums, low fever, night sweats, irritability, poor sleep, dry mouth, constipation. T: red, no coat P: thin and rapid	Nourish Yin, remove Fire, cool Blood, stop bleeding	SP6 (SYJ), KD3 (tai xi), REN4 (guan yuan), KD2 (ran gu), BL17 (ge shu), SP10 (xue hai)	

Retardation and Flaccidity (wu chi wu ruan)

Definition:
Refers to developmental delays in childhood. The five delays are: standing, walking, talking, teeth and hair growth. The five flaccidities are: drooling, weak neck, weak legs and arms, and general softness of the muscles.

Western Medicine Relevant Conditions:
In Western Medicine, these patterns relate to a range of delays in childhood that could be due to: malnutrition, chromosomal issues (such as Down's Syndrome), cerebral palsy, trauma during birth, exposure to toxins, maternal diseases or exposure to toxins, or intellectual disabilities.
In Western medicine, retardation is called intellectual disability (ID). ID is significantly sub-average intellectual functioning present from birth or early infancy, causing limitations in the ability to conduct normal activities of daily living. The previously used term mental retardation has acquired an undesirable social stigma, so health care practitioners have replaced it with the term intellectual disability.

People with ID have significantly below average intellectual functioning that limits their ability to cope with one or more areas of normal daily living (adaptive skills) to such a degree that they require ongoing support. Adaptive skills may be categorized into several areas including: conceptual, social, and practical.
A wide variety of medical and environmental conditions can cause intellectual disability. Some are genetic. Some are present before or at the time of conception, and others occur during pregnancy, during birth, or after birth. The common factor is that something interferes with the growth and development of the brain. Even with recent advances in genetics, especially techniques of chromosome analysis, a specific cause of ID often cannot be identified.

(from http://www.merckmanuals.com/home/children-s-health-issues/learning-and-developmental-disorders/intellectual-disability)

Etiology and Pathogenesis:
- Pre-natal Jing deficiency due to parents with weak Jing or to poor nutrition during pregnancy could lead to delays.
- Post-natal deficiencies due to trauma, chronic illness or malnutrition could cause organ deficiencies and related delays: kidney deficiency will result in late standing, or slow teeth and hair growth; Heart deficiency will result in slow speech; Liver deficiency will result in late standing and problems walking; and, Spleen deficiency will result in a weak body (muscles not nourished).

TCM Differentiation and Treatment:

Pattern	Signs and Symptoms	Treatment Principle	Acupuncture	Formula
	Slow physical development (e.g. standing, teeth growth), poor cognitive ability, dry eyes, sinews and bones weak. T: light red, no coat P: thin and weak	Nourish Liver and Kidneys, strengthen marrow and tendons	KD3 (tai xi), KD6 (zhao hai), BL23 (shen shu), REN4 (guan yuan), REN6 (qi hai), GB39 (xuan zhong), LR8 (qu quan)	
	Mental slowness, delayed speech, listlessness, sallow skin, yellow hair, no crying. T: pale with no coat P: thin and weak	Nourish Heart Blood to nourish intelligence	HT7 (shen men), SP10 (xue hai), PC6 (nei guan, ST36 (ZSL), SP6 (SYJ, REN14 (ju que), REN15 (jiu wei), BL15 (xin shu)	
	History of trauma, deafness, epilepsy, stiff limbs, difficult speech, slow responses. T: deep purple P: deep and choppy	Dispel Blood stasis, open collaterals, open orifices	BL17 (ge shu), SP10 (xue hai), sishencong, LI4-LR3 (4 gates)	
	Low spirit, overweight, epilepsy, developmental delays. T: greasy white coat P: slippery	Drain damp, transform phlegm, open orifices	PC5 (jian shi), BL15 (jiu wei), BL20 (pi shu), BL21 (wei shu), REN12 (zhong wan), ST40 (feng long)	

Rubella (feng sha)

Definition:
Contagious viral infection causing fever, malaise, sore throat, swollen lymph, and a rash that begins on the face and spreads.

Red Flags:
- Rapidly worsening condition or signs of brain infection (encephalitis)

Western Medicine Relevant Conditions:
Rubella (German measles, 3-day measles) is a contagious viral infection that causes mild symptoms, such as joint pain and a rash.

Rubella is a typically mild childhood infection that may, however, have devastating consequences for infants infected before birth. A woman infected during the first 16 weeks (particularly the first 8 to 10 weeks) of pregnancy often passes the infection to the fetus. This fetal infection causes miscarriage, stillbirth, or multiple, severe birth defects (congenital rubella syndrome).

Rubella is spread mainly by breathing in small virus-containing droplets of moisture that have been coughed into the air by an infected person. Close contact with an infected person can also spread the infection. People who have rubella are contagious from 1 week before to 1 week after the rash appears, but most spread occurs when the rash is present. An infant infected before birth can spread the infection for many months after birth. A person who has had rubella develops immunity and cannot contract it again.
Rubella symptoms differ depending on the age of the affected person. Symptoms of rubella begin about 14 to 21 days after infection. Adults and a few children feel mildly ill for a few days, with a low fever and irritated eyes. But in most children, the first sign is the characteristic rash. The rash of rubella is similar to the rash caused by measles, but is not as extensive and does not merge to form large red areas. The rash begins on the face and neck and quickly spreads to the trunk, arms, and legs. As the rash appears, a mild reddening of the skin (flush) occurs, particularly on the face. Painless spots appear on the roof of the mouth. These spots later merge with each other into a red blush extending over the back of the throat. The rash lasts about 3 to 5 days.

People with rubella usually do not feel very ill, but some have joint pain. Some children may have swollen lymph nodes in the neck and back of the head. In rare instances, people develop a middle ear infection or a low platelet count. Brain infection is a very rare but occasionally fatal complication.

Etiology and pathogenesis:
- Zheng Qi weak in children plus wind heat attacking and combating with Qi and Blood leads to rubella.

TCM Differentiation and Treatment:

Pattern	Signs and Symptoms	Treatment Principle	Acupuncture	Formula
	Fever, sneezing, nasal discharge, cough, thirst, poor appetite, rash that is small and scattered, swollen lymph nodes. T: red, yellow coat P: superficial, rapid	Dispel wind, clear heat, promote eruption	LI4 (he gu), BL13 (fei shu), DU14 (da zhui), SJ5 (wei guan)	
	High fever, discomfort, thirst with desire to drink, dense skin rashes, constipation, dark scanty urine, agitation, dry lips, red face. T: red with yellow coat P: full and rapid	Clear heat, cool Ying and Qi, promote eruptions, clear toxins	LI4 (he gu), DU15 (ya men), BL40 (wei zhong), shi xuan, SP10 (xue hai)	

Scarlatina (dan sha)

Definition:

Red Flags:
- Western medical treatment with antibiotics required; complications are rare, but severe (see below)
- Emergency care required for stridor or other signs of respiratory distress, drooling, muffled voice or visible bulge in pharynx

Western Medicine Relevant Conditions:
Scarlet fever is a syndrome characterized by exudative pharyngitis, fever, and bright-red exanthem. It is caused by streptococcal pyrogenic exotoxins (SPEs) types A, B, and C produced by group A streptococci found in secretions and discharge from the nose, ears, throat, and skin. Scarlet fever may follow streptococcal wound infections or burns, as well as upper respiratory tract infections. Food-borne outbreaks have been reported.

(from http://emedicine.medscape.com/article/1053253-overview#a6)

This bacterial infection is marked by a bright red rash that blanches on pressure, high fever, chills, sore throat, swollen tonsils, vomiting, and abdominal pain. The folds of the skin may be deeper red, and the face may be flushed with a pale ring around the mouth. The rash may feel like sandpaper, with numerous, small, popular elevations. Skin may peel as the rash fades. In the mouth, inflamed papillae may protrude through bright red coating (called "strawberry tongue").

Serious complications include rheumatic fever and heart disease.

Etiology and Pathogenesis:
- Zheng Qi is weak allowing epidemic wind-warm pathogens to attack

TCM Differentiation and Treatment:

Pattern	Signs and Symptoms	Treatment Principle	Acupuncture	Formula
Heat toxin invading the Wei	Fever, aversion to cold, thirst, headache, swollen throat, ulcerative tonsillitis, flushed red skin, bright red rash. T: red with white coat P: superficial, rapid	Clear wind, dispel heat, promote eruption, sooth throat	LI4 (he gu), BL13 (fei shu), SJ5 (wei guan), DU14 (da zhui)	
Heat toxins in the Qi and Ying	High fever, flushed red face, thirst, swelling with ulceration of the throat, densely packed rash, dry stool, scanty urine, possible delirium. T: dark red (strawberry tongue) P: rapid, full	Cool Ying and Qi, clear fire, resolve toxin	DU14 (da zhui), LI11 (qu chi), shi xuan, jin jin, yu ye	
Yin deficiency with Fire flaring	History of disease, low grade fever worse at night, skin rash decreasing, skin peeling, thirst scanty urine. T: red without coat P: thin, rapid	Nourish Yin, engender fluids, clear heat	LI11 (qu chi), SP6 (SYJ), KD6 (zhao hai), LU7 (lie que)	

Sweating (han zheng)

Definition:
Sweating, under normal circumstances, is a physiological function where the body radiates heat and expels pathogens from the superficial layers. Abnormal sweating refers to excessive sweating that is not related to the environment or physical exertion.

Red Flags:
- In severe cases not responding to treatment, refer for Western medical evaluation to rule out serious underlying causes.
- Watch for signs of dehydration.

Western Medicine Relevant Conditions:
In Western medicine, excessive sweating may be caused by a wide range of conditions, including:

Etiology and Pathogenesis:
- Lung Qi deficiency: the Lungs regulate the pores, and distribute Wei Qi. Children's Lungs are immature and Wei Qi is relatively weak, as a result pores may not function well leading to sweating.
- Deficiency heat: pathogens, hot and spicy foods, or constitutional heat may consume Yin. As a result, Yang rises to the surface leading to sweating.
- Excess heat: liver fire, food stagnation, or too much sweet and greasy food may cause excess heat (or damp heat). This flares upward disturbing fluids, opening pores, and causing sweating.

TCM Differentiation and Treatment:

Pattern	Signs and Symptoms	Treatment Principle	Acupuncture	Formula
Lung Qi deficiency	Spontaneous sweating, worse with exertion, fatigue, shortness of breath, easily catch colds, pale complexion. T: pale, thin coat P: thin, weak	Tonify Qi to consolidate exterior	LU9 (tai yuan), BL13 (fei shu), KD7 (fu liu)-LI4 (he gu), ST36 (ZSL)	
Damp heat accumulation	Sticky sweat,, irritable, bitter taste, thirst with no desire to drink, constipation, scanty urine. T: red, thick yellow coat P: slippery, wiry, rapid	Clear heat, drain damp	KD7 (fu liu)-LI4 (he gu), GB34 (yang ling quan), GB41 (zu lin qi), GB24 (ri yue), LR3 (tai chong)	
Excess heat flaring	Excessive sweating on the head, irritable, restless, heat in chest, thirst, constipation, scanty urine. T: red, yellow coat P: slippery, rapid, forceful	Clear heat, drain fire	KD7 (fu liu)-LI4 (he gu), LR2 (xing jian), ST44 (nei ting), LI1 (shang yang)	
Yin deficiency	Night sweating, worse on back of head/neck, late afternoon sweating, insomnia, five center heat, malar flush, dry mouth and throat, emaciation. T: red, no coat P: thin and rapid	Nourish Yin, clear fire	KD7 (fu liu)-LI4 (he gu), HT6 (yin xi), SP6 (SYJ), REN4 (guan yuan), REN6 (qi hai), LR2 (xing jian)	

Thrush (e kou chuang)

Definition:
Thrush refers to an overgrowth of fungus in the mouth. It typically causes creamy or milky patches on the tongue or insides of the mouth, with inflammation and possibly erosion of underlying tissues. This is a common condition in babies up to 2 months old.

Red Flags:
- Condition not improving
- Signs of dehydration

Western Medicine Relevant Conditions:
Candida yeast is a normal resident of the mouth, digestive tract, and vagina that usually causes no harm. Under certain conditions, however, *Candida* can overgrow on mucous membranes and moist areas of the skin. Typical areas affected are the lining of the mouth, the groin, the armpits, the spaces between fingers and toes, on an uncircumcised penis, the skin-fold under the breasts, the nails, and the skin-folds of the stomach.
Thrush is candidiasis inside the mouth. The creamy white patches typical of thrush cling to the tongue and sides of the mouth and may be painful. The patches can be scraped off with a finger or blunt object and may bleed when scraped. Thrush in otherwise healthy children is not unusual.

Etiology and Pathogenesis:
- Spleen Qi is weak plus overeating leads to food stagnation and accumulation. This creates Stomach heat that flares up to the mouth.
- Weak Yin constitution (or long term illness consumes Yin) causes empty heat to flare up resulting in mouth ulcers.
- Excess cold and raw foods lead to cold damp accumulation that rises to the mouth.

TCM Differentiation and Treatment:

Pattern	Signs and Symptoms	Treatment Principle	Acupuncture	Formula
Spleen and Stomach accumulation and heat	If heat is pronounced, numerous sores and lesions in the mouth with red borders, local pain, refusal to eat, agitation, crying foul mouth odor, dark yellow urine, dry stools, possible red face. If damp is more pronounced, may be a white, slimy coating or membrane over the mouth and excessive drooling. T: red, yellow coat P: slippery and rapid	Clear heat and resolve toxins, drain damp	REN23 (lian quan), HT6 (yin xi), ST5 (da ying), ST36 (ZSL), ST44 (nei ting), ST7 (xia guan), LI4 (he gu), Si Feng	
Stomach Yin deficiency	Few white, yellow, or grey spots, red bleeding under, weight loss, lack of desire to drink. P: thin and rapid	Nourish Yin, clear heat	Si Feng, ST36 (ZSL), ST5, (da ying) ST7 (xia guan), LI4 (he gu), REN23 (lian quan), KD3 (tai xi), KD6 (zhoa hai), REN4 (guan yuan)	
Cold Damp	White or yellow patches, mild redness, pale complexion, weak, loose stools. P: weak or slippery	Tonify Spleen, resolve damp	SP6 (SYJ), ST36 (ZSL), REN12 (zhong wan), ST5, (da ying) ST7 (xia guan), LI4 (he gu),	

Whooping cough (dun ke)

Definition:
Whooping cough is a pediatric infectious respiratory disease characterized by recurring spasmodic cough marked by the sound made during inspiration, which resembles a rooster's crow.

Red Flags:
- Whooping cough is an infectious disease requiring antibiotic treatment; seriously ill infants with breathing difficulties may require hospitalization

Western Medicine Relevant Conditions:
Pertussis (whooping cough) is a highly contagious infection caused by the bacteria Bordetella pertussis, which results in fits of coughing that usually end in a prolonged, high-pitched, deeply indrawn breath (the whoop).

Pertussis is most serious in children younger than 2 years, and nearly all deaths occur in children younger than 6 months. Most deaths are caused by pneumonia and complications affecting the brain.

An infected person spreads pertussis bacteria into the air in droplets of moisture produced by coughing. Anyone nearby may inhale these droplets and become infected. Pertussis usually is not contagious after the third week of the infection.

The illness begins about 1 or 2 weeks after exposure. It lasts about 6 to 10 weeks, progressing through three stages:

- Cold like symptoms include: sneezing, runny nose, loss of appetite, listlessness, a hacking cough at night, and a general feeling of illness (malaise). People may be hoarse but rarely have a fever.
- Coughing fits develop after 10 or 14 days. These fits typically consist of 5 or more rapidly consecutive forceful coughs followed by the whoop. After a fit, breathing is normal, but another coughing fit follows shortly thereafter. The cough often produces large amounts of thick mucus (usually swallowed by infants and children or seen as large bubbles from the nose). In younger children, vomiting often follows a prolonged fit of coughing. In infants, choking spells and pauses in breathing (apnea), possibly causing the skin to turn blue, may be more common than the whoops.

About one fourth of children develop pneumonia, resulting in difficulty breathing. Otitis media also frequently develops. Rarely, pertussis affects the brain in infants. Bleeding, swelling, or inflammation of the brain may cause seizures, confusion, brain damage, and intellectual disability. Seizures are common among infants but rare in older children.

After several weeks, the coughing fits gradually subside, but for many weeks or even months, children have a lingering, persistent cough.

(from http://www.merckmanuals.com/home/infections/bacterial-infections/pertussis)

Etiology and Pathogenesis:
- The major cause of whooping cough is attack by seasonal external pathogens resulting in phlegm-turbidity. This results in dysfunction of the Lung, obstruction of the Lung function of descending and dispersing, and counter flow of Lung Qi resulting in cough.
- Categorized in three stages:
    - Initial stage, presents as external pattern of wind invading the Wei Qi
    - With development, coughing becomes more severe with seasonal evils accumulating and transforming into phlegm heat
    - In the recovery stage, evils have been dispelled, but the Qi and Yin are depleted

TCM Differentiation and Treatment:

Pattern	Signs and Symptoms	Treatment Principle	Acupuncture	Formula
	Coughing, phlegm, fever, sneezing, runny nose, headache, sore throat, slight aversion to cold, yellow mucus. T: red, yellow coat P: superficial, rapid	Expel wind, clear heat	DU14 (da zhui), LI4 (he gu), SJ5 (wei guan), GB20 (feng chi), LI11 (qu chi), BL12 (feng men)	
	Whooping cough, pain in chest, possible vomiting, sticky yellow phlegm. T: red, yellow coat P: rapid, slippery	Clear heat, drain lungs, stop cough, transform phlegm	ST40 (feng long), SP9 (yin ling quan), LI4 (he gu), LI11 (qu chi), LU5 (chi ze), PC6 (nei guan), REN17 (dan zhong), REN22 (tian tu)	
	Cough improving, tired, weak, red cheeks, night sweats. T: red, peeled coat P: thin and weak	Tonify Qi, nourish Yin	LU9 (tai yuan), SP6 (SYJ), ST36 (ZSL), BL13 (fei shu), BL20 (pi shu), REN4 (guan yuan), REN6 (qi hai), REN17 (dan zhong)	

Infantile edema (xiao er shui zhong)

Definition:
Accumulation of fluids in the body.

Red Flags:
- Refer for Western medical evaluation to rule out serious underlying causes (see below)
- See also red flags for edema (shui zhong) in Internal Medicine section.

Western Medicine Relevant Conditions:
See also edema (shui zhong) in Internal Medicine section.

In children, relevant Western medical conditions include: renal failure (acute or chronic nephritis), and nephrotic syndrome.

Renal failure is the inability of the kidneys to adequately filter metabolic waste products from the blood. It has many possible causes. Some lead to a rapid decline in kidney function (acute renal failure). Others lead to a gradual decline in kidney function (chronic renal failure). In addition to the kidneys being unable to filter metabolic waste products (such as creatinine and urea nitrogen) from the blood, the kidneys are less able to control the fluid, electrolyte and acid balance in the body.

Acute kidney injury can result from any condition that decreases the blood supply to the kidneys, any disease or toxic substances (also called toxins) affecting the kidneys themselves, or any condition that obstructs urine flow anywhere along the urinary tract. In many people, no cause of acute kidney injury can be identified. Symptoms include edema on the face, low urine output, and dark urine.

If both kidneys function normally, damage to one kidney (for example, due to blockage by a kidney stone) does not usually cause major problems because the remaining good kidney can compensate and usually maintain near-normal laboratory measurements of kidney function. Thus, acute kidney injury may be hard for doctors to detect. For acute kidney injury to cause significant problems, usually both kidneys must be damaged or function abnormally.

Chronic kidney disease is a slowly progressive (months to years) decline in the kidneys' ability to filter metabolic waste products from the blood. Many diseases can irreversibly damage or injure the kidneys. Acute kidney disease becomes chronic kidney disease if kidney function does not recover after treatment and lasts more than three months. Therefore, anything that can cause acute kidney injury can cause chronic kidney disease. In Western countries, the most common causes of chronic kidney disease are: diabetes mellitus or hypertension.
(from http://www.merckmanuals.com/home/kidney-and-urinary-tract-disorders/kidney-failure/overview-of-kidney-failure)

Nephrotic syndrome is a disorder of the glomeruli (clusters of microscopic blood vessels in the kidneys that have small pores through which blood is filtered) in which excessive amounts of protein are excreted in the urine. Excessive protein excretion typically leads to edema and low levels of the protein albumin and high levels of fats in the blood.

Nephrotic syndrome can develop gradually or suddenly. Nephrotic syndrome can occur at any age. In children, it is most common between the ages of 18 months and 4 years, and more boys than girls are affected.

Nephrotic syndrome can be caused by:
- Primary, originating in the kidneys
- Secondary, caused by a vast array of other disorders

The secondary causes may involve other parts of the body. The most common disorders causing nephrotic syndrome are: diabetes mellitus, systemic lupus erythematosus, and certain viral infections. The syndrome may be caused by certain allergies, including allergies to insect bites and to poison ivy or poison oak. Some types of nephrotic syndrome are hereditary.

(from http://www.merckmanuals.com/home/kidney-and-urinary-tract-disorders/kidney-filtering-disorders/nephrotic-syndrome)

Etiology and Pathogenesis:
- Zheng Qi deficiency plus external pathogenic invasion blocks Lung, disrupts dispersion and descending of fluids, edema results.
- Improper diet, taxation, illness can deplete the Spleen and Kidney leading to impaired water metabolism and edema.
- Long-term illness can consume Qi and Yin and deplete the Liver and Kidney leading to failed water metabolism and edema.

TCM Differentiation and Treatment:

Pattern	Signs and Symptoms	Treatment Principle	Acupuncture	Formula
	Acute edema beginning in eyelids and moving to face, scanty urine, fever, aversion to wind, cough. P: floating	Expel wind, induce urination	LU7 (lie que), LI4 (he gu), LI6 (pian li), SP9 (yin ling quan), BL39 (wei yang), DU26 (shui gou), SJ5 (wei guan), REN3 (zhong ji)	
	Edema of the limbs and body, dark and scanty urine, fever, thirst, chest oppression, poor appetite, nausea. T: red, yellow coat P: slippery, rapid	Clear heat, drain damp, relieve edema	As above, except DU26 (shui gou) and add LI11 (qu chi)	
	Mild edema, profuse seating, pale and lusterless complexion, fatigue, shortness of breath, poor appetite. T: pale P: slow, weak	Tonify Lung and Spleen, resolve edema	BL20 (pi shu), BL13 (fei shu), BL23 (shen shu), SP9 (yin ling quan), SP6 (SYJ), ST36 (ZSL), REN4 (guan yuan), REN6 (qi hai), REN9 (shui fen)	
	Severe pitting edema, especially below the waste, cold limbs, fatigue, cough with shortness of breath, decreased urination, pale complexion, low back and limbs weak. T: pale P: deep, weak	Warm Yang, tonify Spleen and Kidney, resolve edema	SP9 (yin ling quan), ST36 (ZSL), REN9 (shui fen), BL23 (shen shu), BL20 (pi shu), BL28 (pang guang shu), REN3 (zhong ji), REN4 (guan yuan), DU4 (ming men)	
	Edema on face and lower limbs, dizziness, tinnitus, low-grade fever, night sweats, insomnia. T: red, possibly peeled P: thin, wiry	Tonify Liver and Kidney, suppress Yang	BL18 (gan shu), BL20 (pi shu), BL23 (shen shu), LR2 (xing jian), SP5 (shang qiu), ST36 (ZSL), SP6 (SYJ), REN4 (guan yuan), REN6 (qi hai), KD3 (tai xi)	

Orthopedics and Traumatology (Gu Shang Ke)

Achilles Tendon Injury (gen jian sun shang)

Definition:
A repetitive stress injury characterized by pain, inflammation, and swelling of the Achilles tendon and its sheath. The entire calf muscle group may be affected.

Red Flags:
- A tendon tear (sudden snap and extreme pain) requires Western medical assessment and treatment

Western Medicine:
Achilles tendon injuries include inflammation of the paratenon (fatty areolar tissue that surrounds the tendon), and partial or complete tears.

Achilles tendinitis is very common among running athletes. The calf muscles attach to the calcaneus via the Achilles tendon. During running, the calf muscles help with the lift-off phase of gait. Repetitive forces from running combined with insufficient recovery time can initially cause inflammation in the tendon paratenon. A complete tear of the Achilles tendon is a serious injury, usually resulting from sudden, forceful stress.

The primary symptom of Achilles tendon inflammation is pain in the back of the heel, which initially increases when exercise starts and often lessens as exercise continues. A complete tear of the Achilles tendon typically occurs with a sudden forceful change in direction when running or playing tennis.

Etiology and Pathogenesis:
- Trauma or repetitive strain cause Qi and Blood stagnation in the channels and collaterals
- Bladder and Kidney are the primary meridians involved, but may also involve Liver and Gallbladder channels
- Internal organ imbalances may contribute

TCM Differentiation and Treatment:

Pattern	Signs and Symptoms	Treatment Principle	Acupuncture	Formula
	Pain, inflammation, swelling, and stiffness of the tendon. Most common site is 2-6cm proximal to attachment at calcaneus. Crepitus may be felt on ankle movement. Symptoms worse after rest and relieved with moderate activity, but pain returns during or after more vigorous exercise.	Move Qi and Blood	Local ashi points BL 40 (wei zhong), BL57 (cheng shan), BL58 (fei yang), BL63 (jin men) GB34 (yang ling quan) KD3 (tai xi), KI4, (da zhong) KI5 (shui quan), KI7 (fu liu) BL60 (kun lun) to KD3 (tai xi) (also consider the Dai Mai or Yang Qiao Mai, depending on additional symptoms)	
	May be additional signs and symptoms of Liver Qi stagnation, Liver Yin Deficiency, or Liver Blood Deficiency	Tonify and treat according to pattern	LR3 (tai chong), GB34 (yang ling quan)	
	May be additional signs and symptoms of Kidney Yin or Yang Deficiency	Tonify and treat according to pattern	KD3 (tai xi), BL23 (shen shu)	

Acute Lumbar Muscle Sprain (yao bu niu cuo shang)

Definition:
This condition is an acute muscle strain or sprain of the lower back, often related to the muscles in the area, such as the quadratus lumborum. Pain may radiate to the gluteal region and is often one-sided.

Red Flags:

Western Medicine:
Most acute lower back pain is caused by disorders of the spine and the muscles, ligaments, and nerve roots around it or the disks between vertebrae. Often, no single specific cause can be identified. Any painful disorder of the spine may cause spasms of the muscles around the spine. This spasm worsens the existing pain. Stress may worsen low back pain.

The most common cause of low back pain is muscle strains and ligament sprains. These may result from lifting, exercising, or moving in an unexpected way. The lower back is more likely to be injured when a person's physical conditioning is poor and the supporting muscles of the back are weak. Having poor posture, lifting incorrectly, being overweight, and being tired also contribute.

Other common causes of low back pain include the following, but these more commonly cause chronic pain:
- Osteoarthritis
- Compression fractures
- A ruptured or herniated disk
- Lumbar spinal stenosis
- Spondylolisthesis
- Fibromyalgia

Less common causes that are serious include:
- Spinal infections
- Spinal tumors
- An abdominal aortic aneurysm
- Certain digestive disorders, such as a perforated peptic ulcer, diverticulitis, and pancreatitis
- Certain urinary tract disorders, such as kidney infections, kidney stones, and prostate infections
- Certain disorders involving the pelvis, such as ectopic pregnancy, pelvic inflammatory disease, and cancer of the ovaries or other reproductive organs

(from http://www.merckmanuals.com/home/bone,-joint,-and-muscle-disorders/low-back-and-neck-pain/low-back-pain)

Etiology and Pathogenesis:
- Overuse, injury, poor posture can lead to Qi and Blood stagnation in the channels and collaterals (Bladder and Gallbladder meridians, in particular).
- Internal organ issues may also contribute (e.g. Kidney deficiency is a common cause of lower back pain; or, Liver Yin or Blood deficiency), but these often cause chronic issues.

TCM Differentiation and Treatment:

Pattern	Signs and Symptoms	Treatment Principle	Acupuncture	Formula
Qi and Blood Stagnation	Acute lower back pain and spasm, spine may feel locked, pain may be one-sided, pain may radiate toward the gluteal region, additional symptoms according to etiology. (if disc protrusion-pain may be immbolizing)	Move Qi and Blood, resolve pain	Local ashi points and Jiaji points + Yaoyan, Pigen, Shiqizhuixia, BL40 (wei zhong), GB29 (ju liao), GB30 (huan tiao), BL60 (kun lun) BL67 (zhi yin), GB44 (zu qiao yin) Yao tong xue Ling gu and Dai bai SI3 (hou xi) and BL62 (shen mai) or GB41 (zu lin qi) and SJ5 (wei guan) BL63 (jin men), BL17 (ge shu)	

Bone Fracture (ju zhe)

Definition:
Refers to any break in a bone, for example, due to impact or crushing injuries. These may occur more frequently in old age, cases of deficiency, or diseases affecting the bone.

Red Flags:
- Watch for signs of shock or severe bleeding and use first aid protocol, if necessary
- Refer for Western medical evaluation and treatment

Western Medicine Relevant Diseases:
A fracture is a break in a bone. Most involve a single, significant force applied to normal bone.

In a closed fracture, the overlying skin is intact. In an open fracture, the overlying skin is disrupted and the broken bone is in communication with the environment.

Pathologic fractures occur when mild or minimal force fractures an area of bone weakened by a disorder (eg, osteoporosis, cancer, infection, bone cyst). When the disorder is osteoporosis, they are often called insufficiency or fragility fractures.

Stress fractures result from repetitive application of moderate force, as may occur in long-distance runners or in soldiers marching while carrying a heavy load. Normally, bone damaged by microtrauma from moderate force self-repairs during periods of rest, but repeated application of force to the same location predisposes to further injury and causes the microtrauma to propagate.

(from http://www.merckmanuals.com/professional/injuries-poisoning/fractures,-dislocations,-and-sprains/overview-of-fractures,-dislocations,-and-sprains)

Etiology and Pathogenesis:
- Trauma or repetitive strain may cause bone to fracture
- Aging or chronic illness may weaken the Kidneys and the bone, predisposing patients to bone fractures

TCM Differentiation and Treatment:

Pattern	Signs and Symptoms	Treatment Principle	Acupuncture	Formula
Qi and Blood Stasis	Characterized by local swelling, pain, displacement, deformity, or abnormal movement. P: wiry or choppy	Quicken Qi and Blood, transform stasis, disperse swelling, relieve pain		

Calcaneodynia (gen tong zheng)

Definition:
Refers to pain and stiffness of the heel and the plantar aspect of the foot. This is repetitive stress injury characterized by inflammation and irritation of the plantar fascia. Symptoms are often experienced after prolonged rest, and are alleviated after moderate activity (returning again during or after more strenuous exercise).

Red Flags:
- Refer for acute, severe heel pain with local swelling to rule out acute fascia tear

Western Medicine Relevant Diseases:
Heel pain most commonly results from plantar fasciosis.

Plantar fasciosis is pain originating from the dense band of tissue called the plantar fascia that extends from the bottom of the heel bone to the base of the toes (ball of the foot). The plantar fascia connects the bottom of the heel bone to the ball of the foot and is essential to walking, running, and giving spring to the step.

Plantar fasciosis is sometimes referred to as plantar fasciitis. However, the term *plantar fasciitis* is not correct. The term *fasciitis* means inflammation of the fascia, but plantar fasciosis is a disorder where the fascia is repeatedly stressed rather than inflamed.

Other terms used to describe plantar fasciosis include calcaneal enthesopathy and calcaneal spur syndrome. A heel spur is a pointed growth of extra bone on the heel bone. It is caused over time by a combination of increased pull on the fascia and foot dysfunction. However, a heel spur may or may not be present. Often a small tear results from excessive strain placed on the plantar fascia.

Plantar fasciosis can develop in people who have a sedentary lifestyle, wear high-heeled shoes, have unusually high or low arches in the feet, or have tight calf muscles or a tight Achilles tendon. Sedentary people are usually affected when they suddenly increase their level of activity or wear less supportive shoes such as sandals or flip-flops. Plantar fasciosis is also common among runners and dancers because of increased stress on the fascia, especially if the person also has poor foot posture. The development of this painful disorder occurs more often in people whose occupations involve standing or walking on hard surfaces for prolonged periods.

Disorders that may cause or aggravate plantar fasciosis are obesity, rheumatoid arthritis, and other types of arthritis. Too many corticosteroid injections may contribute to the development of plantar fasciosis by damaging the fascia or the fat pad under the heel.

A person with plantar fasciosis may have pain anywhere along the course of the plantar fascia but most commonly where the fascia joins the bottom of the heel bone. The person often feels a great deal of pain with weight bearing, particularly when placing weight on the foot first thing in the morning. The pain temporarily lessens within 5 to 10 minutes but may return later in the day. It is often worse when pushing off of the heel (such as when walking or running) and after periods of rest. In this case, the pain radiates from the bottom of the heel toward the toes. Some people have burning or sticking pain along the inside border of the sole of the foot when walking.

(from http://www.merckmanuals.com/home/bone,-joint,-and-muscle-disorders/foot-problems/plantar-fasciosis)

Etiology and Pathogenesis:
- Accident, trauma, or repetitive stress leads to local Qi and Blood stagnation
- May also be due to pathologies of the Kidney or Bladder meridian, or internal organ imbalances

TCM Differentiation and Treatment:

Pattern	Signs and Symptoms	Treatment Principle	Acupuncture	Formula
Qi and Blood stagnation	History of injury, local pain and stiffness	Move Qi and Blood		
Liver imbalances	Check for signs of Liver Qi stagnation, Liver Yin deficiency, and Liver Blood deficiency	Treat according to pattern	LR3 (tai chong), GB34 (yang ling quan)	
Kidney imbalances	Check for signs of Kidney deficiency	Treat according to pattern	KI3 (tai xi), DU4 (ming men)	

Carpal Tunnel Syndrome (wan guan zong he zheng)

Definition:
This is a Western medical condition; see below.

Western Medicine Relevant Diseases:
Carpal tunnel syndrome is compression of the median nerve as it passes through the carpal tunnel in the wrist. Symptoms of carpal tunnel syndrome include pain of the hand and wrist associated with tingling and numbness, classically distributed along the median nerve (the palmar side of the thumb, the index and middle fingers, and the radial half of the ring finger) but possibly involving the entire hand. Typically, the patient wakes at night with burning or aching pain and with numbness and tingling and shakes the hand to obtain relief and restore sensation. Thenar atrophy and weakness of thumb opposition and abduction may develop late.

(from http://www.merckmanuals.com/professional/musculoskeletal-and-connective-tissue-disorders/hand-disorders/carpal-tunnel-syndrome)

Etiology and Pathogenesis:
- Overwork, chronic disease, pregnancy can cause Qi and Blood deficiency, which leads to malnourishment of sinews and vessels
- Repetitive strain or blood deficiency not nourishing vessels may lead to Qi stagnation and blood stasis
- May be complicated by wind cold damp entering and lodging in channels and vessels causing impediment

TCM Differentiation and Treatment:

Pattern	Signs and Symptoms	Treatment Principle	Acupuncture	Formula
	Tingling and/or numbness of the fingers of one or both hands, thin and pale fingers, pale lips and nails, pale facial complexion, brittle nails, dry skin, dizziness, heart palpitations. T: pale P: fine	Supplement Qi and nourish blood, harmonize vessels	Ba Xie, PC7 (da ling), BL17 (ge shu), BL18 (gan shu), BL20 (pi shu)	
	Wrist pain may be severe, fixed location, worse at night. T: dark, purple P: choppy	Move Qi and Blood, free flow the vessels, stop pain	SP10 (xue hai), PC7 (da ling), SJ4 (yang chi), Ba Xie	
	Wrist pain that comes and goes or migrates, numbness and heaviness of hand, pain worse in cold damp weather. T: pale P: soggy	Dispel wind, eliminate damp, supplement Qi and nourish blood	Ba Xie, PC7 (da ling), LI4 (he gu), SI3 (hou xi), ST36 (ZSL)	

Cervical Spondylosis (jing zhui bing)

Definition:
This is a Western medical condition; see below.

Red Flags:
- Referral for Western medical diagnoses required

Western Medicine Relevant Diseases:
Cervical spondylosis is osteoarthritis of the cervical spine causing stenosis of the canal. It may also result in cervical myelopathy (motor and sensory deficits) due to encroachment of bony osteoarthritic growths (osteophytes) on the lower cervical spinal cord, sometimes with involvement of lower cervical nerve roots (radiculomyelopathy).

Cord compression commonly causes gradual spastic paresis, paresthesias, or both in the hands and feet and may cause hyperreflexia. Neurologic deficits may be asymmetric, nonsegmental, and aggravated by cough. Eventually, muscle atrophy and flaccid paresis may develop in the upper extremities at the level of the lesion, with spasticity below the level of the lesion.

Nerve root compression commonly causes radicular pain; later, there may be weakness, hyporeflexia, and muscle atrophy.

(from http://www.merckmanuals.com/professional/neurologic-disorders/spinal-cord-disorders/cervical-spondylosis-and-spondylotic-cervical-myelopathy)

Etiology and Pathogenesis:
- External invasion by wind, cold, damp evils impedes free flow of Qi and Blood in the channel
- Poor diet leads to Spleen deficiency and to internal dampness; this may transform into phlegm blocking Qi and Blood in the neck and shoulders
- Over-taxation and aging leads to Yin deficiency and lack of moistening and nourishment of the sinews and bones
- Chronic disease or trauma may give rise to Qi and Blood stagnation and Blood stasis

TCM Differentiation and Treatment:

Pattern	Signs and Symptoms	Treatment Principle	Acupuncture	Formula
	Head, neck, shoulder, upper back aching and pain, fixed neck pain, tender points on neck, stiff neck; possible soreness, pain and numbness of limbs, aversion to cold. T: pale P: floating, tight	Dispel wind, scatter cold, unblock the neck and relieve pain	SI3 (hou xi), GB20 (feng chi), LU7 (lie que), BL10 (tian zhu)+ points according to location of pain	
	Head, neck, shoulder and upper back aching and pain, dizziness, heavy head and body, lack of strength, nausea, chest oppression. T: pale, greasy P: slippery	Transform phlegm, dispel dampness, move Qi and Blood, relieve pain	SI3 (hou xi), GB20 (feng chi), DU14 (da zhui), SP9 (yin ling quan), ST40 (feng long) + local Ashi points	
	Head, neck, shoulder and upper back aching, pain, and numbness, pain may be severe, pain in fixed location, may be worse at night. T: dark purple P: choppy	Move Qi and Blood, transform stasis, stop pain	SI3 (hou xi), BL62 (shen mai), LI4 (he gu), SP6 (SYJ), SP10 (xue hai), Ashi points	
	Head and neck pain with limited movement, weak neck and limbs, numb shoulder and arms, general fatigue, insomnia, spontaneous sweat or night sweats, SOB, pale face. T: pale P: weak	Tonify Qi, nourish Blood, move impediment, relieve pain	ST36 (ZSL), BL17 (ge shu), BL18 (gan shu), BL20 (pi shu), SP6 (SYJ), LI4 (he gu)	

| | Neck, shoulder, upper back aching and pain, possible distended pain in head, numbness and lack of strength, low back and knee pain, dizziness, blurred vision, tidal fever, night sweats, dry mouth.
T: red, scanty coat
P: rapid | Tonify Liver and Kidney, nourish Yin, move Blood, stop pain | KI3 (tai xi), BL11 (da zhu), GB39 (xuan zhong), BL23 (shen shu), BL18 (gan shu) | |

Frozen Shoulder (jian guan jie zhou wei yan)

Definition:
A shoulder condition characterized by a dull, diffuse, or aching pain with decreased or restricted range of motion, and often accompanied by stiffness. Onset may be gradual or acute.

Red Flags:
- Refer for Western medical examination if suspect partial or complete tear of rotator cuff tendon

Western Medicine Relevant Diseases:
Adhesive capsulitis and frozen shoulder syndrome (FSS) are two terms that have been used to describe a painful and stiff shoulder. Historically, the criteria for diagnosing an individual with a frozen shoulder have varied, and this has led to inclusion of conditions such as subacromial bursitis, calcifying tendinitis, and partial rotator cuff tears. The current definition of a frozen shoulder by the American Shoulder and Elbow Surgeons is "a condition of uncertain etiology characterized by significant restriction of both active and passive shoulder motion that occurs in the absence of a known intrinsic shoulder disorder."
(from http://emedicine.medscape.com/article/1261598-overview#a6)

Etiology and Pathogenesis:

TCM Differentiation and Treatment:

Pattern	Signs and Symptoms	Treatment Principle	Acupuncture	Formula
External invasion of Wind Cold	Pain in shoulder is relatively mild/dull, local numbness, short course of disease. May also be pain in upper back and neck. Better with warmth and massage. Slight restriction of joint mobility. P: floating	Dispel wind, scatter cold, promote free flow and stop pain	LI15 (jian yu), SJ14 (jian liao), SI9 (jian zhen), LI11 (qu chi), SJ5 (wei guan), ST38 (tiao kou) + local ashi points	
Invasion of Wind Damp	As above, but disease is usually longer course. P: slippery	Dispel wind, scatter cold, drain damp, promote free flow and stop pain	As above, plus SP9 (yin ling quan), ST40 (feng long)	
Blood stasis blocking vessels	Severe, sharp or pricking pain, restricted movement, possible swelling, possible history of injury. T: dark P: choppy	Move Qi and Blood, transform stasis, stop pain	As above, plus SP10 (xue hai) and local Ashi points	
Phlegm Damp Obstructing	Chronic condition, severe pain in sinews and muscles of shoulder, restricted movement, better with warmth, general body heaviness. T: greasy coat P: slippery	Tonify Spleen, dispel damp, transform phlegm, promote free flow and stop pain	As above, plus ST40 (feng long), SP9 (yin ling quan), ST36 (ZSL)	
Qi and Blood deficiency	Aching pain and weakness around the shoulder, worse after taxation, SOB, fatigue, lack of strength. T: pale and teeth marks P: deep, weak	Tonify Qi and nourish Blood, promote free flow and stop pain	As above, plus BL17 (ge shu), BL20 (pi shu), BL21 (wei shu)	

Anterior shoulder distal point – ST38 (tian kou); Posterior shoulder distal point – BL59 (fu yang)

Ganglionic cyst (jian qiao nang zhong)

Definition:
Ganglion cysts are masses or lumps commonly found in the hands, most frequently developing on the back of the wrist. In most cases, the cysts are not cancerous and are relatively harmless, but if they interfere with function, or have an unacceptable appearance.

Red Flags:
- Refer for severe pain, change in skin color, or cysts that are not responding to treatment

Western Medicine Relevant Diseases:
Ganglia, or ganglion cysts, are swellings on the hands and wrists that contain a jellylike fluid.

Ganglia typically spontaneously occur in people between the ages of 20 and 50. Women are affected 3 times more often than men. Ganglia usually develop on the back of the wrist. Ganglia also develop on the front of the wrist and on the back of the finger, a few millimeters behind the cuticle (where they are also called mucous cysts).

Why ganglia develop on the wrist is not known, although they may be related to a previous injury. Ganglia on the back of a finger usually are related to arthritis of the last joint of the finger. However, in most cases, having a ganglion cyst does not mean that arthritis will develop.

Ganglia are firm, smooth, and round or elliptical swellings that rise from the skin surface. They contain a clear, jellylike, and usually sticky fluid. They are usually painless but occasionally cause discomfort.

Most ganglia disappear without treatment.

(from http://www.merckmanuals.com/home/bone,-joint,-and-muscle-disorders/hand-disorders/ganglia)

Etiology and Pathogenesis:
In Chinese Medicine, ganglion cysts are linked to stagnation. Local obstruction of systemic issues that cause Qi stagnation may result in the thickening of fluids and formation of phlegm.

TCM Differentiation and Treatment:

Pattern	Signs and Symptoms	Treatment Principle	Acupuncture	Formula
	Jelly-like lump, typically round or oval, pain possible, restricted movement possible.	Move Qi, dissolve phlegm and stasis	LI4-LR3 (4 gates), SP9 (yin ling quan), ST40 (feng long), plus treat locally	

Joint dislocation (tuo wei)

Definition:
Refers to joints that are taken out of alignment from impact injuries, such as falls, or because of prolonged muscle imbalances. This may cause pain, swelling, and loss of function. Dislocation is commonly seen at the shoulders, knees, fingers, elbows, and jaw.

Red Flags:
- Refer for Western medical evaluation and treatment

Western Medicine Relevant Diseases:
In Western medicine, a dislocation is a complete separation of the 2 bones that form a joint. Subluxation is partial separation. Often, a dislocated joint remains dislocated until reduced (realigned) by a clinician, but sometimes it reduces spontaneously.

Etiology and Pathogenesis:
- Trauma or prolonged muscle imbalances

TCM Differentiation and Treatment:

Pattern	Signs and Symptoms	Treatment Principle	Acupuncture	Formula
	May be pain, swelling, loss of function	Move Qi and Blood, strengthen sinews	LI4-LR3 (4 gates), SP10 (xue hai), GB34 (yang ling quan), GB39 (zuan zhong), plus treat locally and distally based on location of injury	

Knee joint collateral ligament injury (xi guan jie ce fu ren dai sun shang)

Definition:
Acute pain, inflammation, and swelling in the knee due to injury. Most common in the medial collateral ligament or meniscus. From a meridian perspective, three leg yin meridians (Spleen, Liver, and Kidney) should be considered for pain in the medial aspect of the knee joint.

Red Flags:
- Refer for Western medical assessment to rule out tears to the ligament

Western Medicine Relevant Diseases:
Sprains of the external (medial and lateral collateral) or internal (anterior and posterior cruciate) ligaments or injuries of the menisci may result from knee trauma. Symptoms include pain, joint effusion, instability (with severe sprains), and locking (with some meniscal injuries). Diagnosis is by physical examination and sometimes MRI. Treatment is PRICE (protection, rest, ice, compression, elevation) and, for severe injuries, casting or surgical repair.

Signs and symptoms include swelling and muscle spasm progress over the first few hours. With 2nd-degree sprains, pain is typically moderate or severe. With 3rd-degree sprains, pain may be mild, and surprisingly, some patients can walk unaided. Some patients hear or feel a pop when the injury occurs.

(from http://www.merckmanuals.com/professional/injuries-poisoning/fractures,-dislocations,-and-sprains/knee-sprains-and-meniscal-injuries)

Etiology and Pathogenesis:
- Accident or trauma causing Qi and Blood stagnation and injury to the ligaments and tendons
- Liver imbalances may result in susceptibility of the tendons and ligaments to inflammation and injury

TCM Differentiation and Treatment:

Pattern	Signs and Symptoms	Treatment Principle	Acupuncture	Formula
Qi and Blood Stagnation	Pain, swelling, stiffness, reduced joint function.	Move Qi and Blood	LI4-LR3 (4 gates), LR2 (xing jian), LR7 (xi guan), KD6-LU7 (yin qiao mai), SP9 (yin ling quan), SP10 (xue hai), GB34 (yang ling quan) + local ashi points	
Liver imbalances	Check for signs of Liver Qi stagnation, Liver Yin deficiency, or Liver Blood deficieny	Treat according to pattern	LR3 (tai chong), GB34 (yang ling quan), LR8 (qu quan)	

EXAMINATION

Lumbar muscle strain (yao bu lao sun)

Definition:
Lumbar muscle strain may be due to a history of injury or over-exertion (e.g. straining, over stretching of sinews, flexion or rotation beyond normal range), or to an underlying deficiency. If acute lumbar sprain does not resolve or is not treated, it may become chronic.

Red Flags:
See acute lumbar muscle strain.

Western Medicine Relevant Diseases:
See acute lumbar muscle strain.

Etiology and Pathogenesis:
See acute lumbar muscle strain.

TCM Differentiation and Treatment:

Pattern	Signs and Symptoms	Treatment Principle	Acupuncture	Formula
	Severe, stabbing and fixed pain, worse with pressure and movement, swelling T: may have purple P: wiry, choppy	Move Qi and Blood, loosen the sinews and unblock the channels	DU3 (yao yang guan), DU4 (ming men), BL23 (shen shu), BL52 (zhi shi), BL25 (da chang shu), SI3 (hou xi), BL40 (wei zhong) + local ashi points -BL17 (ge shu), LI4-LR3 (4 gates)	
	Check for signs of underlying Kidney deficiency (see patterns under prolapse of lumbar intervertebral disc) Repeated dull lumbar pain, aggravated by poor weather, aches and weakness in the waist and knees. T: pale P: deep, thready	Treat according to pattern	KI3 (tai xi), DU4 (ming men), Yao tong xue, ling gu dai bai, BL40 (wei zhong), BL60 (kun lun), SI6 (yang lao), BL63 (jin men), BL58 (fei yang)	

Meniscal injury (ban yue ban sun shang)

Definition:
The menisci are pads of cartilage that act as cushions between the femur and larger lower leg bone tibia, which form part of the knee joint. The menisci can be damaged when people have their weight on a foot and their knee twists as it is injured. Signs and symptoms include swelling, pain, loss of range of motion, and possible muscle atrophy.

Red Flags:
- Refer for Western medical assessment to rule out infections, fractures, or dislocations.

Western Medicine Relevant Diseases:
A meniscus tear is a common knee injury. The meniscus is a rubbery, C-shaped disc that cushions the knee. Each knee has two menisci, one at the outer edge of the knee and one at the inner edge. The menisci keep the knee steady by balancing weight across the knee.

A meniscus tear is usually caused by twisting or turning quickly, often with the foot planted while the knee is bent. Meniscus tears can occur when lifting something heavy or playing sports. With age, the meniscus gets worn which can make it tear more easily.

A minor tear might cause slight pain and swelling. This usually goes away in 2 or 3 weeks. A moderate tear can cause pain at the side or center of the knee. Swelling slowly gets worse over 2 or 3 days. This may make the knee feel stiff and limit range of motion. In severe tears, pieces of the torn meniscus can move into the joint space. This can make the knee catch, pop, or lock.

(from http://www.webmd.com/fitness-exercise/tc/meniscus-tear-topic-overview?print=true)

Etiology and Pathogenesis:
- Trauma leading to Qi and Blood stasis

TCM Differentiation and Treatment:

Pattern	Signs and Symptoms	Treatment Principle	Acupuncture	Formula
Qi and Blood Stasis	Pain, swelling, limited range of motion.	Move Qi and Blood	LR3 (tai chong), GB37, (guang ming) SP3 (tai bai), KI10 (yin gu), SP9 (yin ling quan), xi yan, he ding, ST34 (liang qiu), ST36 (ZSL), SP10 (xue hai), LI4 (he gu)	

EXAMINATION

Prolapse of lumbar intervertebral disc (yao zhui jian pan tu chu zheng)

Definition:
Refers to degenerative changes, with or without trauma, resulting in protrusion or rupture of the intervertebral disks in the lumbar region. Signs and symptoms include: sudden, severe, OR insidious pain paresthesias or numbness, and muscular weakness and atrophy.

Red Flags:
- Refer for Western medical assessment to show location of herniation
- Progressive or severe neurological deficits, pain, urinary retention or incontinence
- Refer if there are signs of Kidney infection

Western Medicine Relevant Diseases:
Herniated nucleus pulposus is prolapse of an intervertebral disk through a tear in the surrounding annulus fibrosus. The tear causes pain; when the disk impinges on an adjacent nerve root, a segmental radiculopathy with paresthesias and weakness in the distribution of the affected root results. Diagnosis is usually by MRI or CT. Treatment of mild cases is with analgesics as needed. Bed rest is rarely indicated. Patients with progressive or severe neurologic deficits, intractable pain, or sphincter dysfunction may require immediate or elective surgery.

(from http://www.merckmanuals.com/professional/neurologic-disorders/peripheral-nervous-system-and-motor-unit-disorders/herniated-nucleus-pulposus)

Etiology and Pathogenesis:
- Traumatic injury may result in blood stasis.
- Invasion by external wind, cold, damp or heat evils may obstruct the channels and vessels traversing the low back inhibiting the flow of Qi and Blood and causing pain.
- Aging, taxation, excessive sexual activity, chronic disease may result in lack of nourishment to the sinews and vessels of the low back. These will become dry and contract, resulting in stiffness and pain.
- Kidney deficiency (Kidney is the mansion of the low back) may lead to lumbar pain.

TCM Differentiation and Treatment:

Pattern	Signs and Symptoms	Treatment Principle	Acupuncture	Formula
	Cold pain in low back, heavy sensation in low back, chilled limbs, lack of strength, points tender on palpation, pain worse with cold. T: pale P: deep, tight	Warm the channels and scatter cold, dispel dampness and stop pain	Jia ji points, local ashi points, DU 3 (yao yang guan), DU4 (ming men), BL22 (san jiao shu), BL23 (shen shu), BL24 (qi hai shu), BL25 (da chang shu), BL26 (guan yuan shu), ST40 (feng long), SP9 (yin ling quan) + damp heat add ST44 (nei ting), LR2 (xing jian), GB34 (yang ling quan) + Qi and Blood stasis add BL40 (wei zhong), LI4-LR3 (4 gates), SP10 (xue hai), SP8 (di ji) + Kidney Yin Xu add	
	Low back pain often accompanied by a hot sensation, soreness and heaviness, inability to bend forward or backward, spontaneous perspiration, thirst, dark urine, loose stools. T: yellow coat P: slippery, rapid	Clear heat and drain damp, diffuse impediment and stop pain		
	Sharp low back pain, fixed location, better during the day and worse at night, pain worse with pressure, history of traumatic injury. T: dark P: choppy	Move Qi and Blood, dispel stasis		

	Dull low back pain, may hinder walking, worse with fatigue, better with rest and pressure, five center heat, tidal fever, night sweats, dry mouth. T: red, scanty coat P: fine, rapid	Tonify Kidneys, nourish Yin, clear heat, stop pain	KI3, (tai xi) KI7 (fu liu), SP6 (SYJ) + Kidney Yang xu add DU4 (ming men), KI3 (tai xi), KI7 (fu liu)	
	Dull, lingering low back pain, worse with overwork, better with rest and warmth, weak lower limbs, cold hands and feet, white complexion. T: pale P: deep, fine	Tonify Kidneys, invigorate Yang, scatter cold		

Piriformis Syndrome (li zhuang ji zong he zhang)

Definition:

Red Flags:
- Refer for Western medical examination to rule out disk herniation

Western Medicine Relevant Diseases:
Piriformis syndrome is compression of the sciatic nerve by the piriformis muscle in the posterior pelvis, causing pain in the buttocks and occasionally sciatica.
The piriformis muscle extends from the pelvic surface of the sacrum to the upper border of the greater trochanter of the femur. During running or sitting, this muscle can compress the sciatic nerve at the site where it emerges from under the piriformis to pass over the hip rotator muscles.

In piriformis syndrome, a chronic nagging ache, pain, tingling, or numbness starts in the buttocks and can extend along the course of the sciatic nerve, down the entire back of the thigh and calf, and sometimes into the foot. Pain worsens when the piriformis is pressed against the sciatic nerve (e.g., while sitting on a toilet, a car seat, or a narrow bicycle seat or while running).
(from http://www.merckmanuals.com/professional/injuries-poisoning/sports-injury/piriformis-syndrome)

Etiology and Pathogenesis:
- External injury or over-taxation – causes blood stasis and qi stagnation in the channels and vessels – results in pain
- Aging or constitution – malnourishment of the sinews and vessels
- Wind damp cold impediment hindering free flow of qi and blood – pain (see Impediment Syndrome in Internal Medicine)

TCM Differentiation and Treatment:

Pattern	Signs and Symptoms	Treatment Principle	Acupuncture	Formula
Qi Stagnation and Blood Stasis	History of injury to low back or hip region, severe pain, pain in fixed location, worse at night, may extend to thigh, other symptoms of qi stagnation and blood stasis possible, e.g. irritability, menstrual issues, dark facial complexion. T: dark, purple P: choppy	Move qi and blood, dispel stasis	SP10 (xue hai), BL54 (zhi bian), BL40 (wei zhong), Ashi points locally (GB30 (huan tiao)	
Liver Qi Stagnation with Blood Deficiency	Pain in hip and thigh, better with exercise, irritability, fatigue, loose stools or constipation, ABD distension, possible menstrual issues. T: pale P: fine	Sooth the Liver, nourish Qi and Blood	LR3 (tai chong), BL17 (ge shu), BL18, (gan shu) BL54 (zhi bian), BL40 (wei zhong), local Ashi points (also, if SP deficient, BL20 (pi shu), ST36 (ZSL))	
Liver and Kidney Yin Deficiency with Blood Stasis	Chronic disease, pain less severe, pain worse in evening, pain prefers pressure, dizziness, tinnitus, insomnia, dry skin, joints sore. T: red, scanty coat P: fine, rapid	Supplement and nourish Liver and Kidneys, move Qi and Blood	SP10 (xue hai), SP6 (SYJ), KI7 (fu liu), BL54 (zhi bian), BL40 (wei zhong), local Ashi points	

Sprained Ankle (huai guan jie niu cuo shang)

Definition:
The tern sprain describes injury to soft tissue surrounding the ankle joint. The soft tissues include fascia, tendons, ligaments, parts of muscles, subcutaneous tissues, joint capsules, and articular cartilage. Clinical manifestations include swelling and pain, and restricted movement.

Red Flags:
- Refer if evidence of complete tearing of ligament or tendon, or fracture

Western Medicine Relevant Diseases:
Ankle sprains are very common, most often resulting from turning the foot inward (inversion). Common findings are pain, swelling, and tenderness, which are maximal at the anterolateral ankle.
The most important ankle ligaments are the deltoid (the strong, medial ligament), the anterior and posterior talofibular (lateral ligaments), and the calcaneofibular
Inversion (turning the foot inward) tears the lateral ligaments, usually beginning with the anterior talofibular ligament. Severe 2nd- and 3rd-degree sprains sometimes cause chronic joint instability and predispose to additional sprains. Inversion can also cause talar dome fractures, with or without an ankle sprain.

Eversion (turning the foot outward) stresses the joint medially. This stress often causes an avulsion fracture of the medial malleolus rather than a ligament sprain because the deltoid ligament is so strong. However, eversion can also cause a sprain. Eversion also compresses the joint laterally; this compression, often combined with dorsiflexion, may fracture the distal fibula or tear the syndesmotic ligaments between the tibia and fibula just proximal to the ankle (called a high ankle sprain). Sometimes eversion forces are transmitted up the fibula, fracturing the fibular head just below the knee (called a Maisonneuve fracture).

Ankle sprains cause pain and swelling. The location of pain and swelling varies with the type of injury:

Generally, tenderness is maximal over the damaged ligaments rather than over the bone; tenderness that is greater over bone than over ligaments suggests fracture.
(from http://www.merckmanuals.com/professional/injuries-poisoning/fractures,-dislocations,-and-sprains/ankle-sprains)
Etiology and Pathogenesis:
- Strenuous exercise, external blows, collisions, falls, forceful stretching, overburdening or twisting of joints – lead to local Qi and Blood stagnation
- Conditions of local deficiency following sprains may allow the invasion of eternal wind, cold, and damp adding to severity of injury and prolonging illness
- In cases of chronic sprain, refer to Bi patterns

TCM Differentiation and Treatment:

Pattern	Signs and Symptoms	Treatment Principle	Acupuncture	Formula
Qi and Blood Stagnation	Local distention, swelling and pain, sometimes with redness or dark purple discoloration, and restricted movement. In chronic cases, symptoms are aggravated by overwork or exposure to cold.	Rectify Qi, quicken Blood, sooth soft tissues and clear the connections	Local Ashi points + ST41 (jie xi), BL60 (kun lun), GB40 (qiu xu), xi-cleft points	

Strained Neck (lou zhen)

Definition:
This includes patterns of acute, uncomplicated stiffness and pain of the neck where normal movement is restricted. Stiff neck is most common during spring and winter.

Red Flags:
In people with neck pain, certain signs merit referral for Western medical evaluation:
- Loss of strength or sensation—possibly a symptom of nerve damage
- Fever or severe night sweats
- Severe and sudden onset headache
- Lethargy or confusion
- Chest discomfort
- Sudden sweating, difficulty breathing, or swallowing
- Stiff neck with vomiting

Western Medicine Relevant Diseases:
Neck pain is common and becomes more common as people age.

Neck pain can involve damage to bones, muscles, disks, or ligaments, but pain can also be caused by damage to nerves or the spinal cord. A spinal nerve root can be compressed when the spine is injured, resulting in pain and sometimes weakness, numbness, and tingling in an arm. Compression of the spinal cord can cause numbness and weakness of both arms and both legs and sometimes loss of bladder and bowel control.

Most of the disorders that can cause low back pain can also cause neck pain, and most involve the spine, the tissues that support it, or both.

The most common cause of neck pain is muscle and ligament sprains or tears. In such cases, neck pain usually resolves completely.

Other common causes include
- Muscle spasms
- Arthritis (usually osteoarthritis – see internal medicine for review)
- Cervical spondylosis: condition where the vertebrae in the neck and the disks between them degenerate, usually because of osteoarthritis. As a result, the nerves that emerge through the vertebrae may be pinched. Sometimes the spinal canal is narrowed (cervical spinal stenosis), and the spinal cord is compressed.
- A ruptured or herniated disk The disks between each of the vertebrae have a tough covering and a soft, jelly-like interior. If a disk is suddenly squeezed by the vertebrae above and below it, the covering may tear, causing pain. The interior of the disk can herniate. The bulging disk can push on or even damage the spinal nerve root next to it. Rarely, the disk compresses the spinal cord.
- Fibromyalgia (see internal medicine for review)

Less common causes that are serious include
- A tear in the lining of a neck artery (dissection)
- Meningitis
- A spinal tumor or infection
- A heart attack or angina (chest pain due to an inadequate blood supply to the heart muscle)

Spasmodic torticollis is also a less common cause, but is not as serious as some causes. It is a severe type of spasm that causes the head to tilt and rotate into an abnormal position. Sometimes the spasms are rhythmic, causing the head to jerk. The cause may be unknown or may be due to certain drugs or hereditary disorders.

(from http://www.merckmanuals.com/home/bone,-joint,-and-muscle-disorders/low-back-and-neck-pain/neck-pain)

Etiology and Pathogenesis:
- Involves improper sleeping posture (head too high or too low or excessive rotation), or mild injury (e.g. from sports) – strains muscles
- Invasion of the back of the neck by wind cold pathogens – obstruct Qi and Blood – cause pain and restricted movement

TCM Differentiation and Treatment:

Pattern	Signs and Symptoms	Treatment Principle	Acupuncture	Formula
Qi Stagnation and Blood Stasis	Stiffness and pain of the neck, inclination of head toward affected side, limited movement of head, tightening of the muscles on the back of the neck, possible palpable masses cord-like in shape and local painful pressure points, better with heat. T: thin coat P: wiry	Move Qi and Blood, stop pain	Ashi points, luo zhen, BL10 (tian zhu), SI3 (hou xi), GB39 (xuan zhong), LU7 (lie que)	
Invasion by Wind Cold	Stiffness and pain of the neck, external patterns such as aversion to cold and wind, slight fever, H/A. T: thin white coat P: floating, tight	Dispel wind, dissipate cold, stop pain	Ashi points, luo zhen, LI4 (he gu), SJ5 (wei guan), BL10 (tian zhu), SI3 (hou xi), GB39 (xuan zhong)	

Tennis Elbow (hong gu wais han ke yan)

Definition:
A repetitive stress injury involving pain at the elbow at the lateral epicondyle and distally along the Yang surface (extensor tendon and muscles of the arm).

Red Flags:
- If associated with trauma, refer to rule out elbow fracture
- Tendon tears may require surgery

Western Medicine:
This condition is known as Lateral Epicondylitis in Western medicine. Lateral epicondylitis is inflammation and micro-tearing of fibers in the extensor tendons of the forearm. Symptoms include pain at the lateral epicondyle of the elbow, which can radiate into the forearm.

Lateral epicondylitis can be caused by repetitive backhand returns in tennis. Other activities (for example, rowing and doing forearm curls while holding weights or repeatedly and forcefully turning a screwdriver) can also cause lateral epicondylitis.

Factors that increase the chance of developing lateral epicondylitis among tennis players include having weak shoulder and forearm muscles, playing with a racket that is too tightly strung or too short, hitting the ball off center on the racket (out of the sweet spot), and hitting heavy, wet balls. Hitting backhanded and allowing the wrist to bend increase the chance of developing lateral epicondylitis.

Pain occurs in the outside of the forearm when the wrist is extended away from the palm. Pain can extend from around the elbow to the middle of the forearm. Pain may be increased by firm gripping (handshaking) or even turning doorknobs. Continuing to stress the forearm muscles can worsen this condition and result in pain even when the forearm is not being used.

(from http://www.merckmanuals.com/home/injuries-and-poisoning/sports-injuries/lateral-epicondylitis)

Etiology and Pathogenesis:
- Repetitive stress and overuse – lead to Qi and Blood stagnation in the channels and collaterals
- Consider the Large Intestine and San Jiao meridians, in particular, as these encompass the region

TCM Differentiation and Treatment:

Pattern	Signs and Symptoms	Treatment Principle	Acupuncture	Formula
Qi and Blood Stagnation	Pain in the lateral elbow, pain and stiffness may radiate distally down the forearm, onset is often gradual, pain may be dull and intermittent, activity aggravates pain.	Move Qi and Blood, relieve pain		

Pharmacology

General

Pharmacology: A drug can be broadly defined as an chemical that affects the processes of a living organism. Pharmacology is the study or science of drugs. Drugs have a least two names. The generic name; given by Health Canada under the Food and Drug Act which is the official name used in formal drug lists. And the trade name; or proprietary name, indicates a registered trademark and is used for commercial purposes. For the purposes of this section they will be listed together as generic (trade). A non-drug related example of this would be tissue (Kleenex).

Pharmacodynamics: How drugs produce their effects within the body (their mechanism of action, or MOA). Drugs can exert their actions in 3 basic ways; receptor interactions, enzyme interactions, and nonselective interactions.
 Receptor interactions; Agonist (the drug does something), Antagonist (the drug blocks something), or Agonist-antagonist (the drug does both).
 Enzyme interactions: some drugs can inhibit or enhance the action of specific enzymes
 Nonselective interactions: drugs that physically interfere with or chemically alter cellular structure or process

Pharmacokinetics: How drugs move through the body, what actually happens form the time the drug enters the body until it leaves the body (how they are absorbed, distributed, metabolised, and excreted).
 Absorption: the movement of a drug from its site of administration into the bloodstream for distribution. **Bioavailability** expresses the extent of drug absorption. Several factors such as; food or fluids ingested, dosage, rate of blood flow, stomach acidity, GI motility, and route of administration affect the rate of drug absorption.
 Distribution: the transport of a drug in the body by the bloodstream to its site of action. Areas of rapid distribution include; the heart, liver, kidneys, and brain. Areas of slower distribution are muscle, skin, and fat.
 Metabolism: biochemical alteration of a drug into a more soluble compound, the conversion of a drug from its inactive to active from. The organ most responsible for metabolism is the Liver.
 Excretion: the elimination of drugs from the body. Primary organs responsible are the kidneys

Routes of Administration: Different routes of administration are considered based on pharmacokinetics (speed of absorption, diffusion barriers, lipid solubility) and patient preference.
 Enteral: the drug is absorbed into systemic circulation through the mucosa of the stomach or small intestine. Involves oral ingestion, sublingual (under the tongue), or buccal (through the cheek) administration. When ingested orally, some of the drug is inactivated in the liver before absorbed, also known as first-pass effect.
 Parenteral: for most medications, this is the fastest route a drug can be absorbed. Most commonly refers to injection by any method; intravenous(IV), intramuscular(IM), subcutaneous, or intradermal are the most common routes.
 Topical: application of drugs to body surfaces. Can be applied to skin, eyes, ears, nose, lungs, rectum, and vagina. Delivers a steadier amount of drug over a longer period of time, but the effects are usually slower. (eg. ointments)
 Transdermal: drug delivery through adhesive patches. Commonly used for systemic drugs, delivers a constant amount of drug per unit of time over a specified time period. (eg. nicotine patch)
 Inhalation: delivered to the lungs as small particles in order for the drug to be delivered to the alveoli in the lungs. Particularly useful for drugs treating pulmonary diseases.

Effective dose: The amount of a drug that produces the desired effect in 50% of the population. The amount needed to produce therapeutic effects.
Toxic dose: Amount of a drug that produces adverse effects 50% of the population (note: every substance has a toxic dose; the aim of therapeutic dosing is to achieve drugs effects using the minimal dose without producing negative side effects).
Drug storage sites: Some drugs are preferentially stored in adipose tissue (lipid-soluble drugs tend to remain in the body a long time), bone (e.g., heavy metals), muscle (specific muscle-binding drugs that have action at the muscles), or organs (such as the liver and kidneys).

Common Drugs

The following section highlights drug categories and the key parts you must know for the exam and for your clinical practice. While you won't be prescribing drugs (and therefore don't need to know each drug in detail), it is important to understand the main functions of each drug category, common examples and possible adverse effects. That way, in practice, you will be able to recognise when symptoms might be connected to a drug adverse effect.

Autonomic Nervous System

Adrenergic
adrenergic agonists.

i. Mechanism of Action
- Stimulate the sympathetic nervous system (SNS)
- Mimic the effects of norepinephrine and epinephrine, and dopamine
- 2 main groups of adrenergic receptors: α-adrenergic and β-adrenergic receptors.

Used to treat a variety of illnesses and conditions (Respiratory, ophthalmic, and cardiovascular indications)

ii. Adverse Effects
α-adrenergic drugs – headache, restlessness, excitement, insomnia, and euphoria
ß-adrenergic drugs – adversely stimulate CNS, causing mild tremors, headache, nervousness, and dizziness.

iii. Examples
There are 4 frequently used therapeutic classes of adrenergic drugs;
<u>Bronchodilators:</u> Salbutamol (Ventolin), Salmeterol (Serevent)
<u>Nasal Decongestants:</u> Pseudoephedrine hydrochloride (Sudafed)
<u>Ophthalmic Decongestants:</u> Tetrahydrozoline (Visine)
<u>Vasoactive Adrenergics:</u> Dobutamine, Dopamine, Epinephrine (Twinject, Adrenalin), Norepinephrine (Levophed)

Antiadrenergic
adrenergic-blockers, or adrenergic antagonists

<u>A-adrenergic-blockers</u>
i. Mechanism of Action
- block stimulation of the SNS through direct competition with neurotransmitters; leads to vasodilation, decreased blood pressure, and constriction of pupils

ii. Adverse Effects
- palpitations, orthostatic hypotension, tachycardia, dizziness, headache, nausea, vomiting

iii. Examples
Phentolamine (Regitine), Prazosin (Minipress)

<u>ß-adrenergic-blockers</u>
i. Mechanism of Action
- block stimulation of the SNS by competing with catecholamines
- this effect reduces myocardial stimulation, reduces heart rate and contractility, constricts smooth muscle in the airways, promotes production of glucose and causes release of fatty acids.

Used in the treatment of angina, hypertension, and arrhythmias

ii. Adverse Effects
- bradycardia, heart failure, dizziness, nausea, dry mouth, thrombocytopenia

iii. Examples
Atenolol (Tenormin), Carvedilol (Coreg), Labetalol (Trandate), Metoprolol (Lopressor), Propranolol (Inderal)

Cholinergic
Cholinergic agonists

i. Mechanism of Action
- stimulate the parasympathetic nervous system (PSNS)
- mimic the effect of Acetylcholine (ACh)
- stimulate the intestine and bladder; increasing gastric secretions, GI motility and urinary frequency. Decreased heart rate, vasodilation, and bronchoconstriction. They also stimulate pupil constriction, salivation and sweating.

Used for glaucoma, to treat atony of the bladder and GI tract, myasthenia gravis

ii. Adverse Effects
- bradycardia, hypotension, headache, dizziness, abdominal cramps, bronchospasms, sweating, salivation

iii. Examples
Bethanechol chloride (Duvoid), Pyridostigmine bromide (Mestinon)

Anticholinergic
Cholinergic blockers, or antimuscarinics

i. Mechanism of Action
- block the actions of ACh at the muscarinic receptors in the PSNS. Blocking PSNS allows the SNS to dominate (cholinergic blockers may have the same effects as adrenergics)
- major sites of action are the heart, respiratory tract, GI tract, bladder, eye and exocrine glands

Cause decreased gastric motility and secretions, pupil dilation, increased heart rate, urinary retention, reduced sweating and dry mucous membranes, bronchodilation

iii. Adverse Effects
- increased heart rate, dysrhythmias, restlessness, irritability, disorientation, dry mouth

iii. Examples
atropine sulfate, dicyclomine hydrochloride (Bentylol), glycopyrrolate

Central Nervous System

Analgesics
Used to alleviate moderate to severe pain, chronic pain, dyspnea, anxiety, and cough

Opioids
i. Mechanism of Action
- Agonists: binds to pain receptor in the brain, causes analgesic effect reducing pain sensation
- Partial agonists: binds to pain receptor, but causes a weaker response.
- Antagonists: binds to pain receptors but DOES NOT reduce pain signals, reverses the effects of agonist and partial agonist drugs at the site

ii. Adverse Effects
- hypotension, palpitations, sedation, disorientation, nausea, vomiting, constipation, itching, respiratory depression
- opioid tolerance and physical or psychological dependence

iii. Examples
there are 3 chemical classifications of opioids
- Meperidine-like drugs: Meperidine (Demerol), Fentanyl and Sufentanil

- Methadone- like drugs: Methadone
- Morphine-like drugs: Morphine, Heroin, Hydromorphone (Dilaudid), Codeine, Hydrocodone (Hydocan), and Oxycodone (OxyContin)

Opioid antagonist
- Naloxone hydrochloride (Narcan)

Nonopiods
Used for pain management

i. Mechanism of Action
- blocks peripheral pain impulses by inhibiting prostaglandin synthesis, antipyretic properties

ii. Adverse Effects
- rash, nausea and vomiting

iii. Examples
Acetaminophen (Tylenol), Tramadol hydrochloride (Ralivia)

Antiepileptics
Used to prevent or control seizures while maintaining a reasonable quality of life

i. Mechanism of Action
- exact mechanism is unknown
- increase the threshold of activity in the brain, depress the spread of seizure discharge from its origin, decrease speed of nerve impulse conduction

ii. Adverse Effects
- associated with many adverse effects which often limit their usefulness
- each antiepileptic has its own diverse adverse effects

iii. Examples
Phenobarbital, Phenytoin (Dilantin), Valproic acid (Divalproex), Gabapentin (Neurotin), Levetiracetam (Keppra), Pregabalin (Lyrica), Topiramate (Topamax), Diazepam (Valium), Lorazepam (Ativan)

Antiparkinsonians
There are 3 main types of therapies used in treating Parkinson's Disease (PD) symptoms

Selective Monoamine Oxidase Inhibitor Therapy
- breaks down catecholamines and serotonin, causing an increase in the levels of dopaminergic stimulation in the CNS. Counters the deficiencies that arise from PD
- Selegiline hydrochloride (Anipril): can cause nausea, abdominal pain, insomnia and confusion

Dopaminergic Therapy
- provides an exogenous replacement of lost dopamine
- levodopa-carbidopa (Sinemet): can cause palpitations, orthostatic hypotension, agitation, anxiety and blurred vision

Anticholinergic Therapy
- useful in treating associated tremors and muscle rigidity caused by excessive cholinergic activity
- Benztropine mesylate: can cause drowsiness, confusion, hallucinations, constipation urinary retention and blurred vision

CNS Stimulants
Broad class of drugs that stimulate specific areas of the brain or spinal cord. Elevate mood, produce a sense of increased energy and alertness, decrease appetite, and enhance task performance

i. Mechanism of Action
- Act by stimulating the excitatory neurons in the brain and enhancing the activity of one or more excitatory neurotransmitters (dopamine, norepinephrine, and serotonin).
- CNS stimulants can be classified based on their chemical structure, their site of therapeutic action, and their therapeutic usage (anti-attention deficit, antinarcoleptic, anorexiant, antimigraine, and analeptic).

ii. Examples
ADHD: Amphetamine salts (Adderall), Methylphenidate (Concerta, Ritalin)
Narcolepsy: Caffeine, Modafinil (Alertec)
Migraine: Rizatriptan (Maxalt), Eletriptan hydrobromide (Relpax)
Obesity: Orlistat (Xenical)

Psychotherapeutics
Treatment of emotional and mental health disorders

Antianxiety Medications
i. Mechanism of Action
- reduce anxiety by diminishing over-activity of the CNS
- Benzodiazepines increase the action of GABA (results in anxiolytic effect, sedation, muscle relaxation)
- Antihistamines can be used as anxiolytics; Hydroxyzine (Atarax)

ii. Adverse Effects
- paradoxical reaction, addiction, hypotension, drowsiness, sedation, nausea, vomiting, constipation, blurred vision

iii. Examples
Diazepam (Valium), Lorazepam (Ativan), Alprazolam (Xanax), Clonazepam (Clonapam), Midazolam (Versed)

Antimanic Medications
- **Lithium (Lithobid):** drug of choice to alleviate major symptoms of mania and maintenance of Bipolar Disorer
MOA: reduces catecholamine neurotransmitters
- **Quetiapine (Seroquel):** management of acute mania
- **Lamotrigine (Lamictal), Topiramate (Topomax):** 3rd generation anticonvulsants

Antidepressants
Treatment for major depressive disorders

- Selective Serotonin Reuptake Inhibitors (SSRIs)
  i. Mechanism of Action
  - inhibition of serotonin reuptake

  ii. Adverse Effects
  - headache, dizziness, weight loss or gain, nausea, sweating, insomnia

  iii. Examples
  Citalopram (Celexa), Escitalopram (Cipralex), Fluoxetime (Prozac), Sertraline (Zoloft), Venlexafine (Effexor), Duloxetine (Cymbalta)

- Tricyclic Antidepressants
  i. Mechanism of Action
  - block the reuptake of neurotransmitters, increases concentration of neurotransmitters correct abnormally low levels

  ii. Adverse Effects
  - tremors, tachycardia, orthostatic hypotension, anxiety, confusion, sedation, blurred vision, nausea, constipation

  iii. Examples
  Amitriptyline (Elavil), Imipramine (Tofranil), Nortriptyline (Aventyl)

- Monoamine Oxidase Inhibitors (MAOIs)
  i. Mechanism of Action
  - inhibit MAO enzyme in CNS resulting in higher levels in the brain, results in alleviation of depressive symptoms
  ii. Adverse Effects

- orthostatic hypotension, tachycardia, palpitations, dizziness, drowsiness, anorexia, cramps, blurred vision, insomnia

iii. Examples
Phenelzine sulfate (Nardil), Tranylcypromine sulfate (Parnate)

Antipsychotics
Used to treat serious mental health issues, behavioural problems, and psychotic disorders

i. Mechanism of Action
- block dopamine receptors in the brain responsible for hallucinations, delusions, and paranoia
- decreased levels of dopamine causes a tranquilizing effect

ii. Adverse Effects
-sedation, delirium, syncope, dizziness, photosensitivity, rash, urinary retention, increased appetite, polydipsia, dry mouth, constipation

iii. Examples
Halperidol (Haldol), Loxapine (Loxapac), Olanzapine (Zyorexa), Risperidone (Risperdal)

CNS Depressants
Sedatives – reduce nervousness, excitability, and irritability without causing sleep
Hypnotics – cause sleep
Many medications can act in the body as either a sedative or a hypnotic, hence the term sedative-hypnotic

Sedative-Hypnotics
- Barbiturates
  ### i. Mechanism of Action
  - potentiates the action of GABA, and reduces nerve impulses to the cerebral cortex
  - stimulates liver enzymes responsible for metabolism

  ### ii. Adverse Effects
  - drowsiness, lethargy, dizziness, paradoxical restlessness, deprive people of REM sleep

  ### iii. Examples
  Phenobarbitol, Butalbital, Thiopental

- Benzodiazepines
  ### i. Mechanism of Action
  - potentiates GABA, inhibition of hyperexcitable nerves in the CNS

  ### ii. Adverse Effects
  - headache, drowsiness, paradoxical excitement, vertigo, lethargy

  ### iii. Examples
  Diazepam (Valium), Lorazepam (Ativan), Alprazolam (Xanax), Clonazepam (Clonapam), Midazolam (Versed)

Cardiovascular System

Antianginal

Nitrates
Most commonly given in a sublingual or translingual spray
i. Mechanism of Action
- dilate and relax all blood vessels including coronary arteries

ii. Adverse Effects
- hypotension, headache, tachycardia

iii. Examples
Nitroglycerin, Isosorbide dinitrate (Apo-DSN)

ß-Blockers
i. Mechanism of Action
- decrease heart rate so that myocardial oxygen need is decreased

ii. Adverse Effects
- bradycardia, decreased cardiac output, bronchoconstriction, dysrhythmias, fatigue, insomnia, hypotension

iii. Examples
Atenolol, Metoprolol (Lopressor), Dipyridamole (Persantine), Propanolol (Inderal)

Calcium Channel Blockers
i. Mechanism of Action
- relaxation of smooth muscle surrounding vessels, vasodilation
- increases blood flow and oxygen supply to myocardium

ii. Adverse Effects
- hypotension, palpitations, tachycardia, bradycardia, constipation, nausea

iii. Examples
Amlodipine (Norvasc), Diltiazem (Cardizem), Nifedipine (Adalat), Felopidine (Plendil), Verapamil (Covera-HS)

Antidysrhythmic
Treat dysrhythmias, divided into 4 classes and miscellaneous

Class I
i. Mechanism of Action
- membrane-stabilizing drugs, fast sodium channel blockers

ii. Examples
Disopyramide, Procainamide, Quinidine, Lidocaine (Xylocaine), Mexiletine, Phenytoin, Flecainide (Tambocor), Propafeone (Rhythmol)

Class II
ß-Blockers; see above section

Class III
i. Mechanism of Action
- increase the action potential duration by prolonging repolarization

ii. Examples
- Amiodarone, Ibutilide (Corvert), Dofetilide (Tikosyn), Sotalol

Class IV
Calcium Channel Blockers, see above section

Miscellaneous
Antidysrhythmic drugs that have the properties of several classes and therefore cannot be placed in one particular class
i. Examples
Adenosine, Digoxin, Atropine

Antihypertensives
Numerous drug categories have antihypertensive effects

Angiotensin-converting enzyme (ACE) inhibitors
i. Mechanism of Action

- prevents the conversion of angiotensin I to angiotensin II
- results in decreased systemic vascular resistance and vasodilation

ii. Adverse Effects
- fatigue, dizziness, mood changes, dry cough, hyperkalemia, hypotension

iii. Examples
Captopril (Capoten), Enalipril (Vasotec), Ramipril (Altace)

Angiotensin II receptor blockers (ARBs)
i. Mechanism of Action
- blocks receptors that receive angiotensin II in the adrenal cortex
- blocks release of aldosterone and vasoconstriction

ii. Adverse Effects
- upper respiratory tract infections, headache, dizziness, insomnia, dyspnea

iii. Examples
Losartan potassium (Cozaar), Eprosartan mesylate (Teveten), Valsartan (Diovan), Candesartan cilexetil (Atacand)

Calcium Channel Blockers
See above section

Diuretics
Decrease the plasma and extracellular fluid volumes with an overall effect of decreasing the workload of the heart and decreasing blood pressure
Thiazide diuretics are most commonly used for hypertension (See Diuretic Section)

Vasodilators
i. Mechanism of Action
- directly relax arteriolar and venous smooth muscle

ii. Adverse Effects (drug dependent)
- dizziness, headache, tachycardia, bradycardia, hypotension

iii. Examples
Hydralazine, Minoxidil, Nitroprusside

Cardiac Gycosides
Effective for treating heart failure and controlling atrial fibrillation and flutter

i. Mechanism of Action
- increased force of contraction, decreased heart rate, increased stroke volume, increases coronary circulation, and improved diuresis

ii. Adverse Effects
- any type of dysrhythmia, headache, fatigue, malaise, convulsions, colored vision

iii. Examples
Digoxin (Lanoxin)

Diuretics

Loop Diuretics
i. Mechanism of Action
- acts in the ascending loop of Henle to block reabsorption

ii. Adverse Effects
- fluid and electrolyte imbalances, dehydration, hypotension, hypokalemia, high uric acids

iii. Examples
    Furosemide (Lasix)

Thiazide Diuretics
i. Mechanism of Action
    - blocks reabsorption of sodium and chloride in the distal convoluted tubules, highly dependent on adequate kidney function

ii. Adverse Effects
    - fluid and electrolyte imbalances, dehydration, hypotension, hypokalemia, high uric acids

iii. Examples
    Hydrochlorothiazide (Hydrodiuril), Metolazone (Zaroxolyn)

Potassium-sparing Diuretics
Rarely used alone
i. Mechanism of Action
    - blocks action of aldosterone in the distal convoluted tubule

ii. Adverse Effects
    - hyperkalemia, endocrine effects, tumors (at high dose)

iii. Examples
    Spironolactone (Aldactone)

Osmotic Diuretics
i. Mechanism of Action
    - pulls fluid from surrounding tissues into the renal tubules; results in rapid profound diuresis

ii. Adverse Effects
    - headache, nausea, vomiting, precipitate underlying heart disease

iii. Examples
    Mannitol (Osmitrol)

Antilipemics
Drugs that reduce lipid levels

Hydroxymethylglutaryl (HMG) – CoA Reductase Inhibitors
i. Mechanism of Action
    - inhibits enzyme HMG-CoA from producing cholesterol, reduces LDL levels

ii. Adverse Effects
    - GI disturbances, rash, headache

iii. Examples
    Simvastatin (Zocor), Atorvastatin (Lipitor), Rosuvastatin (Crestor)

Bile-Acid Sequestrants (BAS)
i. Mechanism of Action
    - bind to bile acids, cholesterol, and triglycerides then moved into intestines and excreted in feces
    - lower LDL concentrations, increase HDL

ii. Adverse Effects
    - no systemic effects; constipation, nausea and indigestion

iii. Examples

Cholestyramine (Novo-Cholamine), Colestipol hydrochloride (Colestid)

Fibric Acid Derivatives
i. Mechanism of Action
- eliminates triglycerides out of the blood stream and into muscles and adipose tissue

ii. Adverse Effects
- rash, GI disturbances, gallstones, liver injury

iii. Examples
Gemfibrozil (Lopid), Fenofibrate (Tricor), Fenobibric Acid (TriLipix)

Hematologic Pharmacology

Anticoagulants
i. Mechanism of Action
- Suppresses clotting factors and therefore clot formation

ii. Adverse Effects
- Bleeding, bruising, headache

iii. Examples
Warfarin (Coumadin), Heparin (Hapalean)

Antiplatelets
i. Mechanism of Action
- suppresses platelet aggregation, blood clot prevention

ii. Adverse Effects
- increased risk of GI bleed

iii. Examples
Acetylsalicylic Acid (Aspirin)

Gastrointestinal System

Antidiarrheal and Laxatives

Antidiarrheal Medications
- Adsorbents
  i. Mechanism of Action
  - coat the walls of the GI tract, bind the causative toxin and defecate out

  ii. Adverse Effects
  - increased bleeding time, dark stools, darkening of tongue

  iii. Examples
  Attapulgite (Kaopectate), Bismuth Subsalicylate (Maalox, Pepto-bismol)

- Antimotility Drugs (Anticholinergics)
  i. Mechanism of Action
  - work to slow peristalsis by reducing rhythmic contractions and smooth muscle tone of GI tract

  ii. Adverse Effects
  - urinary retention, impotence, dizziness, dry mouth, blurred vision, photophobia

  iii. Examples

Atropine, Hyoscyamine, Hyoscine

- **Antimotility Drugs (Opioids)**
  i. Mechanism of Action
  - decrease bowel motility and relieve painful rectal spasms, decreases transit time through the bowel
  - decrease stool frequency

  ii. Adverse Effects
  - drowsiness, sedation, respiratory depression, hypotension

  iii. Examples
  Codeine, Diphenoxylate (Lomotil), Loperamide (Imodium)

- **Intestinal Flora Modifiers**
  i. Mechanism of Action
  - probiotics or bacterial replacement medications
  - supply missing bacteria to GI tract, suppress growth of diarrhea causing bacteria

  ii. Adverse Effects
  - none significant

  iii. Examples
  Lactobacillus acidophilus

Laxatives

- **Bulk Forming Laxatives**
  i. Mechanism of Action
  - water absorption, increases bulk, distends bowel, initiates peristaltic reflex

  ii. Adverse Effects
  - impaction, fluid overload, esophageal blockage

  iii. Examples
  Psyllium (Metamucil)

- **Emollient Laxatives**
  i. Mechanism of Action
  - stool softeners and lubricants, promotes more water/fat absorption into the stool and intestine

  ii. Adverse Effects
  - not significant

  iii. Examples
  Docusate salts (Colace), Mineral oil (Fleet enema mineral oil)

- **Hyperosmotic Laxatives**
  i. Mechanism of Action
  - site of action limited to large intestine
  - increases fecal water content

  ii. Adverse Effects
  - abdominal bloating, electrolyte imbalances, rectal irritation

  iii. Examples
  Polyethylene Glycol (PEG, PegLyte), Glycerin, Lactulose

- **Saline Laxatives**
  i. Mechanism of Actions
  - inhibits water absorption causing more water and electrolytes to be secreted from the bowel wall

  ii. Adverse Effects

- magnesium toxicity, cramping, diarrhea, increased thirst

iii. Examples
magnesium sulfate (Epsom salts), Sodium phosphate

- Stimulant Laxatives
  ### i. Mechanism of Action
  - increase peristalsis, increase fluid in the colon which increases bulk and softens the stool

  ### ii. Adverse Effects
  - nutrient malabsorption, skin rashes, rectal and gastric irritation, abdominal discomfort

  ### iii. Examples
  Castor oil, Senna (Senekot), Cascara Sagrada, Biscodyl

Antinausea and Antiemetics
i. Mechanism of Action
- block various neurotransmitters (dependent on drug class), inhibiting stimulation in the Chemoreceptor Trigger Zone and thus stopping messages to the Vomiting Centre

Anticholinergic Drugs
ii. Adverse Effects
- tachycardia, dizziness, drowsiness, disorientation, blurred vision, dry mouth

iii. Examples
Scopolamine (Transderm-V)

Antihistamines
ii. Adverse Effects
- dizziness, drowsiness, confusion, blurred vision

iii. Examples
Dimenhydrinate (Gravol), Diphenhydramine (Benadryl)

Neuroleptics
ii. Adverse Effects
- orthostatic hypotension, blurred vision, dry mouth, anorexia, constipation, urinary retention

iii. Examples
Prochlorperazine (Nu-Prochlor), Promethazine

Prokinetic Drugs
ii. Adverse Effects
- hypotension, tachycardia, sedation, fatigue, restlessness

iii. Examples
Metoclopramide (Reglan)

Serotonin Blockers
ii. Adverse Effects
- headache, diarrhea, rash, bronchospasm

iii. Examples
Dolasetron (Anzemet), Ondansetron (Zofran)

Tetrahydrocannabinol (THC)
ii. Adverse Effects
- drowsiness, dizziness, anxiety, visual disturbances

iii. Examples
Dronabinol (Marinol), Nabilone (Cesamex)

Acid-Controlling Medications
i. Mechanism of Action
- work by either; neutralizing gastric acid secretions, reducing acid secretions in the stomach, or completely preventing the production of hydrochloric acid in the stomach

Antacids
ii. Examples
Calcium Carbonate (Maalox), Hydroxide salts (Milk of Magnesia), Calcium Carbonate (Tums), Simethicone (Oval Drops)

Histamine Antagonists
ii. Examples
Famotidine (Pepcid), Ranitidie (Zantac)

Proton Pump Inhibitors
ii. Examples
Pantoprazole (Pantoloc)

Respiratory System

Bronchodilators
i. Mechanism of Action
- relax bronchial smooth muscle bands to dilate the bronchi ad bronchioles that become narrowed as a result of airway disease such as; asthma and COPD

ii. Adverse Effects
- Insomnia, restlessness, tachycardia, tremors, dry mouth, nausea and vomiting
-

iii. Examples
Formoterol (Oxeze), Salbumatol (Ventolin), Salmeterol (Serevent), Ipratropium bromide (Atrovent)

Corticosteroids
i. Mechanism of Action
- reduce inflammation in the airway and increase the responsiveness of bronchial smooth muscle, exact mechanism is unknown

ii. Adverse Effects
- coughing, dry mouth, and oral fungal infections

iii. Examples
Budesonide (Pulmicort), Fluticasone (Flovent), Methylprednisolone (Solu-Medrol)

Endocrine

Adrenal Medications
i. Mechanism of Action
- influence carbohydrate metabolism, or modulate salt and water balance

Glucocorticoids
Decrease inflammation, varied metabolic effects
ii. Examples

Hydrocortisone (Cortef), Dexamethasone (Dexasone), Prednisone (Winpred), Cortisone, Prednisolone (Millipred)

Mineralcorticoids
Influence renal processing of sodium and potassium, have direct effects on the heart and blood vessels
ii. Examples
Fludrocortisone

Antidiabetics

Insulin
Used in the treatment of type 1 and type 2 diabetes mellitus
- Fast Acting
  i. Examples
  Lispro (Humalog), Aspart (Novolog), Regular insulin (Humalin R)
- Intermediate Acting
  i. Examples
  NPH insulin (Humalin N)
- Slow Acting
  i. Examples
  Glargine (Lantus)

Oral Medications
- Biguinides
  i. Mechanism of Action
  - inhibit glucose production by the liver, reduce intestinal absorption of glucose, sensitize insulin receptors on target tissues
  ii. Adverse Effects
  - nausea, diarrhea, cramping, weight loss
  iii. Examples
  Metformin (Glucophage)

- Sulfonylureas
  i. Mechanism of Action
  - stimulates the pancreas cells to release insulin
  ii. Adverse Effects
  - hypoglycemia, should be avoided during pregnancy
  iii. Examples
  Gliclazide (Diamicron), Glyburide (Diabeta)

Thyroid Hormones
i. Mechanism of Action
- increase metabolic rates, used for thyroid replacement

ii. Adverse Effects
- insomnia, tremors, tachycardia, palpitations and weight loss

iii. Examples
levothyroxine (Synthroid)

Anti-Infective

Antibiotics

Macrolides
i. Mechanism of Action
- impede bacterial replication by impairing protein synthesis

ii. Adverse Effects
- GI upset, liver damage

iii. Examples
Erythromycin (Romycin), Clarithromycin (Biaxin), Azithromycin (Zithromax)

Tetracyclines
i. Mechanism of Action
- inhibit protein synthesis and therefore bacterial replication

ii. Adverse Effects
- GI upset, sus sensitivity, esophageal damage

iii. Examples
Tetracycline (Apo-Tetra, Sumycin), Doxycycline (Vibramycin), Minocycline (Minocin)

Penicillins
i. Mechanism of Action
- inhibit cell wall synthesis, homeostasis is disrupted and the cell is destroyed

ii. Adverse Effects
- diarrhea, nausea, c. difficile

iii. Examples
Penicillin V (Apo-Pen-VK, Penicillin VK), Amoxicillin (Moxatag)

Sulfonamides
i. Mechanism of Action
- impair DNA synthesis and stop bacterial replication

ii. Adverse Effects
- rash, fever, nausea, photosensitivity

iii. Examples
Sulfasalazine (Salazopyrin, Azulfidine)

Antivirals
i. Mechanism of Action
- interfere with DNA synthesis that is needed for viral replication

ii. Adverse Effects
- nausea, vomiting, headache, anorexia, and diarrhea

iii. Examples
Acyclovir (Zorvirax), Oseltamivir (Tamiflu), Ribavirin (Virazole, Rebetol)

Antituberculars
i. Mechanism of Action
- inhibit RNA or DNA, or by interfering with lipid and protein synthesis therefore decreasing replication

ii. Adverse Effects
- nausea, vomiting, anorexia and rash

iii. Examples
Rifampin (Rofact, Rifadin), Rifabutin (Mycobutin), Pyrazinamide (Tebrazid)

Antineoplastic Drugs

i. Mechanism of Action
- divided into Alkylating agents, antimetabolites, antibiotic agents, and hormonal agents
- all aimed at inhibiting cell replication

ii. Adverse Effects
- hair loss, nausea, vomiting, diarrhea, myelosuppression, anemia

iii. Examples
Methotrexate (Apo-Methotrexate, Trexall), Fluorouracil (5-FU), Carboplatin, Cisplatin, Doxorubicin (Myocet), Estramustine

Bibliography

1. Michael T. Murray, N. (1996). *Encyclopedia of Nutritional Supplements: The Essential Guide for Improving Your Health Naturally* (Vol. 1). Roseville, CA, USA: Prima Publishing.
2. Bob Flaws, Philippe Sionneau. (2005). *The Treatment of Modern Western Diseases* (2nd Edition). Boulder, CO, USA: Blue Poppy Press.
3. Giovannia Maciocia (1994). *The Practice of Chinese Medicine.* New York, N.Y. USA. Churchill Livingstone.
4. Simon Becker, Bob Flaws, Robert Casanas (2005). *The Treatment of Cardiovascular Diseases with Chinese Medicine.* Boulder, CO, USA: Blue Poppy Press.
5. Lewis, S., Barry, M., Goldsworthy, S., & Goodridge, D. (2014). *Medical-surgical nursing in Canada* (2nd ed.). Toronto: Elsevier.
6. Potter, P., Kerr, J., & Potter, P. (2014). *Canadian fundamentals of nursing* (5th ed.). Toronto: Elsevier.
7. *Taber's Cyclopedic Medical Dictionary.* (2005) (21st ed.). Philadelphia: F.A. Davis Company.
8. Martini, F., Nath, J., & Bartholomew, E. (2012). *Fundamentals of anatomy & physiology* (9th ed.). San Francisco: Pearson/Benjamin Cummings.
9. *Types of Seizures – Epilepsy Ontario.* (2017). *Epilepsyontario.org.* http://epilepsyontario.org/about-epilepsy/types-of-seizures/
10. Mayo Clinic. (2017). *Mayoclinic.org.* http://www.mayoclinic.org/
11. *Diseases & Conditions - Medscape Reference.* (2017). *Emedicine.medscape.com.* http://emedicine.medscape.com/

Cardiovascular Disorders:

Angina Pectoris: http://www.merckmanuals.com/en-ca/professional/cardiovascular-disorders/coronary-artery-disease/angina-pectoris

Atherosclerosis: http://www.merckmanuals.com/en-ca/professional/cardiovascular-disorders/arteriosclerosis/atherosclerosis

Aortic Aneurysm: http://www.webmd.com/heart-disease/tc/aortic-aneurysm-symptoms

Afib: http://www.mayoclinic.org/diseases-conditions/atrial-fibrillation/diagnosis-treatment/treatment/txc-20164944

Buerger's Disease: http://patient.info/doctor/buergers-disease-pro

Cor Pulmonale: http://www.merckmanuals.com/en-ca/professional/cardiovascular-disorders/heart-failure/cor-pulmonale#v936546

Infective Endocarditis: http://www.merckmanuals.com/en-ca/professional/cardiovascular-disorders/endocarditis/infective-endocarditis

Myocardial Infarction: http://www.merckmanuals.com/en-ca/professional/cardiovascular-disorders/coronary-artery-disease/acute-myocardial-infarction-mi

Tachycardia: http://www.mayoclinic.org/diseases-conditions/tachycardia/diagnosis-treatment/treatment/txc-20253978

Bradycardia: http://www.mayoclinic.org/diseases-conditions/bradycardia/basics/treatment/con-20028373

Viral myocarditis: http://www.myocarditisfoundation.org/wp-content/uploads/MF_QuadfoldBro_Adult3-2015.pdf

PAD: http://www.merckmanuals.com/en-ca/professional/cardiovascular-disorders/peripheral-arterial-disorders/peripheral-arterial-disease

Chronic Cardiomyopathy: https://www.nhlbi.nih.gov/health/health-topics/topics/cm/treatment

Orthostatic Hypotension: http://www.merckmanuals.com/en-ca/professional/cardiovascular-disorders/symptoms-of-cardiovascular-disorders/orthostatic-hypotension

Thrombophlebitis: http://www.mayoclinic.org/diseases-conditions/thrombophlebitis/diagnosis-treatment/treatment/txc-20251896

Cerebrovascular Disorders:

http://www.medicalnewstoday.com/articles/184601.php

ALS: http://www.mayoclinic.org/diseases-conditions/amyotrophic-lateral-sclerosis/symptoms-causes/dxc-20247211

Brain Cancer: http://www.webmd.com/cancer/brain-cancer-treatment#1-2

MS: https://mssociety.ca/about-ms/what-is-ms

Parkinson's: http://www.mayoclinic.org/diseases-conditions/parkinsons-disease/basics/treatment/con-20028488

Peripheral Neuropathy: http://www.mayoclinic.org/diseases-conditions/peripheral-neuropathy/home/ovc-20204944

Trigeminal Neuralgia: http://www.mayoclinic.org/diseases-conditions/trigeminal-neuralgia/basics/tests-diagnosis/con-20043802

Viral encephalitis: http://www.mayoclinic.org/diseases-conditions/encephalitis/basics/treatment/con-20021917

Blood Disorders:
Aplastic anemia: http://www.mayoclinic.org/diseases-conditions/aplastic-anemia/basics/causes/con-20019296
Hodgkins' Disease: http://www.cancer.org/cancer/hodgkindisease/detailedguide/hodgkin-disease-what-is-hodgkin-disease
http://www.healthline.com/health/hodgkins-lymphoma#Overview1
Thrombocytopenia: http://www.webmd.com/a-to-z-guides/thrombocytopenia-symptoms-causes-treatments#2-3
Bleeding Disorders: http://www.healthline.com/health/bleeding-disorders#Types3
Hemolytic Anemia: http://www.healthline.com/health/hemolytic-anemia#Treatment7

ENT:
Cataracts: http://www.medicinenet.com/cataracts/page4.htm
Macular Degeneration: http://www.allaboutvision.com/conditions/amd.htm
Serous Otitis Media: http://www.earsurgery.org/conditions/serous-otitis-media-fluid-in-the-middle-ear/

Infectious Diseases:
Allergies: http://www.news-medical.net/health/Different-Types-of-Allergies.aspx
Malaria: http://www.who.int/mediacentre/factsheets/fs094/en/
Epidemic Encephalitis: https://en.wikipedia.org/wiki/Encephalitis_lethargica
Schistosomiasis: http://www.who.int/mediacentre/factsheets/fs115/en/
Typhoid Fever: http://www.webmd.com/a-to-z-guides/typhoid-fever#2-4

merckmanuals.com

Chest Impediment: http://www.heart.org/HEARTORG/Conditions/HeartAttack/WarningSignsofaHeartAttack/Heart-Attack-Symptoms-in-Women_UCM_436448_Article.jsp#.WNVANxSE43Q

Constipation: http://www.merckmanuals.com/professional/gastrointestinal-disorders/symptoms-of-gi-disorders/constipation

Diabetes: http://www.merckmanuals.com/home/hormonal-and-metabolic-disorders/diabetes-mellitus-dm-and-disorders-of-blood-sugar-metabolism/diabetes-mellitus-dm

Depression: http://www.acupuncturesociety.org.uk/pdf/BAcC%20Red%20Flags.pdf

Diarrhea: http://www.merckmanuals.com/home/digestive-disorders/symptoms-of-digestive-disorders/diarrhea-in-adults

Dyphagia Occlusion Syndrome: http://www.merckmanuals.com/home/digestive-disorders/symptoms-of-digestive-disorders/difficulty-swallowing

Dyspnea: http://www.merckmanuals.com/home/lung-and-airway-disorders/symptoms-of-lung-disorders/shortness-of-breath.
http://www.merckmanuals.com/professional/pulmonary-disorders/symptoms-of-pulmonary-disorders/dyspnea.

Edema: http://www.merckmanuals.com/professional/cardiovascular-disorders/symptoms-of-cardiovascular-disorders/edema

Epilepsy: http://www.merckmanuals.com/home/brain,-spinal-cord,-and-nerve-disorders/seizure-disorders/seizure-disorders

Fainting: http://www.merckmanuals.com/home/heart-and-blood-vessel-disorders/symptoms-of-heart-and-blood-vessel-disorders/fainting

Goitre: http://www.merckmanuals.com/home/hormonal-and-metabolic-disorders/thyroid-gland-disorders/goiter

Headache: http://www.acupuncturesociety.org.uk/pdf/BAcC%20Red%20Flags.pdf
http://www.merckmanuals.com/home/brain,-spinal-cord,-and-nerve-disorders/headaches/overview-of-headache

Hiccoughing and Belching: http://www.merckmanuals.com/professional/gastrointestinal-disorders/symptoms-of-gi-disorders/hiccups

Hypochondrial Pain: http://www.acupuncturesociety.org.uk/pdf/BAcC%20Red%20Flags.pdf

Impediment Syndrome: http://www.acupuncturesociety.org.uk/pdf/BAcC%20Red%20Flags.pdf

Impotence: http://www.merckmanuals.com/home/men-s-health-issues/sexual-dysfunction-in-men/erectile-dysfunction-ed

Internal Damage Fever: http://www.merckmanuals.com/home/infections/biology-of-infectious-disease/fever-in-adults

Ischuria: http://www.merckmanuals.com/home/kidney-and-urinary-tract-disorders/disorders-of-urination/urinary-retention

Jaundice: http://www.merckmanuals.com/home/liver-and-gallbladder-disorders/manifestations-of-liver-disease/jaundice-in-adults

Lung Disease: http://www.merckmanuals.com/home/lung-and-airway-disorders/chronic-obstructive-pulmonary-disease-copd/chronic-obstructive-pulmonary-disease-chronic-bronchitis-emphysema

Malaria: http://www.merckmanuals.com/home/infections/parasitic-infections/malaria

Mania: http://www.merckmanuals.com/home/mental-health-disorders

Palpitation: http://www.merckmanuals.com/professional/cardiovascular-disorders/symptoms-of-cardiovascular-disorders/palpitations

Pulmonary Absess: http://www.merckmanuals.com/home/lung-and-airway-disorders/abscess-in-the-lungs/abscess-in-the-lungs

Pulmonary TB: http://emedicine.medscape.com/article/230802-overview#a3
http://www.merckmanuals.com/home/infections/tuberculosis-and-leprosy/tuberculosis-tb

Spontaneous/Night Sweats: http://www.merckmanuals.com/home/skin-disorders/sweating-disorders/excessive-sweating)

Stranguria: http://www.acupuncturesociety.org.uk/pdf/BAcC%20Red%20Flags.pdf
http://www.merckmanuals.com/home/kidney-and-urinary-tract-disorders/urinary-tract-infections-uti/overview-of-urinary-tract-infections-utis and http://www.merckmanuals.com/home/kidney-and-urinary-tract-disorders/stones-in-the-urinary-tract/stones-in-the-urinary-tract

Tinnitus and Deafness: http://www.acupuncturesociety.org.uk/pdf/BAcC%20Red%20Flags.pdf

http://www.merckmanuals.com/home/ear,-nose,-and-throat-disorders

Vertigo: http://www.merckmanuals.com/home/ear,-nose,-and-throat-disorders/symptoms-of-ear-disorders/dizziness-and-vertigo

Vomiting: http://www.merckmanuals.com/home/digestive-disorders/symptoms-of-digestive-disorders/nausea-and-vomiting-in-adults

Wheezing Syndrome: http://www.merckmanuals.com/home/lung-and-airway-disorders/asthma/asthma

Acne: http://emedicine.medscape.com/article/1069804-overview#a1

Alopecia Areata: http://www.merckmanuals.com/home/skin-disorders/hair-disorders/alopecia-areata

Anal Fissure: http://emedicine.medscape.com/article/196297-overview#a9

Bedsore: http://www.merckmanuals.com/home/skin-disorders/pressure-sores/pressure-sores

Boil: http://www.merckmanuals.com/professional/dermatologic-disorders/bacterial-skin-infections/furuncles-and-carbuncles

Breast Cancer: http://www.merckmanuals.com/professional/gynecology-and-obstetrics/breast-disorders/breast-cancer#v1065825
http://www.tcmpage.com/hpbreastcan.html

Breast Lump: http://www.merckmanuals.com/home/women-s-health-issues/breast-disorders/breast-lumps

Carbuncle: http://www.tcmwindow.com/diseases/Skin-Diseases/Carbuncle-treatment.shtml

Contact Dermatitis: http://acuherb.us/contact-dermatitis/ + http://acuherb.us/contact-dermatitis/)

Digital Gangrene: http://www.webmd.com/skin-problems-and-treatments/guide/gangrene-causes-symptoms-treatments#2-5

Drug Rash: http://www.merckmanuals.com/home/skin-disorders/hypersensitivity-and-inflammatory-skin-disorders/drug-rashes + http://www.tcmwindow.com/diseases/Skin-Diseases/Drug-Rash-treatment.shtml

Eczema: http://www.merckmanuals.com/professional/dermatologic-disorders/dermatitis/atopic-dermatitis-eczema

Goitre: http://www.merckmanuals.com/professional/endocrine-and-metabolic-disorders/thyroid-disorders/hyperthyroidism + http://www.merckmanuals.com/professional/endocrine-and-metabolic-disorders/thyroid-disorders/hashimoto-thyroiditis + http://www.merckmanuals.com/professional/endocrine-and-metabolic-disorders/thyroid-disorders/hyperthyroidism

Haemorrhoid: http://www.merckmanuals.com/professional/gastrointestinal-disorders/anorectal-disorders/hemorrhoids

Herpes Zoster: http://www.merckmanuals.com/professional/infectious-diseases/herpesviruses/herpes-zoster

BPH: http://www.merckmanuals.com/home/men-s-health-issues/benign-prostate-disorders/benign-prostatic-hyperplasia-bph
http://www.tcmwindow.com/diseases/diseasesList-5.aspx

Prostatitis: http://www.merckmanuals.com/home/men-s-health-issues/benign-prostate-disorders/prostatitis
http://www.tcmwindow.com/diseases/diseasesList-5.aspx)

Scrofula: http://www.merckmanuals.com/professional/infectious-diseases/mycobacteria/extrapulmonary-tuberculosis

Sebaceous Cyst: http://www.merckmanuals.com/professional/dermatologic-disorders/benign-skin-tumors,-growths,-and-vascular-lesions/cutaneous-cysts

Uritcaria: http://www.merckmanuals.com/professional/dermatologic-disorders/approach-to-the-dermatologic-patient/urticaria

Varicose Veins: http://www.merckmanuals.com/professional/cardiovascular-disorders/peripheral-venous-disorders/varicose-veins
http://chinesenaturecure.com

143 Illnesses

References

Traditional Chinese Medicine and Acupuncture:
Cheng, X. (chief editor), *Chinese Acupuncture and Moxibustion 2nd Edition*, Foreign Language Press, Beijing, 2005.
Crockett, Conrad, *Manual of Orthopedic Acupuncture 4th Edition*, 2013
Deadman, P., Al-Khafaji M., Baker, K, *A Manual of Acupuncture*, Journal of Chinese Medicine Publications, 2007.
Flaws, B., *A Handbook of TCM Pediatrics 2nd Edition*, Blue Poppy Press, Colorado, 2006.
Flaws, B., Sionneau, P. *The Treatment of Western Medical Diseases with Chinese Medicine*, Blue Poppy Press, Colorado, 2005.

Liang J., , *A Handbook of Traditional Chinese Dermatology,* Blue Poppy Press, Colorado, 1993.
Liu Z.W., Liu L. (editors), *Essentials of Chinese Medicine: Volume 3*, Springer-Verlag London Ltd., 2009.
Maciocia, G. *The Practice of Chinese Medicine: The Treatment of Diseases with Acupuncture and Chinese Herbs*, Churchill Livingstone, 1994.
Maciocia, G. *Obstetrics and Gynecology in Chinese Medicine.* Churchill Livingstone, 2008.
Norris, Acupuncture: *Treatment of Musculoskeletal Conditions*, Reed Educational and Professional Publishing Ltd., 2001.
Reaves, Whitfield, *The Acupuncture Handbook of Sports Injuries and Pain*, Hidden Needle Press, Colorado, 2009.
Shi and Zeng, *Essentials of Chinese Medicine Internal Medicine 2nd Edition*, Bridge Publishing Group, 2011.
Sionneau, P., Gang, L., *The Treatment of Disease in TCM Volume 4: Diseases of the Neck, Shoulder, Back, and Limbs*, Blue Poppy Press, Colorado, 2007.
Sionneau, P., Gang, L., *The Treatment of Disease in TCM Volume 6: Diseases of the Urogenital System and Proctology*, Blue Poppy Press, Colorado, 1999.
Xie J., Li M., Han C., *Chinese Internal Medicine,* People's Medicine Publishing House, 2013.
Yan W., Fischer W., *Practical Therapeutics of Traditional Chinese Medicine,* Paradigm Publications, 1997.
www.tcmwindow.com, 2017
http://chinesenaturecure.com/wp/, 2017

Class notes from Pacific Rim College (2014-2016):
- Gynecology and obstetrics, Dr. Jing Zhang
- Orthopedic acupuncture, Dr. Conrad Crockett
- Pediatrics, Dr. Ali Jopp
- External medicine, Dr. Jing Zhang
- Internal medicine, Dr. Kai Chen

Red flags:
www.acupuncturesociety.org.uk, *Red Flag Conditions: A guide for acupuncturists,* 2008
www.merckmanuals.com, 2017
www.webmd.com, 2017
www.medscape.com, 2017

Western Medicine:
www.merckmanuals.com, 2017
www.medscape.com, 2017
www.webmd.com, 2017
Gould, B., Dyer, R., *Pathophysiology for the Health Professions 4th edition*, Saunders Elsevier, 2011.
Maciocia, *The Practice of Chinese Medicine: The Treatment of Diseases with Acupuncture and Chinese Herbs*, Churchill Livingstone, 1994.

Pharmacology

Lilley, L., Harrington, S., Snyder, J., Swart, B., & Lilley, L. (2011). *Pharmacology for Canadian health care practice* (1st ed.). Toronto: Mosby/Elsevier.

Skidmore-Roth, L. (2014). *Mosby's 2014 nursing drug reference* (1st ed.). St. Louis, MO: Elsevier Mosby.

*A large amount of research came from 'Class notes: Biomedical Clinical Diagnosis. Chuck Alsberg. 2000.'

LIFT Education
Disclaimer

Please note that although you have received instruction from Lift Education to prepare you for your Acupuncture Board Exams, the ultimate result of your Exams rest with you (i.e. GET STUDYING!). Lift Education and its representatives or subsidiaries will not be held accountable in the event of an unfavourable result.

All content is subject to copyright and may not be reproduced in any form without express written consent of the author.

Manufactured by Amazon.ca
Bolton, ON